Nutrition
and
Neurotransmitters

Prentice Hall Advanced Reference Series

Physical and Life Sciences

Nutrition
and
Neurotransmitters

The Nutrient Bases
of Behavior

Michael D. Chafetz

University of New Orleans
New Orleans, Louisiana

Prentice Hall, Englewood Cliffs, New Jersey 07632

Library of Congress Cataloging-in-Publication Data

CHAFETZ, MICHAEL D.
  Nutrition and neurotransmitters: the nutrient bases of behavior /
Michael D. Chafetz.
      p.   cm.
  Includes bibliographies and index.
  ISBN 0-13-627860-4-
  1. Neurotransmitters—Metabolism—Regulation.   2. Nutrition.
3. Neuropsychology.   I. Title.
  [DNLM: 1. Behavior—physiology.   2. Diet.   3. Neuroregulators—
physiology.   4. Nutrition.   WL 102 C433n]
QP364.7.C47   1990
152—dc20
DNLM/DLC
for Library of Congress   89-3980
                                                           CIP

Editorial/production supervision: *Jean Lapidus*
Cover design: *Wanda Lubelska Design*
Manufacturing buyer: *Mary Ann Gloriande*

 © 1990 by Prentice-Hall, Inc.
A Division of Simon & Schuster
Englewood Cliffs, New Jersey 07632

This book can be made available to businesses
and organizations at a special discount when
ordered in large quantities. For more information
contact:

Prentice-Hall, Inc.
Special Sales and Markets
College Division
Englewood Cliffs, N.J. 07632

Printed in the United States of America
10 9 8 7 6 5 4 3 2 1

ISBN 0-13-627860-4

PRENTICE-HALL INTERNATIONAL (UK) LIMITED, *London*
PRENTICE-HALL OF AUSTRALIA PTY. LIMITED, *Sydney*
PRENTICE-HALL CANADA INC., *Toronto*
PRENTICE-HALL HISPANOAMERICANA, S.A., *Mexico*
PRENTICE-HALL OF INDIA PRIVATE LIMITED, *New Delhi*
PRENTICE-HALL OF JAPAN, INC., *Tokyo*
SIMON & SCHUSTER ASIA PTE. LTD., *Singapore*
EDITORA PRENTICE-HALL DO BRASIL, LTDA., *Rio de Janeiro*

For
Marjorie

Contents

Foreword

by Curt Richter
and
David Olton

T he development of my work on dietary self-selection was spontaneous and rapid. The basic principle was that animals could choose their diets through behavior. Everywhere I looked, I found more and more illustrations of this fact.

Hopkins was really a wonderful place at that time. My instructor at Harvard, Yerkes, had strongly recommended that I go to work with John Watson at Hopkins. When I arrived, Watson gave me some clear instructions. He was interested in a good place of scientific work, and did not care about a particular plan of graduate education. He gave me a group of rats, told me to go do significant research, and report the results back to him.

This type of research endeavor suited me very well. I had been brought up to be independent when I was young, and had spent time working in a factory. My experiences had taught me the skills necessary to produce the hardware for my experiments, and by temperament, I was a doer, not a reader.

I followed some general principles in those experiments. One was to keep things simple. Consequently, the experiments often gave the animals pure substances, or ones that differed along a single dimension. This approach ensured that there would be no confusion, and that the results would come out right, easy to interpret. The object was to identify an important variable, manipulate it, find out its effects on behavior, and then carry on.

Two examples are appropriate. In one experiment, I manipulated the type of corn in the diet and got a clear preference for yellow corn. Consequently, all other variables were held constant, and the results could be attributed directly to the type of corn used. In another experiment, only one sugar was given, and this brought out precise differences in behavior indicating clearly how the animals got along.

A second principle was the importance of charts as a means of displaying data. At the time, many of the experiments recorded data on smoked paper. I had ovens and other paraphernalia necessary to produce these sheets scattered throughout the laboratory, and went through copious amounts of it during the experiment. I have always found the results of experiments to be interpreted most easily in the forms of charts, rather than in words. Charts recorded data, reported it in publications, and guided the next research project.

A third principle was to have the highest regard for the selections made by the animals in the study. I always relied on what the animals did, and was impressed by the accuracy and consistency of their consumption. When the experiment was kept simple, it brought out differences that were so precise that I knew I was getting down to the real facts. The behavior of the animals often indicated that the experiment had hit things right on the button.

At the time, life at Hopkins was simple. Adolf Meyer gave me virtually everything I needed to conduct the work. Neither he nor Watson interfered with my progress. An orderly in the hospital gave me all the information that I needed to know about places to go in Baltimore to buy the many different small items that I needed in my experiments. Grant applications were unknown, and I was able to spend my time doing research rather than writing a continual flow of proposals.

The experiments themselves went well. They just seemed to happen and occurred spontaneously without my speculation about specific outcomes. My previous experiences had prepared me to be an independent entrepreneur, and I was able to build all the apparatus that I needed right in the laboratory. I just followed the direction of the animals without any preconceived notions, and the results just happened. Often, significant results appeared in the first day of an experiment. This type of single handed progress with inexpensive components contrasts markedly with the high technology that is often required with current neuroscience.

Dietary self-selection has proven to be a potent influence on animal's behavior, and is found with both specific substances (such as a vitamin) and whole foods (such as corn). The phenomena were there to be discovered, and were demonstrated clearly through these experiments. There are obviously many questions yet to be addressed in this area. However, my experiments have always been guided by the results at hand, rather than grand theories or speculation about underlying causes. Consequently, I am unwilling to make a specific prediction about the direction that future research may pursue. However, a logical development is the emphasis on neuroscience, represented by the contributions of Richard Wurtman in this volume. The behavioral data from the dietary self-regulation experiments demonstrate that animals must have a means to sense dietary variables, realize their significance, and alter their behavior in an adaptive way to respond to dietary alternatives. It is comforting to know that neuroscience is now beginning to look at some of the intervening neural mechanisms, and give us information about how those behavioral changes take place.

The work with behavioral regulation that I carried out was exciting and pleasurable, and I recall it with fondness. Let's all hope that the individuals pursuing neuroscience today will have the same feelings about their work when they have reached the same stage in their lives and I am in mine.

Johns Hopkins University   *Curt Richter*
Baltimore, Maryland   *David Olton*

Foreword

by Richard J. Wurtman

At first thought—and probably second, as well—it seems surprising that the chemical composition of the brain should be affected by what we choose to eat, all the more so when we contemplate that the brain chemicals so affected include some of its neurotransmitters, the signals that transmit information from one neuron to another. Surely this is not the case for chemical signals originating *outside* the brain: For example, no one would suggest that eating cholesterol-rich foods stimulates the production of hormones like testosterone or estradiol, which are formed from cholesterol. How can this be? If we believe in the "wisdom of the body" and the good judgment of Natural Selection, the biologic marketplace, *why* should this be?

This book attempts to explain how and suggest why. It teaches that, in the final analysis, the ability of nutrients to control the rates of key neuro-

chemical reactions is simply a function of the kinetic properties of enzymes
and related macromolecules (like those which transport amino acids and other
electrically-charged compounds across the blood-brain barrier): If one of these
macromolecules happens to have a low affinity for its ligand, and if that ligand
happens to be a nutrient—and if plasma levels of that nutrient are not hom-
eostatically regulated (as happens to be the case), such that these levels are
"allowed" to rise when the nutrient has been ingested—then eating a food
which provides the brain with more of that nutrient will, quite mechanically,
cause its neurons to synthesize more of its neurotransmitter product. Of
course, the brain needn't have worked this way: One could perfectly well
have anticipated that the enzymes and other macromolecules responsible for
the syntheses of dopamine, serotonin, acetylcholine, and the other nutrient-
dependent brain constituents would have been endowed with high-affinity
kinetic properties. But they weren't, and the phenomenon of "precursor-
control" follows as a direct consequence. It turns out that a high proportion
of the brain's enzymes apparently share this kinetic property (i.e., poor affinity
for their substrates), hence it seems likely that many additional brain compounds besides the neurotransmitters examined thus far will turn out to be
affected to some degree by the availability of their precursors (and thus,
potentially, by eating).

But why should the brain have evolved in this manner? Clearly, not simply
to provide physicians with additional compounds for modulating neurotransmitter release. One physiologic consequence of the ability of some foods to
affect brain composition—the ability of serotonin-forming neurons to distinguish between high-carbohydrate and high-protein meals seems to relate to
the maintenance of nutritional balance, i.e., the propensity of normal people
to consume a fairly constant proportion of protein in their diets, without being
conscious of doing so. One anticipates that other consequences may exist,
and may, with time, reveal themselves to the clever and fortunate investigator.

"This volume constitutes, to my knowledge, the first attempt by a single
author to summarize the large body of information relevant to the effects of
nutrients on the brain. As such, it should do much to encourage the application
and expansion of this knowledge."

Massachusetts Institute of Technology   *Richard J. Wurtman*
Cambridge, Massachusetts

Preface

This work juxtaposes the research legacy of two pioneers: Curt P. Richter and Richard J. Wurtman. Richter developed the line of research showing how nutrient intake is regulated by total organismic (behavioral and physiological) processes. Wurtman pioneered the ongoing research showing how central nervous system processes monitor and organize nutrient balance.

Since the work of these two individuals was first published, numerous researchers have added breadth and depth to the principal findings. We now know, for example, how neurotransmitter mechanisms monitor and control nutrient intake, and where in the brain some of these chemicals are acting, though controversy still exists as to whether natural regulatory behavior is indeed controlled by these mechanisms. We also know more about which of the regulatory behaviors are innate, and which are acquired through the subtle processes of conditioning.

Viewed one way, the principal findings of these individuals are worlds apart. After all, the research *Zeitgeist* was separated by at least two decades. The methodologies are not comparable, and the language of the research communications is in grossly different dialects. But what has impressed me about these two bodies of work is that their essential ideas imply the necessity of understanding each other. We are enriched by understanding total organismic regulation in terms of neural processes, just as we are enlightened by understanding neural mechanisms of nutrient balance in terms of behavior.

It is in this spirit of "joining" that this book was conceived. In the introduction I have tried to draw the broad outlines of theory on neural processes and behavior as they impinge upon nutrient regulation. Because much of what is known about nutrient/brain interactions involves brain circuits. I have also included an introductory chapter on neuroanatomy. I hope this chapter will facilitate an understanding of nutrients and behavior by describing the relevant circuits involved. The reader well-versed in neuroanatomy can safely skip this section without lacking in an understanding of the work.

The book is divided into two parts: One focuses on neurotransmitters, the other on nutrients. In the neurotransmitter section, nutrient regulation and behavior are viewed from their position in "classical" transmitter function. The "classical" neurotransmitters provide the principal forum because they have been the most widely researched in terms of nutrients. In each of these "transmitter" chapters, physiology and anatomy are first presented, followed by an account of their relevant influences on behavior. This provides the basis for the ensuing discussion on the ways in which diet affects brain and behavior, including pathology.

In the nutrient section, the emphasis is reversed. Neural (and visceral) mechanisms are discussed in terms of their primary interactions with particular nutrients. Biochemical and physiological considerations focus on the nutrient. Anatomical descriptions are based on nutrient binding or uptake sites. Behavior, in this section, is discussed from the point of view of feeding and nutrient regulation. Thus, there is still much to be discussed of the ways in which diet affects brain and behavior, but nutrients rather than transmitters are in focus.

Four nutrients were chosen for this section—two macro- and two micronutrients. Salt (sodium) and glucose are the two macronutrients; zinc and vitamins C and B1 (together) are the micronutrients. I am well aware that other logical representatives of each category exist, but in each case the choices were made for historical or theoretical reasons.

There are volumes of research on salt and glucose. These complement each other, both historically and theoretically, but each alone would not do the topic justice. Together, they illustrate most of the theoretical and empirical work on nutrient regulation and feeding behavior. Of the possible trace metals, zinc was chosen because of current, intense research on its behavioral and neural influences. This research far surpasses that of the other trace metals. As for vitamins, thiamine (B1) was chosen primarily for historical reasons. It was one of the focal nutrients of Richter's work, and has been the nutrient-of-choice in subsequent work showing behavioral mechanisms of nutrient regulation. Ascorbic acid (C) was chosen because of recent intense research activity on its interaction with neurotransmitter systems. It is hoped that these choices, though not complete, will provide a necessary framework for the joining of these two important research areas.

Finally, it should be noted that this is more than a book of facts. The joining of nutrients and behavioral function into one research area is such a new proposition that this is of necessity also a book of ideas. Many of these ideas are "in the air," but it is hoped that current research will quickly turn them into facts.

New Orleans, Louisiana   *Michael D. Chafetz*

Acknowledgments

I am indebted to the many students and colleagues who have enriched my thinking through discussions of these topics. I wish to thank Pat Loughlin for his special library work. I am also grateful to the staffs of the medical school libraries at Tulane University and Louisiana State University for assistance with research material.

I am also most grateful to David Olton, who acted as my liaison with Professor Richter and who expended much time and effort with him on his foreword. For writing the forewords and providing many additional helpful comments, I thank Professors Wurtman and Richter.

The reviewers of this work helped me to see many of its initial shortcomings. I would like to thank Donald Novin, Bruce King, B. Glenn Stanley, Jay Schulkin, Micah Leshem, Jesse Rosenthal, and Randall Sakai for pushing me through to the other side of my logic. I am also indebted for the craftsmanship in production by Jean Lapidus, whose patience and attention to details elevated the quality of the project. I alone am responsible for any shortcomings.

Nutrition and Neurotransmitters

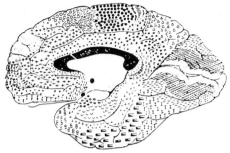

Part **I**

Introduction

Chapter **1**

The Interactions of Diet, Brain, and Behavior

T his book is about how nutrients influence behavior. These nutrient influences can accrue slowly over several years of development, or they can happen quickly, like the effects of a psychoactive drug shortly after ingestion.

Nutrients that affect behavior are found in common foods. For example, tryptophan is found in many proteins, and virtually any source of carbohydrate can, through an indirect mechanism, affect the amount of tryptophan that is taken up by the brain. Once in the brain, tryptophan is converted into serotonin, which has profound behavioral effects. Another example of a common nutrient that influences behavior is salt. Variations in the salt content of the diet have a major influence on the foods a person chooses to eat.

That food can act quickly as a psychoactive drug is certainly not surprising if a drug is found in the food. An old Materia Medica (Bartholow, 1986) prescribes wine rich in ethers as especially useful for treating nervous restlessness, wakefulness, and cardiac depression. The caffeine in coffee or tea was prescribed as useful when "circulation is depressed from various causes" or as a "stomachic tonic."

Foods that contain psychoactive agents such as alcohol or caffeine, however, will not be discussed here because information on these drugs can be found in standard references on pharmacology (see Rall, 1980). Chocoholics are forewarned: your favorite substance of abuse contains caffeine and theobromine (a xanthine similar to caffeine) and is therefore out of bounds.

The common nutrients we will discuss are important to consider because they have *direct* effects on neural or visceral activity in known systems. General metabolic effects that may alter activity in the entire nervous system will be only briefly mentioned because of the lack of specificity; it is difficult to pinpoint a direct effect on behavior without knowing which neural system has been activated. The scope of the work is thus limited to relatively direct and clear effects.

It is also beyond the scope to consider every nutrient that could possibly have an effect on brain or behavior. General principles of interaction, however, do exist. By considering nutrients whose effects illuminate these principles, a framework can be built to facilitate the acquisition of greater knowledge of nutrient effects on behavior.

The purposes of this book are thus to describe effects of foods on behavior, and to describe how behavior in turn can influence the acquisition of nutrients. Although data on nutrient influences provide the scientist with antecedents for an analysis of behavioral control, a discussion at the level of specific neural and visceral systems is still required. However, two major questions remain: How do we achieve a focus on neural and visceral systems? How do we achieve a focus on behavior?

Neural and Visceral Systems

Each behavior in our repertoire is controlled by neurochemicals acting on and acted upon by neurons. Some of the larger neurochemicals are proteins, which have both structural and functional roles in the nervous system. Functionally, proteins may act as receptors, gates, channels, or pumps. The status and relative effectiveness of each of these roles depend upon the regulation of the protein itself, as well as the milieu in which the protein is operating. That milieu may be partially composed of neurotransmitters, peptides, steroid hormones, components of intermediary metabolism, and elements of the diet dissolved in the plasma and absorbed or actively transported into the brain.

For a book on diet's influence on behavior, a focus on proteins–even receptor proteins–and their milieu, or other large molecular constituents of the nervous system, would not go far enough. Not only are there few data on these causal links, but, more importantly, the constituents of the diet that influence behavior are broken down into, or already exist in, smaller units before they can gain access to the brain. Moreover, many of these dietary constituents influence behavior by controlling the activity or amounts of "small" neurotransmitters. It is therefore useful to focus on smaller neurochemicals, such as neurotransmitters, in the description of dietary effects.

Richard Wurtman (1979) has proposed a tripartite classification of neurotransmitters based upon mechanisms of synthesis that could be altered by dietary influences. The first grouping includes those neurotransmitters synthesized from circulating precursors provided or influenced by the diet. Examples include serotonin (from tryptophan), catecholamines (from phenylalanine or tyrosine), and acetylcholine (from choline and an activated acetate group). The second grouping is comprised of peptides synthesized on polyribosomes from circulating amino acids. Examples include somatostatin, luteinizing hormone-releasing hormone, and substance P. The third grouping is composed of nonessential amino acids, such as glutamate, aspartate, and gamma-amino butyric acid (GABA).

For the first grouping, Wurtman has further specified requirements for plasma precursors to affect neurotransmitter synthesis. First, precursor levels in plasma must be able to change, due either to diet or other physiological effects. Second, the brain must be unable to synthesize as much precursor as it needs. Third, a low-affinity transport system must mediate uptake at the blood-brain barrier, effectively providing a filter between brain and blood that allows precursor changes in the blood to affect the amount of precursor transported into the brain. Finally, a low-affinity enzyme must catalyze the key step in converting the precursor to the transmitter, also effectively providing a filter that allows precursor changes to affect the amount of transmitter produced.

Beyond these groupings lie other dietary substances that have neurochemical effects. Some of these include *trace metals* (which have an uneven distribution in the brain and well-studied behavioral effects) and *vitamins,* whose dietary alterations have important behavioral implications. Then there are other nutrients, such as sodium and glucose, which have such fundamental roles in the nervous system and in intermediary metabolism that they are distributed throughout the organism. These nutrients also have such important roles in behavioral control that special neural and visceral mechanisms exist to regulate and monitor their intake.

Although dynamic nutritional influences provide immediate antecedents for behavioral control, it may sometimes be difficult to understand how early nutritional influences alter adult behavior. How could present behavior–moods, sex, food consumption–be influenced by a diet consumed in infancy? Is it a difficult intellectual feat to extend the immediate influences of diet across the expanses of organismic time? Such an historical causation would require permanent storage in a retrievable neural file. The question thus becomes whether components of an infant or maternal diet can alter the developing nervous system to change adult behavior.

In the psychological sciences this is not such a radical idea. Freudians invoke historical causation to say that adult behavior is determined by the infant's experiences impinging on its natural development. Unconscious adult memories of these childhood events express themselves later in our adult defenses.

In the neural sciences, the notion that an early life event can alter the brain so as to alter adult behavior has considerable grounding. The studies by Rosenzweig and colleagues (Bennett et al., 1964) have shown that by enriching an animal's early environment, one can radically influence the course of brain development. This is seen in increased dendritic branching, acetylcholinesterase activity, and the size of synaptic contact areas. An early manipulation as subtle as placing a rat pup in a separate container for a few moments also has profound consequences for its adult behavior. The studies by Victor Denenberg (1972) show that "held" pups, compared to pups left untouched by human hands, seek more tactual variation, and are more active and less fearful when tested as adults.

One of the subpurposes of this book is to describe early nutritional effects on behavioral development. Although a vast literature on behavioral and neural effects of early protein malnutrition exists, our discussion is constrained by the framework of describing *specific* neural systems mediating *specific* behaviors.

*B*ehavioral Theory

Data on nutritional effects are accumulating rapidly despite the difficulty of proving direct effects on behavior. This is said with some trepidation because almost any movement an animal makes could be measured and regarded as "behavior." What could be more straightforward than the measurement of a "behavior" after manipulation of a dietary component with a specific effect on the nervous system?

Indeed, it would seem easy to accept a behavioral consequence if one kind of malnourishment deprived the developing nervous system of an entire set of neurons dependent on the missing nutrient. All one has to do is to identify behaviors controlled by those missing neurons.

Unfortunately, this is not as easy as it sounds. The problem is similar to finding the individual behavioral contribution of each of the components in a radio. If a part were left out in its manufacturing, and the radio hissed when it was turned on, no one would claim that the missing part was a "hiss suppressor." The figure/ground problem also comes into play when one considers that the hiss is a function of the action of the remainder of the radio, without the part. It would take an analysis from several converging sources of measurement and manipulation to identify the integrated function of the missing part (especially if the analyzer is not the radio's manufacturer). Therefore, to provide such converging evidence, each discussion of a dietary influence on behavior is set within the context of data from anatomic, neurochemical, and pharmacologic findings.

But there is another problem. An animal deprived of a nutrient that serves as a precursor to a neurotransmitter may change its behavior. By extension, does the original behavior result from an appropriate level of the neurotransmitter? This is no simple extrapolation from the "hiss suppressor" problem. The same problem occurs if one considers an argument about depression: If depression is the result of too little norepinephrine, then "normal" moods generally are a function of "normal" levels of norepinephrine activity. In this case, behavior has been linked to neuronal function by converging evidence, but something is still missing. That "something" is a strong theoretical framework to help explain the brain-behavior relationships.

Two frameworks are considered here. One is *optimal foraging theory*, which helps explain the behavioral acquisition of these nutrients. The other is *control theory*, which provides a mechanistic account of the effects of nutrients.

*O*ptimal Foraging Theory

Natural selection should favor those individuals in a population best suited biochemically, anatomically, or behaviorally to adapt to local ecological conditions. These individuals will contribute the most to subsequent generations. Accordingly, there should be a change in average foraging behavior over time toward those behaviors that enable individuals to adapt to ecologic conditions. "Fitness" is said to be maximized when those behaviors lead to the production of viable offspring. If fitness is linked directly to reproductive success, the "best" or the "optimal" foraging strategies would include those feeding behaviors that give animals the best chance of producing viable offspring.

This sounds simple enough, but the concept of optimality does not always translate into an easy prediction of behavior. If you could assume that the basic strategy of any animal is to maximize its net rate of energy intake, you could identify at least two kinds of behavior, according to Pyke, et al. (1977). If the animal has a fixed energy requirement, its "fitness" is greatest when it minimizes time required to obtain the fixed amount of energy and uses the remaining time to perform other activities. ("Fitness" is in quotes because it remains to be demonstrated that the animal actually used the leftover time to perform activities that lead to more offspring). These animals are called *time minimizers.*

The other kind of behavior occurs if the animal has a fixed amount of time in which to forage. In this case, "fitness" generally increases as the animal obtains more energy. The maximum "fitness" occurs when the animal obtains the maximum amount of energy in the allotted time. This kind of animal is called an *energy maximizer.*

This simple view of a world populated by time minimizers and energy maximizers changes rapidly when one considers nutrition. The quality of foods, especially for generalist omnivores such chickens, rats, or humans, is diverse enough to force these animals to make choices about nutrition. In this sense, one could identify an optimal strategy based upon diet choice. But, it is not clear that any such strategy would be used at the expense of calorie intake. The conditions under which compromises occur between obtaining calories and optimizing diet would have to be described. For these animals who have a relatively constant energy budget, a time-minimizing strategy would probably be imposed as an overlay on optimal diet choice.

This view of optimization implies a hierarchy of behaviors, especially in generalist feeders. The drive for calories is asserted to be the "bottom line" of foraging behavior, and there are two ways to achieve that goal. One is to maximize calories; the other is to minimize foraging time. But animals need not always forage for calories. Under appropriate conditions, the optimal strategy may involve behaviors related to diet choice or timing. In this regard, it will be helpful to consider a few examples.

In a research report on the economics of food choice in domestic chickens, Rovee-Collier et al. (1982) considered that the fledgling chick, as a generalist omnivore, is faced with at least two problems. One is to obtain a balanced diet from items that vary widely in nutritional composition and caloric density. The other problem is deciding when to feed.

Since previous observations had revealed high variability in feeding times, it was considered that the typical diurnal feeding in chicks may be an optimizing strategy rather than a physiological necessity. These investigators therefore predicted that growing chicks should adopt a pattern of nocturnal feeding when the benefits of eating at night outweighed the costs. To increase the costs of diurnal feeding, a high-protein (low-carbohydrate) or a low-protein (high-carbohydrate) diet was made available in the day. To increase the benefits of nocturnal feeding, a diet containing an optimum protein/carbohydrate ratio was made available at night.

The chicks offered the costly daytime diets containing either a surfeit of or inadequate protein changed to a pattern of day and night feeding. This is not a typical feeding schedule for these animals. Keep in mind that the high-protein diet contained inadequate carbohydrates and that the low-protein diet malnourished the animals for proteins. Both the low-protein and low-carbohydrate chicks improved their conditions by supplementing daytime diets with the alternative component at night. These data show that a change in calorie strategy is not the only choice for chicks faced with a nutritional challenge. Chicks are apparently sensitive enough to the quality of foods and flexible enough in their foraging times to adopt an alternative nocturnal strategy when the benefits outweigh the costs.

When the pressure to obtain calories is not intense, the necessity for generalist feeders to strike a compromise between nutrition and calorie foraging appears to be minimal. Kenneth Glander's (1981) observations of mantled howling monkeys illustrate nicely how an optimal diet might be acquired.

Mantled howling monkeys forage in Costa Rica for different parts of selected trees. They eat mature leaves, new leaves, fruit, and flower parts. These animals do not select food from all the tree species in the home range; they use at most 62 of the 96 tree species. In fact, the top 15 tree species accounted for 81% of the feeding time. If you count all the available trees, 79% of the feeding time took place in 5% of the available trees. This highly selective behavior was not a result of greater availability of the selected trees. Indeed, feeding time appeared to correlate negatively with tree abundance; the more common a tree species was, the less inclined the animals were to spend time with that tree species.

A chemical analysis of the tree parts eaten in various amounts by the howlers revealed important insights. Because of their preference for fruits and flowers, the monkeys made it clear they were maximizing their energy intake. These animals were also maximizing intake of water, total protein, and all amino acids except isoleucine. When a digestibility coefficient, which takes into account crude fiber, was computed for the mature leaves, it was reliably higher for the leaves eaten than for those not eaten. The animals were apparently maximizing the digestibility of their foods. Furthermore, the animals balanced their diets in terms of carbohydrates and specific amino acids.

The analysis also revealed insights into secondary compounds in these plants. Tannins will inhibit protein, starch, and cellulose digestion, and alkaloids found in many plants can be toxic. The animals in this study tended to minimize their intake of these compounds by carefully selecting leaves without tannins or by selecting new rather than mature leaves on some trees. This strategy may involve conditioned taste aversions and quite clearly demonstrates that optimal diet choice involves a minimizing as well as a maximizing strategy.

The image is of a monkey making sophisticated choices about its diet by tasting its foods very carefully; Glander observed this exact behavior. Usually a single adult would enter a tree, take one or two mouthfuls, and then leave that tree within 3 minutes.

Perhaps this kind of analysis cannot be used in humans who have such culturally enriched habits that the typical assumptions may not apply. But consider the optimal diet model. The main assumption of this model is that the forager will continue to gather or hunt foods that increase the ratio of calorie returns relative to foraging costs. The costs of foraging are usually measured in the time it takes to hunt or search for food and in the handling time for various foods. All of the foods in the forager's diet are ranked according to the ratio of returns (calories) to costs (handling or processing time). The "best" (optimal) strategy is to acquire those foods for which this ratio is higher than the total benefit/cost ratio and to ignore those foods for which the ratio is lower, because foods having higher benefit/cost ratios than the net total ratio elevate that total ratio. Foods with lower benefit/cost ratios decrease the total.

Using this model, one should predict that the abundance of a particular food item is beside the point. An item that is out of the optimal diet is out, no matter how abundant it becomes, and an item that is in the optimal diet is not excluded no matter how rare it becomes.

Foraging in the hunter-gatherer society of the Aché of eastern Paraguay was observed by Hawkes et al. (1982). The choice of foods taken from the variety encountered is consistent with predictions from the optimal diet model. If the resources taken by the Aché are ranked in order of benefit/cost ratios, these ratios are higher than the net total ratios for any set of items (Figure 1.1). In this analysis, it was quite clear that foods were not chosen by abundance. The choice depended only on the benefit/cost ratio.

This same model has been used to predict choice of prey in Amazonian hunting societies. Once again, prey were not taken according to their abundance, but for their caloric benefits relative to costs. More recently, the model has been successfully applied to the prediction of horticultural production among a native Amazonian population of southeastern Peru.

In the laboratory, similarly sophisticated dietary choices are made. For example, raw soybeans are markedly inferior in nutritional quality to properly heated soybeans. In fact, when properly processed, the nutritional value of soybean approaches that of meat or milk. Rats show a strong preference for a diet containing processed soybean over raw soybean flakes. This preference is apparent after a brief exposure, which indicates a measure of involvement of sensory factors such a taste, smell, or texture, rather than post-ingestional factors.

The fundamentals of dietary choice as a means of total organismic regulation were set forth by Richter and his collaborators (1938). To simplify the experiment, these investigators decided to restrict selections to the most representative nutrients of those known at the time to play an important part in the nutrition of the rat. Rather than make a priori selections on the basis of theoretical knowledge, they let the rat's survival time be a measure of the nutritional value of the foodstuffs.

The rats were fed a single foodstuff from each of the major groups. Of the six fats tested (olive oil, lard, wheat germ oil, cod liver oil, peanut oil, and perilla oil), olive oil provided the longest survival time, allowing animals

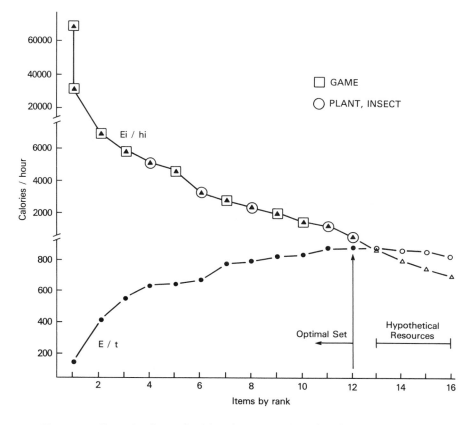

Figure 1.1 Data showing optimal foraging among the Aché of Paraguay. If you rank the food items according to calorie returns per cost (handling time), you see that all the food items taken have higher returns per cost (upper line) than the total returns/total costs for all the foods at that point (lower line). These people thus increase their total returns/costs for each food item, and they only hunt those prey for which such a profit exists. (From Hawkes, et al., 1982. © American Ethnologist Society.)

about 46.5 days on the substance. Of the six carbohydrates tested (dextrose, sucrose, starch, levulose, lactose, and galactose), dextrose provided the most sustenance, giving animals about 57 days. Of the proteins (casein, desiccated blood fibrin, egg albumin, lactalbumin, hemoglobin, and dialyzed egg albumin), casein was the most sustaining, giving animals 38.5 days survival. Thus, olive oil and casein were chosen for the selection experiment. Sucrose, having both glucose and fructose, and giving the second longest survival time of the carbohydrates (43 days), was chosen as the carbohydrate.

In the selection experiment, animals were offered olive oil, casein, sucrose, sodium chloride, calcium lactate, dibasic sodium phosphate, potassium chloride, yeast (as a source of vitamin B complex), cod liver oil (vitamins D and A), wheat germ oil (vitamin E), and water. The growth of the animals on the self-selection regimen was rapid, paralleling the growth of animals on the composite McCollum diet. The estrus cycles of the females on the self-selection regimen, however, studied by obtaining vaginal smears, showed far more regularity than those of animals on the McCollum diet. The activity levels of both sets of animals were essentially identical.

The animals' selections were remarkably similar, except for sucrose and olive oil. Two animals chose larger amounts of sucrose ("sugar burners"), while six animals chose larger amounts of oil ("oil burners"). After several months, however, the "sugar burners" became "oil burners". The animals consistently sampled small amounts of each of the other nutrients. The investigators concluded that despite the fact that nutrients rarely appear separately in natural foods, animals are able to recognize them in isolated forms.

In summary, foraging theory is used to predict behaviors related to the acquisition of specific nutrients. The most powerful foraging models predict the acquisition of calories without taking into account a fine-grained analysis of specific nutrients. When specific nutrients are analyzed, animals show a strategy of optimal diet choice. Because energy requirements dominate every metabolic function, calorie acquisition is probably the bottom line of foraging. If there were ever a choice between selecting calories and optimizing a nutrient mix, the animal would probably obtain calories first. If calorie benefits were equal, however, the animal would probably choose foods that contain the optimal mix of nutrients. These "trade-offs" still need to be determined under actual foraging conditions.

Control Theory

Even if an animal's diet selection can be predicted in terms of its calorie or nutrient profit margins, we still need to know how an animal controls this selection. This knowledge involves questions about how an animal senses changes in nutrient levels and modifies its behavior to act on the nutrient information. We are asking: What are the neural and visceral mechanisms of diet selection? This section on control theory provides a framework for answering this question.

In his excellent book, *Brains, Behavior, and Robotics* (1981), James Albus considers the structure of control systems directed toward attainment of specific behavioral goals. The simplest form of goal-seeking device is the servomechanism. This device is composed of a setpoint, or reference command, that provides the device with a value to control. Feedback from a sensor monitors the action of the device and compares the results of that action with the value of the reference command. An error signal is generated if there is any discrepancy between the commanded action and the results. This error signal directs the action of the device such that the resulting feedback matches the reference command. This entire system operates continuously so that the system will act to match the setpoint value. In behavioral terms, we can say that the system seeks the goal set by the reference command.

You are already familiar with the actions of controlled systems. Consider the state of your hunger. You would like to maintain enough energy to do all the things you need to do. This energy value can be viewed as the reference command. In your environment, you undergo various changes in energy expenditure. On some days, you might be more active or anxious, and you expend more energy. On other days, you are not as active, and you do not expend as much energy.

Your body is somehow monitoring these changes in energy expenditure (for the present, we will not specify how). When there is a difference between the reference command and the state of your energy supply, a signal is generated so that you can act to correct this imbalance. If you have too little energy, the signal involves hunger; you feel like consuming additional fuels. If you consume a surfeit of utilizable fuels, the signal involves a shutting off of further consumption.

To describe your maintenance of energy supply in simple servomechanism terms, however, is to deny the elegance of all your interacting control systems. The feedback questions "Too much?, Too little?" can be juxtaposed with other relevant questions: "Nutrient levels too high? Too low?" At other levels, relevant feedback questions relate to whether the correct balance of nutrients exists. At yet other levels, feedback relates to nerve impulses and neurotransmitter activity.

Feeding behavior often appears to be more flexible than a simple homeostatic concept would predict. This is because an omnivore has to adjust to meet the complex requirements of ever-changing environmental circumstances. These changes can affect the priority of nutrient needs such that a forager may eat one food while skipping another that also provides necessary nutrients. A hierarchy of nutrient controls implies a flexibility that the study of one system of nutrient homeostasis often neglects.

The notion of a hierarchy of controlled systems is thus a key concept. From the top down, the output condition becomes the reference value for the next level of control. From the bottom up, feedback identifies the completion of the immediately relevant subtask. The feedback enters the hierarchy at every level. As we ascend levels of control, feedback provides more highly processed data until the original command is satisfied.

If an engineer were to design a behaving system that even remotely resembled a real-life, goal-directed system, a hierarchy of subsystems would be a necessary inclusion. Consider Albus's design of a robot arm that might be used for a pick and place task that a human operator might perform on an assembly line. The hierarchy of information in the flow diagram would include shoulder lift, shoulder rotate, upper arm rotate, elbow lift, lower arm rotate, wrist flex, and finger pinch. "Fetching" would be an upper-level task that would be broken down into subtasks such as "orienting," "reaching," and "grasping." Feedback from the lowest members in the hierarchy identify completion of the immediately relevant subtask.

What about in a real brain? The diagram in Figure 1.2 shows the hierarchy of motor control in real brains. The results from transection experiments with animals, and observations of humans with brain damage, are consistent with the notion of a hierarchy. If the spinal cord is transected from the brain (cut A-A), most of the basic motor patterns remain, including the flexor reflex and locomotion rhythms.

These rhythms are not coordinated, however, unless the brainstem below the cut B-B remains intact. The control of posture and the sequential coordination necessary for walking requires the area below C-C to be functional. When you are out for a stroll, if you wish to avoid obstacles, you must use

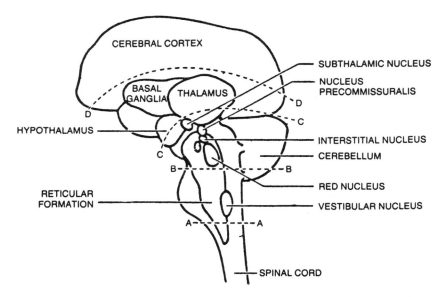

Figure 1.2 A hierarchy of motor control. Primitive flexor reflexes are still observed if the spinal cord is severed from the brain at A-A. The balance and coordination of these reflexes for standing is possible if the intact area includes everything below B-B. Walking requires the area below C-C to be functional. If you want to avoid obstacles while you walk, you need most of the central nervous system below D-D intact. Lengthy purposive tasks probably require functioning of the cerebral cortex above D-D. (From Albus, 1981.)

systems that coordinate head and eye movements and provide processed visual information about objects. For this you need all the nervous system to be intact below D-D. The specific functions above D-D are difficult to identify, but animals with cuts at D-D seem to lack what can only be described as a long-term "purposiveness."

It is curious that as animals recover from brain damage, they seem to re-develop a hierarchical control of behavior. Philip Teitelbaum and colleagues (1984) observed that lateral hypothalamic brain-damaged rats first regain movements in a two-dimensional plane: lateral head scans are about all they are capable of in the earliest stages. Recovery then proceeds through more sophisticated stages of movement from straightforward locomotion to movements in the vertical plane (rearing). Along with having locomotor deficits, animals with lateral hypothalamic damage also refuse to eat. They can be force fed until they begin to feed on their own.

To show further the hierarchical control of behavior, Teitelbaum used a procedure called cortical spreading depression, whereby the functioning of the cortex is inhibited with injections of potassium chloride. When the cortex is depressed this way in a damaged animal that has recovered, the original damaged behaviors re-emerge: the animal stops eating and regresses back to two-dimensional behaviors. Apparently, activity of the cortex was necessary for the recovery of more sophisticated behaviors.

The concept of behavioral hierarchy is not just restricted to findings in the laboratory; behavioral biologists invoke this concept to make sense out of natural behavior. The diagram in Figure 1.3 shows the hierarchy proposed by Niko Tinbergen to account for the behavior of the male three-spined stickleback fish. The dashed line shows the relationship between subtasks for one particular survival goal: reproduction. Several of these subtasks are re-

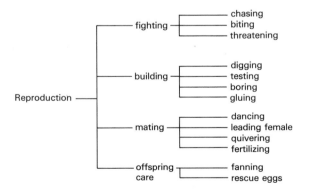

Figure 1.3   Niko Tinbergen's account of a behavior hierarchy in a male stickleback fish. (From Tinbergen, 1951.)

quired for reproduction, including fighting, nest-building, mating, and caring for young. Each requires more specific (lower level) behaviors for completion: e.g. fighting requires chasing, biting, and threatening. Of course, it is possible to extend this hierarchy down through specific motor behaviors required to chase, bite, or threaten.

The hierarchical control model provides a framework for an analysis of food intake from the upper command levels of foraging behavior to lower behavioral levels of diet choice to even lower levels of the actual feeding behavior. Yet many authors treat the control of feeding as if it exists independently of other foraging concepts. Although it is changing, the literature is replete with studies of food intake as if animals always choose one kind of food (lab chow).

One can certainly describe a glucostatic or lipostatic control of feeding without reference to higher-level organismic commands. If one of these control loops is taken in isolation, however, it then becomes difficult to reconcile the explanation with newer data showing links between specific amino acid intake and subsequent carbohydrate selection. In short, it seems difficult to show how an animal can maintain a constant internal environment (obtaining all the essential nutrients) in the face of a highly variable external environment. To describe the behavioral feedback effects of specific nutrients, it will be necessary to adopt an explanation along several levels of the foraging hierarchy.

For example, the separate behavioral effects that occur as a result of deprivation of a specific nutrient–change in taste acuity, increased sensory reactivity, heightened predation–might be viewed in the larger, integrative sense as behaviors that satisfy increased foraging demands for calorie and nutrient optimization. In other words, these are specific (hierarchically arranged) behavioral control mechanisms for the maintenance of energy and nutrient levels. The task before us is to integrate these behavioral control changes by explaining their neural control mechanisms.

Perhaps the most interesting and elegant feature of this task is the requirement that behavior produce consequential feedback detected by the nervous system. Such feedback is not hard to imagine, but difficult to prove. Changes in taste acuity, glucose levels (glucoreception), and insulin levels provide convenient examples of such feedback regulation. These satiety signals have been discussed in terms of the regulation of feeding, but what of the regulation of nutrient intake?

Many of the nutrients that have specific receptors in the nervous system are *essential nutrients*. No biosynthetic process exists to manufacture them; the organism must behave (forage) to acquire them. Even in the case of glucose, which has a biosynthetic sequence, the organism is responsive to the nutrient (glucose) taken in by its foraging. Thus, the consequences of nutrient intake may be feedback signals providing the nervous system with information relative to the particular state of nutrient intake. Because there are direct neural consequences of foraging, the nervous system can provide the organism with behavior appropriate to optimizing these nutrient signals. We thus link the two theoretical concepts of optimal foraging and neural control of behavior.

Concepts of hierarchical control are maintained throughout the discussions in each of the chapters. It is best, however, to remember that the data on any one nutrient did not accrue with this book's organizing principles in mind. It is therefore not possible to maintain an identical pattern of discussion for each nutrient. For example, much of the behavioral work on thiamine developed without concurrent research on the brain. This should be contrasted with research on tryptophan, in which behavioral and neural data were gathered within the same time periods, and often in the same studies.

To facilitate an understanding of the neural control of behavior, the following chapter presents an overview of neuroanatomy. The reader who is well-versed in nervous system structure and function can safely skip this chapter and proceed to the chapters on neurotransmitters and nutrients.

References

Albus, J.S. *Brains, behavior, & robotics,* Peterborough, NH: BYTE, 1981.

Bartholow, R. *A practical treatise on materia medica and therapeutics* (9th Ed.), New York: Appleton & Co., 1896.

Bennett, E.L., Diamond, M.C., Krech, D., & Rosenzweig, M.R. Chemical and anatomical plasticity of brain. *Science, 146,* 1964, 610–618.

Denenberg, V.H. *The development of behavior,* Stamford, Conn.: Sinauer, 1972.

Glander, K.E. Feeding patterns in mantled howling monkeys. In A.C. Kamil & T.D. Sargent (Eds.), *Foraging behavior: Ecological, ethological, and psychological approaches,* New York: Garland Press, 1981, pp. 231–258.

Hawkes, K., Hill, K., & O'Connell, J.F. Why hunters gather: Optimal foraging and the Aché of eastern Paraguay, *American Ethnologist, 9,* 1982, 379–398.

Pyke, G., Pulliam, H., & Charnov, E. Optimal foraging: A selective review of theory and tests, *Quarterly Review of Biology, 52,* 1977, 137–154.

Rall, T.W. Central nervous system stimulants: The xanthines, In A.G. Gilman, L.S. Goodman, & A. Gilman (Eds.), *Goodman and Gilman's the pharmacological basis of therapeutics,* 6th Ed., New York: Macmillan 1980, pp. 592–607.

Richter, C.P., Holt, L.E. Jr., & Barelare, B. Jr. Nutritional requirements for normal growth and reproduction in rats studied by the self-selection method. *American Journal of Physiology, 122,* 1938, 734–744.

Rosenzweig, M.R. Experience, memory, and the brain. *American Psychologist, 39,* 1984, 365–376.

Rovee-Collier, C.K., Clapp, B.A., & Collier, G.H. The economics of food choice in chicks, *Physiology and Behavior, 28,* 1982, 1097–1102.

Teitelbaum, P. The lateral hypothalamic double-disconnection syndrome: A reappraisal and a new theory for recovery of function. In S.H. Hulse, & B.F. Greene, Jr. (Eds.), *100 years of psychological research in America: G. Stanley Hall and The Johns Hopkins tradition,* Baltimore: Johns Hopkins Press, 1984.

Tinbergen, N. *The study of instinct,* Oxford: Clarendon Press, 1951.

Wurtman, R.J. Precursor control of transmitter synthesis. In Barbeau, A., Growdon, J.H., & Wurtman, R.J. (Eds.), *Nutrition and the brain* (Vol 5), New York: Raven Press, 1979, pp. 1–12.

Suggested Readings

Blundell, J.E. Problems and processes underlying the control of food selection and nutrient intake. In R.J. Wurtman & J.J. Wurtman (Eds.), *Nutrition and the brain* (Vol. 6), New York: Raven Press, 1983, pp. 163–222.

Grossman, S.P. *A textbook of physiological psychology,* New York: John Wiley, 1967.

Hames, R.B., & Vickers, W.T. Optimal diet breadth theory as a model to explain variability in Amazonian hunting, *American Ethnologist, 9,* 1982, 358–378.

Keegan, W.F. The optimal foraging analysis of horticultural production. *American Anthropologist, 88,* 1986, 92–107.

Naim, M., Kare, M.R., & Ingle, D.E. Sensory factors which affect the acceptance of raw and heated defatted soybeans by rats. *Journal of Nutrition, 107,* 1977, 1653–1658.

MacArthur, R.H., & Pianka, E.R. On optimal use of a patchy environment, *American Naturalist, 100,* 1966, 603–609.

Chapter *2*

Introduction to Neuroanatomy

Oe of the useful ways of arriving at a conception of the central nervous system (CNS) is to consider that it is composed of seven main parts. If you took a cleaver and cut through the brain right between the eyes (mid-sagittal section), you would see that each of the parts has a bilaterally paired structure on the opposite half of the brain. (In actuality, the brain halves are not completely symmetrical, giving us the basis for handedness.) Refer to Figure 2.1 for the description of the seven main parts of the CNS:

(1) The *spinal cord* receives sensory impulses from the skin and muscle and integrates these with motor commands to the same areas of skin and muscle.

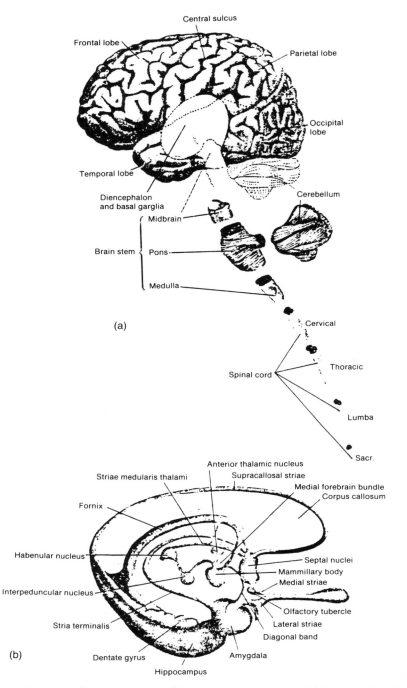

Figure 2.1 Seven major parts of the central nervous system. (a) Spinal cord, brain stem, cerebellum, basal ganglia, diencephalon, and cerebral cortex. (b) Limbic system. (From Kandel and Schwartz, 1981.)

18

(2) The *brainstem* is the rostral extension of the spinal cord. It integrates sensory and motor information for the head and neck and also contains the cell bodies of cranial nerves, which control facial movements and special senses such as balance.

(3) The *cerebellum* is a distinct structure attached to the dorsal surface of the brainstem. The cerebellum classically is concerned with the coordination of somatic motor activity, the regulation of muscle tone, and the maintenance of equilibrium.

(4) The *basal ganglia* are contained laterally within the forebrain and are concerned with control of motor movement.

(5) The *diencephalon* is composed of thalamus, hypothalamus, subthalamus, and epithalamus and is located in the center and ventral aspects of the brain. The thalamus integrates all sensory and motor information at supraspinal levels, while the hypothalamus integrates internal signals for homeostasis.

(6) The *limbic system* is (classically) thought to be involved in affective (emotional) components of behavior. The limbic lobe is the ring of tissue surrounding the central core of the brain.

(7) The *cerebral cortex* is the mantle of tissue comprising the outer regions of the brain and is the convoluted structure we see when we look at a whole brain. The cerebral cortex is involved in perceptual and cognitive processes.

*S*pinal Cord

Next you would take your cleaver and cut the spinal cord coronally (crosswise). What you would see at most levels of the cord is presented in Figure 2.2. The central canal runs nearly the length of the cord and carries the cerebrospinal fluid. The gray cellular matter (it is gray because it does not contain the whitish myelin sheath) can be found forming the shape of a butterfly throughout most of the levels of the cord. The white matter runs longitudinally through the cord and can be found around the outside of the gray matter.

There are 31 "levels" or segments of the spinal cord, each with a pair of dorsal and ventral spinal nerves associated with localized regions of the body. At each level, the dorsal root carries sensory information into the dorsal horn from the skin and muscle groups corresponding to that level. The ventral root carries motor information from cells in the ventral horn out to the appropriate muscles for each segment. For example, the patellar tendon reflex (kneejerk) is controlled by lumbar levels L2–L4.

The size and shape of the gray matter vary as functions of the size of the spinal nerve roots. This depends on the amount of motor control required. For example, cervical segments are enlarged relative to thoracic segments

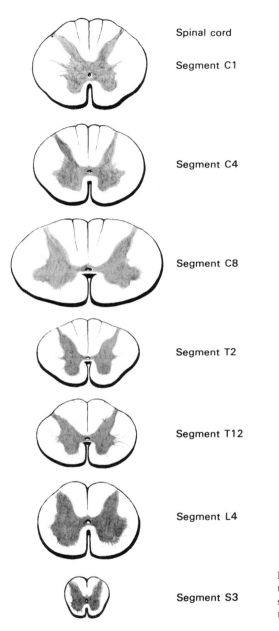

Spinal cord

Segment C1

Segment C4

Segment C8

Segment T2

Segment T12

Segment L4

Segment S3

Figure 2.2   Cross-sections (coronal slices) through different levels of the spinal cord showing the changing relationship of gray to white matter. (From Carpenter, 1972.)

because of the greater amount of control necessary for arms, hands, and fingers than for the chest. The white matter also varies considerably in size along the spinal cord. The increase in size from caudal (lower) to rostral (higher) levels reflects the increasing number of fibers that ascend to higher levels as additional groups of fibers carrying sensory information from each level begin to ascend in the cord.

The spinal cord has three principal functions: (1) to integrate and relay sensory information for processing at higher levels; (2) to receive and process motor commands from higher levels for action at the muscles; and (3) to mediate the lower level integration of motor control.

There are two major ascending systems for somatic sensation: the dorsal column (medial lemniscal system) and the anterolateral system. The medial lemniscal system mediates touch, pressure, and position information. The anterolateral system mediates pain and temperature sensation.

The descending motor systems course through the lateral and anterior aspects of the spinal cord. These systems are concerned with somatic movement, visceral innervation, modification of muscle tone, and segmental reflexes. The corticospinal tract is generally regarded as the descending pathway most concerned with voluntary, discrete, and skilled movements. The tectospinal tract presumably mediates postural adjustments in response to visual stimuli. The rubrospinal, vestibulospinal, and reticulospinal tracts presumably mediate muscle tone and balance.

Cells in the ventral horn respond directly to sensory information (carried by dorsal root fibers) from muscle stretch receptors. Muscle stretch activates these cells to produce motor commands for a contraction in the same muscle. However, actual behavior is much smoother than the simple initiation of a contraction for every stretch. To smooth out a motor response, sensory information from a tendon receptor will produce inhibition of the contraction and a contraction of the antagonistic muscle. This means that even as a muscle contraction (movement) is initiated, feedback mechanisms act to inhibit and slow down the contraction so that the movement is smooth throughout its trajectory. A more detailed look at these feedback mechanisms is given in Figure 2.3.

*B*rainstem

As you move rostrally up the spinal cord, you see that the cord enlarges into the three regions known collectively as the brainstem: medulla, pons, and midbrain. These areas are enlarged as are the cervical levels of the spinal cord for similar reasons: more sensory and motor information and greater recruitment of sensory and motor systems exist in the head and neck. Within the brainstem are cells enmeshed in a network, or "reticulum," of fine fibers. This reticular formation is important for sensory arousal of the rest of the brain. Other discrete nuclei in the brainstem contain specific neurotransmitters that have an influence on virtually every process in the CNS. These are discussed in detail in the chapters on neurotransmitters.

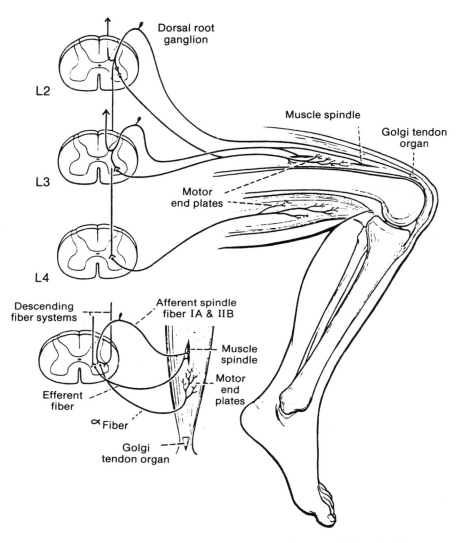

Figure 2.3 Spinal reflex. Stretch receptors in the muscle convey information (impulses) about muscle stretch to the motor neurons in the ventral spinal cord. The motor neurons, once activated, send out impulses to contract the selfsame muscle and inhibit contraction in the antagonistic muscle. The Golgi tendon organ receptors also sense stretch; their impulses inhibit the motor neurons, thereby limiting the contraction. (From Carpenter, 1972.)

Much of your knowledge about the brainstem will come from examining the anatomy and function of the cranial nerves (Figure 2.4). In their original arbitrary order, the cranial nerves are presented with a brief statement of their functions:

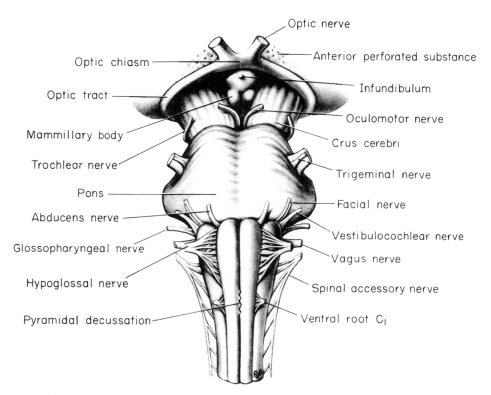

Figure 2.4 The brain stem showing the relation of cranial nerves to the medulla, pons, and midbrain. (From Carpenter, 1972.)

    I. Olfactory: sensory, for smell
   II. Optic: sensory, for vision
  III. Oculomotor: motor, for eye movements
  IV. Trochlear: motor, for eye movements
   V. Trigeminal: sensory, from face; motor, for mastication
  VI. Abducens: motor, for eye movements
 VII. Facial: sensory, for taste (anterior two-thirds of tongue); motor, face movements
VIII. Vestibulocochlear: sensory, for balance and hearing
  IX. Glossopharyngeal: sensory, for taste (posterior one-third tongue); sensory, from upper pharynx
   X. Vagus: sensory, from viscera; motor, parasympathetic
  XI. Spinal accessory: motor, for neck and head muscles
 XII. Hypoglossal: motor, tongue muscles

The cranial nerves associated with the medulla (first enlargement of the brainstem from the spinal cord) are the hypoglossal (XII), spinal accessory (XI), vagus (X), and glossopharyngeal (IX). The medial lemniscus carries touch-pressure sensory information from the spinal cord and decussates (crosses) in the medulla to convey this information to the opposite side of the brain. One of the most conspicuous features upon gross examination of the medulla is the decussation of the corticospinal tract. This tract forms the pyramids on the ventral surface of the medulla, and it is easy to see the interdigitation of fibers as they cross to the opposite side. This crossing means that motor commands arising from cells in your right cerebral cortex might initiate the act of shaking your left leg. Internally, the medulla contains cells that communicate with the cerebellum and spinal cord. The medullary reticular formation contributes projections to the ascending reticular activating system.

The cranial nerves present at the junction between the medulla and pons are abducens (VI), facial (VII), and vestibulocochlear (VIII). Further up, at about the middle level of the pons, is the largest cranial nerve, the trigeminal (V). Three main roots of the trigeminal nerve carry sensory information from three main portions of the face: ophthalmic, maxillary, and mandibular. The motor nucleus of the trigeminal nerve projects to the mandibular muscles. The lateral lemniscus is the primary ascending auditory pathway carrying fibers to the midbrain. The vestibular nuclei are concerned with orientation in three-dimensional space, equilibrium, and muscle tone. The pons has a continuation of the reticular formation and gives rise to fibers in the ascending reticular activating system. Upon gross examination of the ventral surface of the brainstem, it is easy to see the transverse fibers of the pons communicating with the cerebellum, which is attached to the dorsal surface of the brainstem at about the level of the pons.

Quite noticeable when you look at the ventral surface of the midbrain are the massive cerebral peduncles. These are the rostral continuation of the corticospinal tract carrying motor information from the cerebrum to the spinal cord. Two cranial nerves arise at the level of the midbrain: oculomotor (III) and trochlear (IV). If you look at the dorsal surface of the midbrain (Figure 2.5), you see four bumps: two on top (superior colliculi) and two on the bottom (inferior colliculi). The superior colliculi interchange visual and sensory-motor information for visually guided movements and reflexes. The inferior colliculi receive auditory information from the pons and interchange with sensory-motor systems for auditory reflexes.

A conspicuous structure within the midbrain is the red nucleus, so designated because it has a pinkish yellow color on gross examination. This nucleus receives motor control fibers from cerebrum and cerebellum and relays information down to the spinal cord and up to the thalamus. The substantia nigra projects to the basal ganglia and is also involved in motor control. The principal lesion in patients with Parkinson's disease is to the

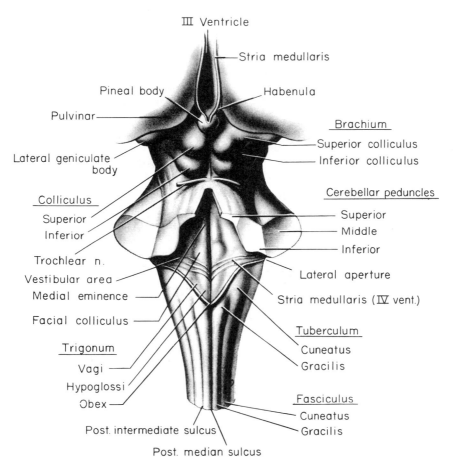

Figure 2.5 Dorsal surface of the midbrain showing the superior and inferior colliculi. (From Carpenter, 1971.)

substantia nigra. One aspect of the brainstem reticular formation ascends from this level, projects widely throughout the brain, and is involved in behavioral arousal and wakefulness.

Cerebellum

The cerebellum lies beneath the cerebrum (in humans) and is attached to the dorsal surface of the pons by three cerebellar peduncles. The cerebellum consists structurally of a gray cellular mantle called the cerebellar cortex, an internal white mass called the medullary substance, and four pairs of intrinsic nuclei embedded in the white matter. The core or medial portion of the cerebellum is called the vermis. The lobes are referred to as the cerebellar hemispheres. The cerebellum is shown in Figure 2.6.

Functionally and embryologically, the cerebellum can be considered to be divided into three main parts: archicerebellum, paleocerebellum, and neocerebellum. The most caudal archicerebellum is associated with the control of posture and balance by virtue of its interconnections with the vestibular system. The most rostral paleocerebellum receives impulses from stretch receptors and is concerned with the regulation of muscle tone. The large neocerebellum—between the other two divisions—is concerned with skilled voluntary and associated movements and is thought to be involved in the planning of movements. Activity of neurons in this part of the cerebellum seems to occur immediately preceding the movement of a limb.

James Albus (1981) has proposed an interesting mathematical model of the cerebellum called the Cerebellar Model Arithmetic Computer (CMAC), based upon known cellular interconnections of the cerebellum. The model proposes that the cerebellar connections form a hierarchical control system (see Chapter 1) involved in the control of movement. The CMAC also predicts that memory should be a function of cerebellar activity. This is quite interesting in view of the recent findings by Richard Thompson (1986), who has shown that cerebellar nuclei are important for the memory of a classically conditioned response. Only the response associated with the conditioned stimulus (memory) is affected by cerebellar damage; the unconditioned response is still observed after such damage.

*B*asal Ganglia

The basal ganglia are usually considered to comprise the caudate nuclei, the putamen, and the globus pallidus, though various authors sometimes include (because of cellular structure and interconnections) the amygdaloid complex and even the thalamus. The present aggregation reflects our incomplete knowledge about the relations between structure and function. For example, the tail of the caudate nucleus is continuous with the caudal amygdala, and the globus pallidus derives in development from the diencephalon. This scheme excludes amygdala as belonging to the limbic system and the thalamus as belonging separately to the diencephalon. The basal ganglia are treated functionally as belonging to the extra-pyramidal motor system, thereby inextricably linking these structures to the midbrain structures: red nucleus and substantia nigra.

The basal ganglia lie in the center of the brain lateral to the lateral ventricles (Figure 2.7). The caudate nucleus has an enlarged anterior portion, or

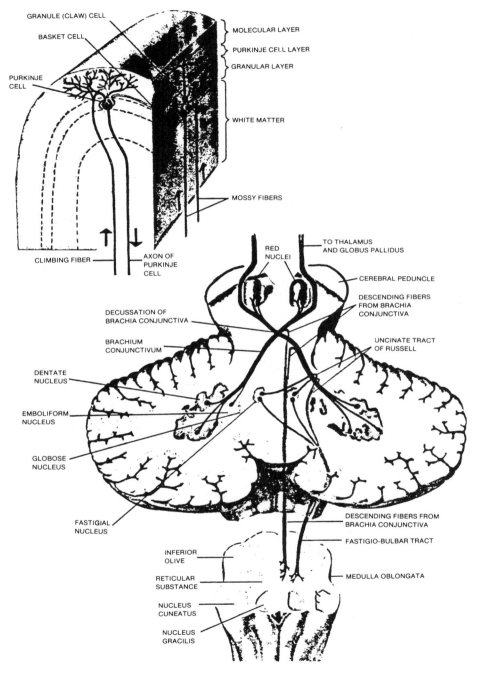

Figure 2.6   Cerebellum. (From Netter, 1972.)

head, and a long caudal portion, or tail, that arches up and runs caudally along the lateral edge of the lateral ventricle, finally looping down and forward to reach the amygdala. The putamen lies lateral to the head of the caudate and is separated from the caudate by the internal capsule, which is the main rostral tract of the corticospinal system. The globus pallidus lies medial and ventral to the putamen, but still lateral to the internal capsule (in humans).

Several areas of neocortex give rise to axons that project directly to the caudate and putamen nuclei. These structures, collectively known as neo-striatum, then project to globus pallidus, which gives rise to major thalamic projections. The neostriatum also projects to the substantia nigra, which has major dopamine projections back to the neostriatum.

Functions of the basal ganglia were elucidated by clinicians who observed characteristic motor disorders associated with isolated damage to each component (see "hiss suppressor" discussion in Chapter 1). The classic basal ganglia disorder is Parkinson's disease, which is associated with a resting tremor and rigidity. This motor disorder is primarily due to degeneration of cells in the substantia nigra that project directly to the neostriatum. Athetosis describes slow, writhing involuntary movements and is typically associated with damage in putamen and globus pallidus. Huntington's disease is associated with chorea: a rapid, graceful series of involuntary movements resembling fragments of purposeful, voluntary movements.

Recent experimental studies (primarily electrical stimulation) have elaborated on the functions of the basal ganglia. On the basis of these studies, Philip Groves (1983) proposed that the neostriatum is involved in the prep-

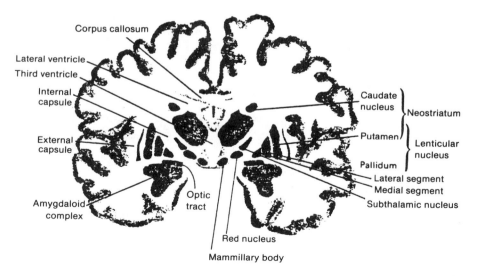

Figure 2.7 Cross-section (coronal slice) of the brain showing the embedded basal ganglia. (From Kandel and Schwartz, 1981.)

aration, execution, and guidance of voluntary movement in response to the analysis and volition of the cortex. Hassler (1978) has concluded that the putamen focuses the attention on a single event by suppressing all other data. Pallidal function, according to Hassler, is horizontal locomotion.

Diencephalon

The diencephalon, at the rostral end of the brainstem, is divisible into four major parts: thalamus, hypothalamus, subthalamus, and epithalamus. The diencephalon is bounded laterally by the lateral ventricle. Medially it is separated by the third ventricle. The thalamus is the most central structure in the brain. The hypothalamus lies ventral to the thalamus at the base of the brain. The subthalamus lies between the thalamus and hypothalamus. The epithalamus is comprised of the habenula at the roof of the third ventricle and the pineal body extending further dorsally and caudally above the superior colliculus.

Thalamus

The nuclei of the thalamus may be considered as classified into three main groups: medial, lateral, and anterior. The pulvinar is a large nuclear mass at the caudal end of the thalamus. These nuclei are separated by white matter laminae, which contain the small intralaminar nuclei. All sensory impulses, with the primary exception of olfaction, are conveyed to the cellular masses of the thalamus. Visual impulses project to the lateral geniculate nucleus, while auditory impulses are conveyed to the medial geniculate cells. Cells in the ventrobasal complex respond to tactile and position sensations. Gustatory information also reaches these cells. This complex, along with the posterior thalamic cells, is concerned with the perceptions of pain. The thalamus can therefore be described as concerned with both the discriminative and affective components of sensation.

The major thalamic projections respect the functional input: medial geniculate auditory input is relayed to auditory cortex. Lateral geniculate visual input is relayed to visual cortex. Somatic sensory input to ventral posterolateral thalamus is relayed to somatic sensory areas in the post-central gyrus of the cortex. Extrapyramidal system projections from substantia nigra and basal ganglia are relayed to the motor cortex in the precentral gyrus. The thalamus might therefore be conceived as a kind of switching station for all sensory and motor information reaching the brain. The connections of the thalamus are shown in Figure 2.8.

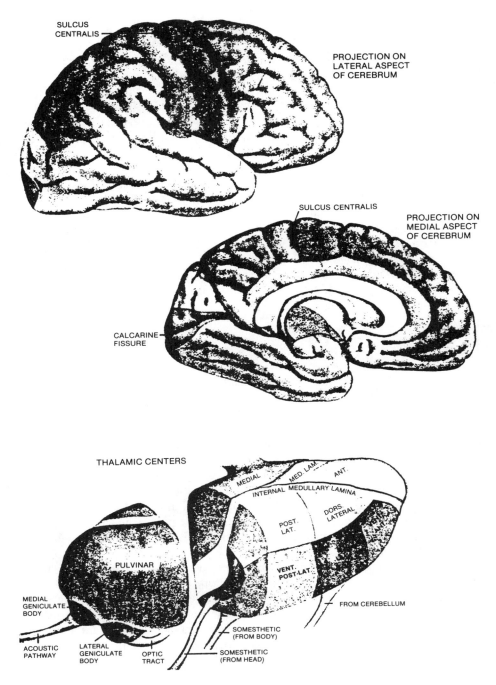

Hypothalamus

The hypothalamus resides ventrally in the center of the brain. If you turn the brain over to look at the underside (ventral surface), you would see the crossing of the optic chiasm (nerve II) as the landmark at the anterior border of the hypothalamus. The mammillary bodies delimit the hypothalamus posteriorly. The other striking feature of this ventral view is the protrusion of the pituitary gland attached to the hypothalamus by the pituitary stalk. The anterior portion of the pituitary is in vascular communication with the hypothalamus. The posterior portion of the pituitary receives neural projections from the hypothalamus. The scheme of the hypothalamus is shown in Figure 2.9.

You might regard the hypothalamus generally as having three broad functions: (1) cells that contain polypeptides regulate endocrine levels (via the pituitary system) and related behaviors; (2) autonomic control: sympathetic and parasympathetic functions; (3) limbic system control (see next section). Because the latter two functions are covered in other sections, only the first function will be discussed here.

In the far anterior (and slightly dorsal) portions of the hypothalamus are cells that contain the peptide luteinizing hormone releasing hormone (LHRH). These LHRH cells project caudally back through the arcuate-median eminence regions of the hypothalamus to release their LHRH contents into the pituitary portal system. This blood-borne releasing hormone stimulates cells in the anterior pituitary to secrete luteinizing hormone (LH), which has an activating (and maintaining) effect on gonadal secretions. Testosterone, for example, is released from the testes when increasing amounts of LH circulate through testicular tissue. Testosterone release is regulated because increasing amounts of blood-borne testosterone *inhibit* LHRH secretion. This continuous feedback inhibition "informs" the hypothalamus of the levels of testosterone release.

Other hypothalamic peptides activate pituitary systems in a similar manner: corticotropin-releasing factor (CRF) stimulates adrenocorticotropin (ACTH) release from the pituitary. ACTH consequently stimulates corticosterone release from the adrenal cortex. Thyrotropin-releasing hormone (TRH) stimulates the pituitary release of thyroid-stimulating hormone (TSH), which activates thyroxin release. Melanocyte-stimulating hormone (MSH) releasing factor (MRF) stimulates pituitary MSH release for melanin production. These are just a few examples.

Magnocellular neurons in the supraoptic and paraventricular nuclei use a different scheme. These cells send axons directly into the posterior pituitary, where they release their contents directly into the general blood circulation. Vasopressin (also called antidiuretic hormone) thus released acts on the collecting ducts of the kidneys to increase their recovery of water. Oxytocin,

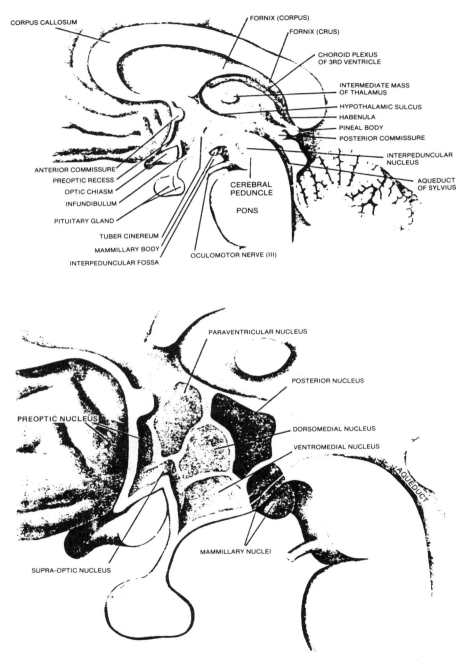

Figure 2.9 A view of the hypothalamus showing its ventral location in the brain and most of its major nuclei. (From Netter, 1972.)

also secreted in this way, increases the amplitude of uterine smooth muscle contraction.

It should be no surprise that motivational behaviors are regulated in the hypothalamus along with their associated hormones. For example, the male pattern of mating behavior (mounting, intromission) requires the integrity of cells in the medial preoptic area. The feedback signals for water regulation (drinking) derive from several sources, but at least one mechanism involves the increased release of vasopressin. Older reports by Hetherington and Ranson (1942) showed that destruction in the ventromedial hypothalamus resulted in voracious eating and severe obesity. Stimulation of this area suppresses feeding. Later, Anand and Brobeck (1951) showed that lesions of the lateral hypothalamus produced the opposite effect: anorexia and loss of appetite. In this regard, it is interesting that stimulation of the lateral hypothalamus elicits feeding. These topics are covered in depth in Chapter 8.

Subthalamus and Epithalamus

The subthalamic region lies lateral and caudal to the hypothalamus, medial to the internal capsule, and ventral to the thalamus. It is comprised primarily of Forel's fields and the zona incerta and is considered to be part of the extrapyramidal motor system. Lesions of this area result in ballism, a set of violent flailing movements.

The epithalamus is composed primarily of the habenular complex–located on the dorsomedial surface of the thalami–and the pineal body, located caudally and dorsally in a region above the superior colliculi. The habenula receives fiber projections from the septal area and anterior hypothalamus and is necessary for mating behavior. The pineal body receives its sole innervation from the sympathetic nervous system and is involved in the circadian and seasonal regulation of hormonal control. The epithalamus is also shown in Figure 2.9.

Limbic System

The concept of *limbic lobe* was introduced by Paul Broca to account for the cellular constancy of the most medial gyrus forming a border (limbus) around the brain stem and diencephalon. In 1937, James Papez proposed that the limbic lobe was actually part of a neural circuit providing the emotional aspect of sensory reactions. His circuit was composed of anterior thalamic nuclei, with projections to the cingulum ("girdle"), a cortical area lying immediately above the corpus callosum. The cingulum has projections to the hippocampus, which curves down ventrally and laterally to end in the temporal lobe near the amygdala (in humans). The hippocampus and septal area (above the rostral hypothalamus and oriented medially) have intimate connections via the fornix, which also projects down to the mammillary bodies of the hypothalamus. The circuit is completed by the large mammillothalamic tract projecting from the mammillary bodies to the anterior thalamic nuclei. It is now considered that other structures such as the olfactory tubercle (from nerve I), amygdala, and habenula (and their interconnections) form integral parts of this circuit (Figure 2.1). The concept of a limbic system has been considerably strengthened by the recent finding that you can raise antibodies to limbic system tissue that will preferentially mark only the limbic system and not other neural areas.

Knowledge that the Papez circuit deals in emotions was derived from clinical observations. For example, the rabies virus has a predilection for the hippocampus (and cerebellum), and because the disease is characterized by intense emotional and convulsive symptoms, this offered a clue to limbic system function. In 1937 and 1939, Kluver and Bucy reported that bilateral removal of the temporal lobe in monkeys (destroying amygdala, ventral hippocampus, and nonlimbic temporal cortex) produced a dramatic behavioral syndrome that included flattened emotions, extreme oral tendencies, and hypersexuality.

These interesting experimental observations were elaborated when Brady and Nauta (1953) showed that specific destruction of the septal area in rats resulted in an extreme rage reaction. More recently, Gage and Olton (1975) showed that the septal rage reaction could be prevented by prior destruction of the communicating tract (the fornix) between the septum and hippocampus. Although this is convincing evidence that limbic areas are involved in emotional behaviors, other behaviors are also involved. For example, it is clear that a spatial working memory seems to involve the hippocampus; destruction of the hippocampus prevents a rat from remembering the places it has recently visited in a maze (Olton & Samuelson, 1976).

Cerebral Cortex

The cerebral cortex forms a large convoluted mantle with an area (in humans) of about 2.5 square feet, only one-third of which is found on the surface (the remainder is hidden within the folds). This is neocortex; other kinds of cortex such as the hippocampus have been previously described.

The neocortex has a distinct lamination, with six layers distinguished by the types and arrangement of their cells. The arrangement of the layers varies, so that the cerebral cortex does not have a homogenous structure throughout. Figure 2.10 shows the widely used Brodmann mapping describing the different areas. Areas 1-3 in the post-central gyrus correspond to the somatic sensory

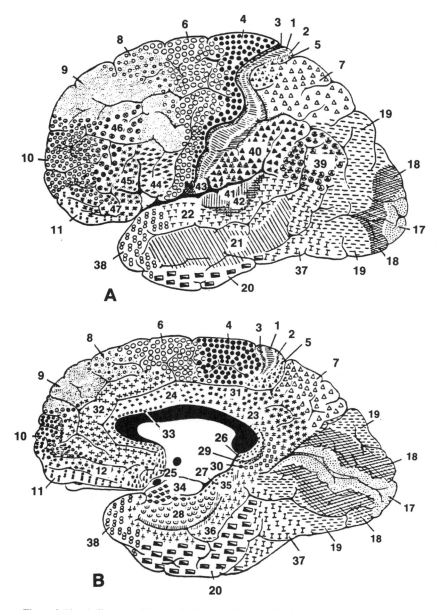

Figure 2.10   A diagram of the cerebral cortex showing Brodmann's mapping scheme. (From Carpenter, 1971.)

projections, which map the body according to the location and amount of somatic sensation. Area 4 in the precentral gyrus contains the motor cells that give rise to the corticospinal tract. These cells have a relatively precise map according to the areas of the body (levels of the spinal cord) they command. Areas 17-19 correspond to the visual cortex projections. These areas receive fibers from the lateral geniculate (thalamus) and project to the superior colliculi in the midbrain.

Lashley's classic study of the rat neocortex in 1929 taught us about the role of neocortex in memory. He experimentally damaged virtually every area of neocortex in varying amounts. The rats were required to learn mazes of differing complexity. It was clear from his study that no one area of neocortex subserved a generalized memory function. More memory was impaired, however, with the more complete destruction of neocortex. From these findings Lashley argued that cortical areas are *equipotential* in housing memory: any one area is as good as any other. *Mass action* was the principle accounting for memory loss; more memory was lost with increasing destruction of cortex.

More recently, other defining principles of the cortex have been discovered. Hubel and Wiesel (1962) showed that the visual cortex is organized into narrow columns running from the surface to the white matter (see Figure 2.11). Each column is about 2 mm deep and 10-30 mm wide. Cells in each column respond to specific linear features of the visual world. For example, one column may contain cells that respond only to a line oriented 30 degrees from the horizon. Within a column, there may be differing complexities of a cell's response. Other cells in the same column may respond to a 30 degree line only when it is moving across the visual field.

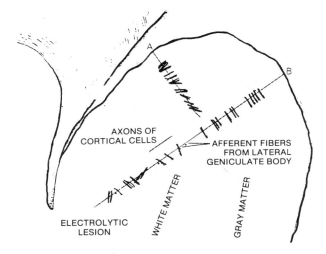

Figure 2.11 Diagram of section of visual cortex showing cortical columns for specific line orientations in the visual world. (From Hubel, 1972.)

Along a perpendicular axis to the orientation columns is another set of columns that respond to eye preference, or ocular dominance. The term *hypercolumn* has been used by Hubel and Wiesel to refer to the set of columns for analyzing lines of all orientations from a particular region in space with both eyes. Because these cortical responses show a different level of visual field organization than their corresponding subcortical cells in the lateral geniculate portion of the visual system, it is easy to see that the cortex provides a different level of feature abstraction from the visual world.

Keep in mind that columnar organization appears to be a principle of cortical organization. Vernon Mountcastle (1975) showed that somatic sensory cortex is also organized into columns, with each column responding to a different sense submodality. For example, one column will respond to joint (position) impulses, while a neighboring column will respond to pressure stimulation. Still another column will respond to body hair stimulation. Given that there appears to be a topographic map of the body throughout the somatic sensory cortex, this area of neocortex is capable of responding to different kinds of sensation from the entire body.

*A*utonomic Nervous System

The autonomic nervous system is composed of *sympathetic* and *parasympathetic* divisions, both of which provide innervation to smooth muscles, blood vessels, heart, glands, and other visceral organs. The sympathetic nervous system consists of 22 pairs of ganglia that lie just outside the spinal cord. These ganglia are often considered to provide thoracic and lumbar outflow, but there are also cervical and sacral ganglia. The thoracolumbar designation does not delimit the sympathetic nervous system; it is meant to distinguish the portion of the sympathetic system that has reflex responses to afferent visceral input.

The parasympathetic nervous system issues from three regions of nerve cells: midbrain, medulla, and the sacral (lowest) region of the spinal cord. The classic descriptor of this nervous system combines the first two regions into a "cranial" outflow, so the designation for the parasympathetic system is cranial-sacral.

The general concept of the autonomic nervous system is that it regulates the activities of organs not under voluntary control. Typically, both sympathetic and parasympathetic fibers innervate an organ, and the divisions are often observed to be physiological antagonists for the activity of that organ. Despite the conventional concept of antagonism, the activities of these two nervous systems may be either different and independent or integrated and interdependent (Mayer, 1980). For example, the activities of the sympathetic and parasympathetic nerves in the heart and in the iris are mutually antagonistic, while the actions on male sexual organs are complementary and integrated to promote sexual function.

Figure 2.12 shows the arrangement of the autonomic nervous system.

Sympathetic Nervous System

The sympathetic trunks lie outside the spinal cord and extend from the base of the cranium to the coccyx. Twenty-two cellular masses, or ganglia, appear as bulges in each trunk. Because the vertebral numbering runs from C1 to C8 (cervical), from T1 to T12 (thoracic), from L1 to L5 (lumbar), and from S1 to S5 (sacral), plus the coccyx, the correspondence with the vertebrae is only approximately segmental. Each ganglion contains nerve cells with axons that project peripherally to the visceral organs. The sympathetic trunks consist of nerve fibers that run longitudinally.

Each sympathetic trunk is connected with every spinal nerve on the same side of the body by bundles of nerve fibers called communicating rami. In the thoracic and rostral lumbar segments there are white and gray rami. In the cervical, lower lumbar, and sacral segments there are only gray rami. The white rami are made up of outgoing preganglionic nerves that project to sympathetic ganglia and incoming visceral nerves that project to cells in the spinal cord. The gray rami are made up of axons of ganglionic neurons that join the peripheral nerve running out to muscles, vessels, and glands of the skin. Figure 2.13 shows this scheme clearly.

Parasympathetic Nervous System

The parasympathetic nervous system arises from cells in the midbrain, medulla, and the sacral region of the spinal cord. Many of the cranial nerves previously described have parasympathetic functions. The cranial nerves with general or special visceral efferent components are oculomotor (III), trigeminal (V), facial (VII), glossopharyngeal (IX), vagus (X), and spinal accessory (XI). The muscles controlling mastication, facial expression, and the larynx and pharynx are innervated by the special visceral efferents. The general visceral efferents synapse upon autonomic ganglia in the head, which innervate glands, blood vessels, and smooth muscle.

The cranial nerves with general or special visceral afferent components are facial (VII), glossopharyngeal (IX), and vagus (X). Sensory innervation to internal organs such as the larynx and pharynx, heart, and abdominal viscera is provided by general visceral afferents. Special visceral afferents mediate the sense of taste.

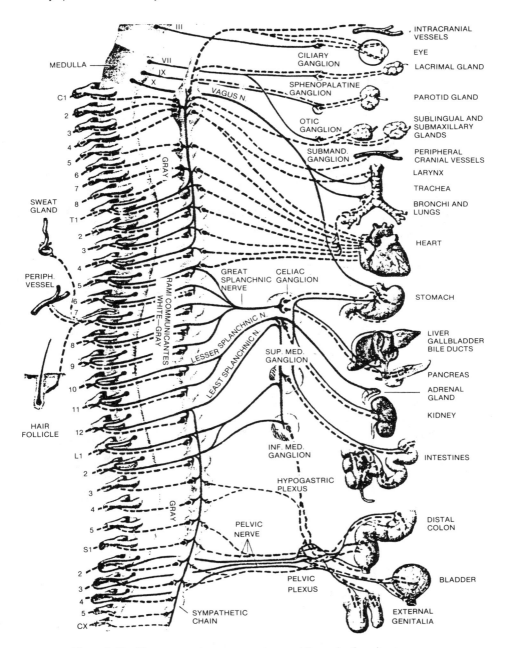

Figure 2.12 The autonomic nervous system and its projection sites.
(From Netter, 1972.)

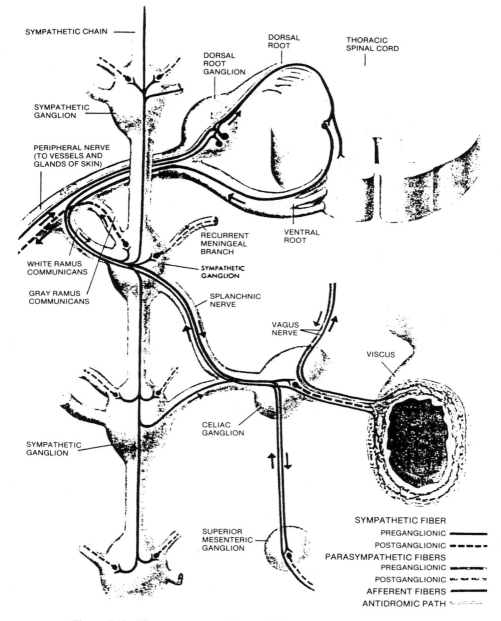

Figure 2.13 The arrangement of sympathetic ganglia to the spinal cord. (From Netter, 1972.)

The vagus nerve (X) may be considered to be the primary parasympathetic innervation of the viscera. It extends through the neck and thorax into the abdomen innervating organs all along the way. The vagus innervates the larynx, trachea, bronchi, and lungs. In the chest there is also vagal innervation of the heart. The vagal fibers descending into the abdomen innervate the stomach, liver, gallbladder, bile ducts, pancreas, kidney, and intestines. Consult Figure 2.14 for an explanation of the innervation of the vagus.

The sacral outflow arises from parasympathetic cells in the second, third, and fourth sacral segments. These preganglionic fibers form the pelvic nerves and synapse in terminal ganglia lying near or within the bladder, rectum, or sexual organs. Parasympathetic outflow to these organs stimulates sexual arousal and the emptying of bladder and bowels.

*A*utonomic Function

In the late 1800s Claude Bernard pointed out that the autonomic nervous system functions to maintain the constancy of the internal environment. This concept of "homeostasis" was later elaborated by Walter Cannon in the 1920s. From the point of view of control systems theory (see Chapter 1), the autonomic nervous system reacts to deviations from the body's internal environment to maintain a constant, internal reference level. This kind of control may be contrasted with the behavioral operations performed on the external environment for the guidance and balance of movement (see Chapter 1) (Van Toller, 1979).

The regulation of body temperature provides a good example. A critical requirement for temperature regulation is to dissipate body heat in the presence of a higher external temperature. Under conditions in which body temperature rises above a critical level, blood vessels in the skin vasodilate (expand), permitting heat to escape. Sweat glands begin a generalized secretion that facilitates heat loss. Arterioles and sweat glands are both innervated by the sympathetic nervous system. When body temperature falls below a critical level, vasoconstriction occurs, thereby preventing further heat loss.

The sympathetic nervous system continuously varies in its level of discharge to the organs it innervates. Under conditions of fight and flight, the sympathoadrenal system is especially active. Normally, for most of its innervated organs, the sympathetic system uses norepinephrine (noradrenalin) as its primary neurotransmitter. When the adrenal gland is activated to secrete epinephrine (adrenalin), organs normally innervated by sympathetic nerves exhibit an increasing degree of activity. The sympathoadrenal system can, in this way, recruit various activities to maintain the organism under extreme conditions: heart rate is accelerated; blood pressure increases, and blood is

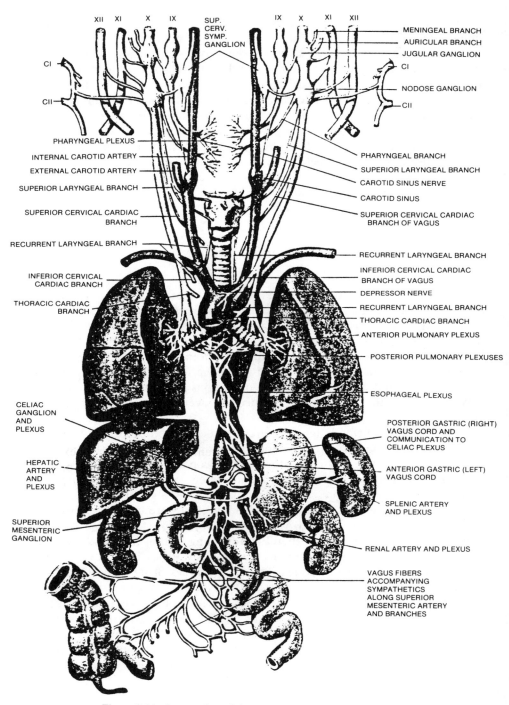

Figure 2.14 Innervation of the vagus nerve. (From Netter, 1972.)

shunted from the viscera and skin to the skeletal muscles; red blood cells empty into the circulation from the spleen; bronchioles dilate for increased respiratory activity; and pupillary dilation occurs. The mobilization of these visceral systems therefore occurs to meet the threat to the organism.

By contrast, the parasympathetic system is concerned primarily with the conservation and restoration of energy rather than with energy expenditure. This system stimulates gastrointestinal movements, lowers blood pressure and slows heart rate, and empties the urinary bladder and rectum. The primary neurotransmitter of this system is acetylcholine.

The antagonism of the two systems can be easily seen when you consider dilation and constriction of the pupil. Norepinephrine liberated by the sympathetic system dilates the pupil. Acetylcholine liberated from the parasympathetic system constricts the pupil. To dilate your eyes, the ophthalmologist has a choice of drugs that take advantage of this antagonism. A drug that stimulates norepinephrine receptors may be used directly to dilate the pupils, or a drug that blocks acetylcholine receptors may be used. In this case, the parasympathetic innervation is prevented from balancing the activity of the sympathetic innervation, thereby permitting sympathetic activity to gain the upper hand for pupillary dilation.

A good example for sympathetic and parasympathetic integration is provided by the reproductive system. Parasympathetic acetylcholine activity is critical for erection of the penis and clitoris. Sympathetic norepinephrine activity, however, is required for ejaculation.

Although the autonomic nervous system may be considered separately from the central nervous system, a moment's reflection will show that some hierarchic integration is required. Conditions of flight or fight must be perceived and interpreted by the central nervous system as extreme conditions before autonomic reactions can come into play. The hypothalamus may be thought of as an interface between limbic system perception of these extreme conditions and autonomic reactions to them. To the extent that it may provide reference commands for the control of autonomic functions, the hypothalamus will be discussed in relation to the autonomic system. However, the hypothalamus is not exclusively autonomic; it is responsible for integration of basic behavioral patterns that involve correlated somatic, autonomic, and endocrine functions.

W.R. Hess (1954) contributed extensively to our knowledge of the relationship between the hypothalamus and the autonomic nervous system. He implanted electrodes into several thousand stimulation points in the hypothalami of cats to study the effects of electrical stimulation of these areas. Stimulation in the more posterior and lateral areas of the hypothalamus produced primarily sympathetic nervous system effects, including pupillary dilation. Hess called these effects ergotropic, which literally means "turning toward work." Stimulation in the more anterior areas produced parasympathetic effects, which were called trophotropic, or "turning toward nourishment."

For example, temperature regulation requires integrated autonomic, endocrine, and skeletomotor responses. Stimulation of the anterior hypothalamus suppresses shivering and results in cutaneous vasodilation. These parasympathetic responses result in a drop in body temperature. Stimulation of the posterior hypothalamus produces a set of opposite sympathetic responses that function to generate or conserve heat.

Thus, two divisions of the autonomic nervous system may have antagonistic or integrated effects. Independent functions also exist. Axons from the superior cervical ganglion (sympathetic nervous system) innervate the choroid plexus where they participate in the manufacturing and release of cerebrospinal fluid. This ganglion also innervates the pineal gland where it is active in converting pineal serotonin to melatonin, which has antigonadal effects. An indirect pathway via the optic nerve and the hypothalamus eventually reaches the superior cervical ganglion (through preganglionic stimulation). This pathway provides the superior cervical ganglion—and through its innervation, the pineal gland—with information about the relative length of daylight. The relative secretion of the antigonadal melatonin can therefore be affected by the length of the day. This is one pathway through which seasonal variation in gonadal activity and mating can be mediated.

References

Albus, J.S. *Brains, behavior, and robotics.* Peterborough, New Hampshire: BYTE, 1981.

Anand, B.K., & Brobeck, J.R. Hypothalamic control of food intake in rats and cats. *Yale Journal of Biology and Medicine, 24,* 1951, 123–140.

Brady, J.V., & Nauta, W.J.H. Subcortical mechanisms in emotional behavior: Affective changes following septal forebrain lesions in the albino rat. *Journal of Comparative and Physiological Psychology, 46,* 1953, 339–346.

Carpenter, M.B. *Core text of neuroanatomy.* Baltimore: Williams & Wilkins, 1972.

Gage, F.H., & Olton, D.S. Hippocampal influence on hyperreactivity induced by septal lesions. *Brain Research, 98,* 1975, 311–325.

Groves, P.M. A theory of the functional organization of the neostriatum and the neostriatal control of voluntary movement. *Brain Research Reviews, 5,* 1983, 109–132.

Hassler, R. Striatal control of locomotion, intentional actions, and of integrating and perceptive activity. *Journal of the Neurological Sciences, 36,* 1978, 187–224.

Hess, W.R. *Diencephalon: Autonomic and pyramidal function.* New York: Grune & Stratton, 1954.

Hetherington, A.W., & Ranson, S.W. The spontaneous activity and food intake of rats with hypothalamic lesions. *American Journal of Physiology, 136,* 1942, 609–617.

Hubel, D. The visual cortex of the brain. *Perception: Mechanisms and models.* San Francisco: Scientific American (Freeman), 1972.

Hubel, D.H., & Wiesel, T.N. Receptive fields, binocular interaction and functional architecture in the cat's visual cortex. *Journal of Physiology (London), 160,* 1962, 106–154.

Kandel, E.R., & Schwartz, J.H. *Principles of neural science.* New York: Elsevier/North-Holland, 1981.

Kluver, H., & Bucy, P.C. Preliminary analysis of functions of the temporal lobes in monkeys. *Archives of Neurology and Psychiatry, 42,* 1939, 979–1000.

Lashley, K. *Brain mechanisms and intelligence,* Chicago: University of Chicago Press, 1929.

Mayer, S.E. Neurohumoral transmission and the autonomic nervous system. In A.G. Gilman, L.S. Goodman, & A. Gilman (Eds.), *Goodman and Gilman's the pharmacological basis of therapeutics.* 6th edition. New York: MacMillan, 1980.

Mountcastle, V.B. The view from within: Pathways to the study of perception. *Johns Hopkins Medical Journal, 136,* 1975, 109–131.

Netter, F.H. *The Ciba collection of medical illustrations,* Vol. 1. *Nervous system,* Summit, New Jersey: Ciba Medical Education, 1972.

Olton, D.S., & Samuelson, R.J. Remembrance of places passed. Spatial memory in rats. *Journal of Experimental Psychology: Animal Behavior Processes, 2,* 1976, 97–116.

Papez, J.W. A proposed mechanism of emotion. *Archives of Neurology and Psychiatry, 38,* 1937, 725–743.

Thompson, R.F. The neurobiology of learning and memory. *Science, 233,* 1986, 941–947.

Van Toller, C. *The nervous body: An introduction to the autonomic nervous system and behavior.* New York: John Wiley, 1979.

Chapter **3**
Serotonin and Behavioral Quieting

Many components of the diet, including carbohydrates and amino acids, modify the activity of this important, and phylogenetically "old," neurotransmitter. Regarding its evolutionary age, serotonin is so biologically conserved that it has been found in invertebrates such as ants, where it has been shown to be physiologically active. Even the growth hormone in many plants—indoleacetic acid—is quite similar structurally to a natural metabolite of the serotonin molecule.

At least 9 and probably 10 nuclei (clusters of neurons) in mammalian brains contain serotonin. These nerve cells have axons that project widely throughout the brain and spinal cord. Most of these axons do not contain the insulating glial sheath called myelin, though recent findings have shown that some primates have a higher proportion of myelinated serotonin axons. Like most other small, unmyelinated axons, serotonin axons conduct nerve impulses slowly (0.5-1.5 m/sec), and they probably release serotonin from bulges or varicosities all along the axon. The released serotonin usually has an inhibitory hyperpolarizing influence on the nerve cells and processes that contain serotonin receptors, but excitatory depolarizing effects have been documented.

Given that serotonin axons are highly branched, that they release serotonin throughout their extent, and that they project widely throughout the central nervous system (CNS), any small change in serotonin activity potentially has amplified consequences throughout the CNS. These many consequences include behavioral activity and reactivity, as well as feeding and diet selection.

*B*iochemistry

Serotonin itself is not easily transported across the blood-brain barrier. This means that serotonin in the brain must be synthesized in serotoninergic nerves and terminals in the brain. The initial substrate for brain serotonin synthesis is the amino acid tryptophan, which is actively transported across the blood-brain barrier from the circulation. It is interesting that brain serotonin neurons project to small blood vessels in the brain. Investigators have also described dendrites of serotonin neurons wrapping around blood vessels. These neurons could function to detect changes in the blood composition of tryptophan.

Although the process of synthesis only consumes about 1% of the total tryptophan in the brain, it is still strongly influenced by tryptophan levels in the blood plasma. In fact, one of the ways of increasing serotonin fluorescence to visualize serotonin neurons is to increase blood plasma levels of tryptophan. Dietary restrictions of tryptophan can severely curtail the levels of brain serotonin.

Examine Figure 3.1 to see the flow of serotonin synthesis. A hydroxyl (OH) group is first added to tryptophan by the enzyme tryptophan hydroxylase. Molecular oxygen and the cofactor BH_4 are also necessary for this conversion. Oxygenation of the blood by exercise could therefore enhance serotonin synthesis.

Some controversy has existed about the level of brain tryptophan and the K_m for tryptophan hydroxylase (the K_m value gives the amount of tryptophan necessary for half-maximal activity of the synthesis enzyme). The K_m value was originally found to be considerably higher than the brain tryptophan amounts, indicating that virtually any change in the amount of tryptophan would result in a change in the amount of serotonin produced. It was later

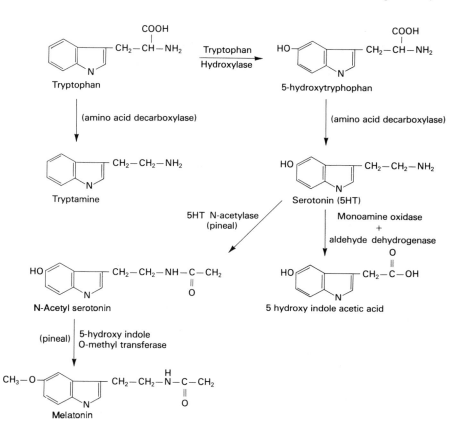

Figure 3.1 Biosynthesis and metabolism of serotonin. (From Cooper, Bloom, and Roth, 1982.)

shown that a more natural cofactor yielded a K_m closer to the value for tryptophan levels, but still slightly higher. In any case, serotonin levels empirically fluctuate with variation in tryptophan levels, so that any dietary alteration changing plasma tryptophan levels can be expected to change brain serotonin levels in the corresponding direction.

Tryptophan hydroxylase converts tryptophan to 5-hydroxytryptophan (5-HTP). Only one step is left for the conversion to 5-hydroxytryptamine (serotonin). Two enzymes are able to mediate the decarboxylation of 5-HTP to serotonin: one is the highly specific 5-HTP decarboxylase; the other is a nonspecific L-amino acid decarboxylase, which is also able to decarboxylate other amino acids, including tryptophan.

This is an important point. Tryptamine is produced as a result of the decarboxylation of tryptophan. Tryptamine probably has its own neurotransmitter action in the spinal cord where it is known to facilitate spinal reflexes.

Changes in tryptophan levels can therefore directly change the synthesis of at least two biochemicals active in regulating behavior.

The major chemical degradation of serotonin follows a two-step process. The first involves the formation of an acetaldehyde. This step is catalyzed by the enzyme monoamine oxidase. The aldehyde is then converted by aldehyde dehydrogenase to 5-hydroxyindoleacetic acid (the compound similar to the plant growth hormone).

In the cells of the pineal gland, a different form of conversion for serotonin exists. Serotonin is acetylated to N-acetylserotonin. This product is then converted to the hormone melatonin, which when released into the bloodstream has an antigonadal effect. Indeed, administration of the precursor 5-hydroxytryptophan to sheep elevates serum melatonin within two hours.

Dietary tryptophan—or any dietary nutrient that alters plasma tryptophan levels—therefore has at least three potential sources of behavioral effects. One is based on the dependence of serotonin levels on synthesis from tryptophan. Two alternatives for behavioral effects that have received little attention include the conversion of tryptophan to tryptamine and the production of melatonin from serotonin.

Tryptophan fluctuations also have another important biochemical consequence. Tryptophan is converted to nicotinic acid (the name *niacin* is now widely used to avoid an unwarranted association with any tobacco product), a vitamin from the B group, at a ratio of 60 mg tryptophan to 1 mg nicotinic acid. Any tryptophan deficiency therefore has the potential of producing a vitamin deficiency, the consequences of which may be similar (behaviorally) to other vitamin deficiences (see Chapter 10 on vitamins).

*A*natomy

Serotonin Cells

Several clusters of serotonin nuclei have been discovered. The nine nuclei originally described by Dahlstrom and Fuxe (1965) are shown in Figure 3.2. As you can see, the most caudal serotonin nuclei (B1-B3) project primarily down the spinal cord, where they are active in sensory/motor integration and automonic regulation. These are called the bulbospinal serotonin nuclei. The midrange serotonin nuclei (B4-B6), located at the level of the pons, project rostrally up into the telencephalon and diencephalon and caudally down the spinal cord. These nuclei also project to other brainstem cells.

The most rostral serotonin cells found by Dahlstrom and Fuxe (B7-B9) are located in the midbrain raphe nuclei (dorsal, median, and central superior). These are thought to provide the most extensive innervation of the

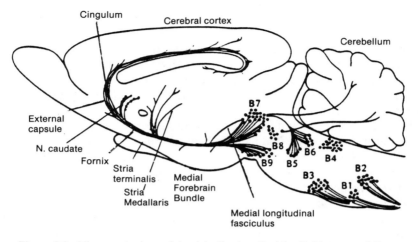

Figure 3.2   Nine serotonin nuclei originally described by Dahlstrom and Fuxe. (From Cooper, Bloom, and Roth, 1982.)

diencephalon and telencephalon. They will therefore form the focus of much of our discussion of forebrain serotonin activity.

Beaudet and Descarries (1979) have also described a cluster of serotonin cells in the dorsomedial hypothalamus. They named this group B10 in accordance with the original naming scheme. Other serotonin neurons have been found in area postrema, in and around the interpeduncular nucleus, and in the caudal locus ceruleus.

Lest you think that all the important serotonin cells have been described, CNS serotonin cells account for only 1-2% of the total body serotonin content. The greatest concentration of serotonin in mammalian cells is in the enterochromaffin cells of the intestine and in the pinealocytes of the pineal gland. This means that dietary changes in tryptophan levels have the potential for affecting one's overall digestive and endocrine physiology.

Serotonin Cell Projections

Descending serotonin fibers reach the cells of the ventral and dorsal horns via anterior and lateral columns of the spinal cord. Some serotonin projections descend in the dorsolateral fasciculus and inhibit dorsal horn interneurons. Some of these serotonin fibers branch off to innervate the preganglionic cells in the lateral horn and thus have an influence on preganglionic activation of the sympathetic nervous system.

Serotonin fibers also project to brain stem nuclei, innervating the lateral part of the dorsal accessory nucleus of the inferior olive. Serotonin projections innervate the spinal trigeminal tract, solitary tract, dorsal vagal, and commissural nuclei. Serotonin fibers project to cerebellum, where they are involved in cerebellar regulation of muscle tone and motor coordination.

The serotonin fibers that ascend in the forebrain arise primarily (80%) from the dorsal (B7) and median (B8) raphe. Figure 3.3 shows a cross section of the midbrain at the level of the dorsal and median raphe. Figure 3.4 shows a diagram of their main projection sites in the brain. The ventrally oriented bundle through which most of the forebrain serotonin fibers pass (DRFT and MRFT circled) is called the medial forebrain bundle. The dorsal raphe (B7) fibers in the lateral aspect of this bundle project mainly to lateral forebrain structures: basal ganglia, amygdala, accumbens, and piriform cortex. The median raphe (B8) fibers in the medial aspect of this bundle innervate medial forebrain structures: septum, cingulate cortex, and hippocampus.

The median raphe system thus has primarily a limbic system distribution, with fibers projecting also to mammillary bodies, anterior hypothalamus (pre-

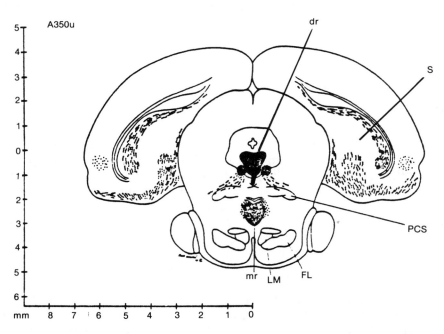

Figure 3.3 Cross section of the midbrain at the level of the dorsal and median raphe. Abbreviations: dr—dorsal raphe; mr—median raphe; LM—medial lemniscus; S—subiculum; FL—longitudinal fasciculus; PCS—superior cerebellar peduncle. (From Azmitia, 1978.)

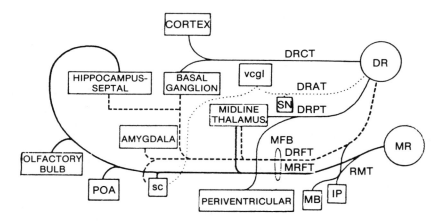

Figure 3.4 Diagram of rostral serotonin projections. (From Azmitia, 1978.)

optic area and suprachiasmatic nuclei), and olfactory bulb. Many "limbic" behaviors (emotionality and activity) are therefore altered by appropriate manipulations of this serotonin system.

*B*ehavior

Serotonin

As a way of introducing yourself to the behavioral activity of serotonin, consider the work of Gaylord Ellison (1977). Ellison provided rats with an environment as relevant to the animals' ecology as he could under laboratory conditions: a large enclosure with sandy floors, burrows on one side, a small tower in the center on which the rats could climb, and a separate feeding enclosure (Figure 3.5). The only way for the animals to get to the feeding areas was to run through pipes that connected the two areas. The tower in the center was the water drinking station. Having several rats in the enclosure permitted Ellison to observe the social behaviors of the animals as well as other relevant activities.

Ellison considered the idea that serotonin and norepinephrine (NE) work antagonistically to modulate behavior. To this end, he performed basically two types of manipulations on the animals in this enclosure. One involved intraventricular injections of the neurotoxin 6-hydroxydopamine. This provided relatively selective lesions of the NE system, leaving the balance in favor of serotonin. The other manipulation involved injections of 5,6 dihydroxytryptamine, which produces relatively selective lesions of serotonin fibers, leaving the balance in favor of NE. (A third manipulation involved

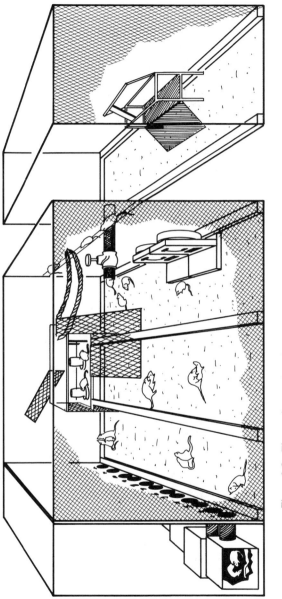
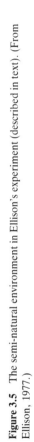

Figure 3.5 The semi-natural environment in Ellison's experiment (described in text). (From Ellison, 1977.)

depletion with both neurotoxins but is not considered here.) For the present discussion it is useful to call the animals receiving the first manipulation the high-serotonin (low NE) animals; the animals receiving the second manipulation will be called the low-serotonin animals.

The high-serotonin animals were less active and reactive. They remained in their burrows longer than the low-serotonin animals, and they interacted less socially. These animals diminished in social dominance, which was in part tested by observing who was first to enter the pipe leading to the food chamber. Fights were also observed in which high-serotonin animals usually came out on the bottom. High-serotonin animals ate less food and did not play as much on the tower in the middle of the chamber. These high-serotonin (low-NE) animals showed in clinical terms the signs of lethargy and depression.

The low-serotonin rats showed just the opposite behavior. They rose in social dominance and ate more food. They were more active and reactive. They stayed out of their burrows longer and played more on the tower. If we could form a continuum with these serotonin manipulations (not really possible with only two manipulations), it seems that increasing serotonin inhibits behavior while decreasing serotonin stimulates behavior. In short, serotonin seems to have an inhibitory effect on behaviors that could be interpreted in some form of behavioral hierarchy (see Chapter 1).

Individual behaviors have been examined more closely. Of the hierarchically higher behaviors, mouse killing (muricide)—a specific form of aggression—appears to be enhanced by lesions of serotonin systems. According to Waldbillig (1979), lesions of the dorsal, but not median, raphe are sufficient to produce muricide in naturally nonkilling rats.

Sex behavior is also among the more organized behaviors studied. Injections of parachlorophenylalanine (PCPA), which inhibits the synthesis of serotonin, induce copulation in male noncopulators and shorten the ejaculation latency in experienced males.

Serotonin activity has also been implicated in the inhibition of gonadotropin release, an activity important in hamsters for seasonal regulation of reproduction and hibernation. Evidence shows that additional tryptophan fed to hamsters kept on short daylengths reduces testicular weights severely, indicating that the increased tryptophan was active in promoting serotonergic-mediated inhibition of gonadotropins. This effect is not seen in hamsters kept on long daylengths.

Extensive depletion of CNS serotonin (with neurotoxins) induces hyperphagia in rats and leads to considerable weight gain. Injections of drugs that increase serotonin activity tend to decrease feeding, although hypothalamic injections of serotonin-releasing drugs produce hyperphagia and weight gain (Blundell & Leshem, 1973). However, energy and protein intake are under separate regulatory controls. Ashley, Coscina, and Anderson (1979) found that three ways of producing brain serotonin depletion—PCPA, neurotoxin, or raphe lesion—all reduced the amount of protein consumed, but did not affect energy intake. It therefore seems clear that different nutrients are under different controls. Studies in the Leibowitz laboratory (Leibowitz & Stanley, 1986) have shown that hypothalamic serotonin injections specifically reduce carbohydrate intake.

Geyer and colleagues (1976) have shown that lesions of the median raphe, which provides serotonin innervation primarily to midline limbic structures, result in behavioral changes characteristic of hippocampal damage. Animals with such lesions are hyperactive and hyperreactive to stimuli designed to startle rats. These animals also fail to alternate spontaneously in a Y maze. These results complement those of Smith (1979), who showed that reactivity is increased when telencephalic serotonin is depleted by PCPA injection, medial forebrain bundle lesion, or septal lesion. Hole and colleagues (1977) also showed that neurotoxic lesions of ascending serotonin pathways reduce habituation to touch and sound stimuli, as well as increase mouse killing.

It is not satisfactory to say that serotonin has an inhibitory role in behavior if the only evidence comes from animals with lesions (see "hiss suppressor" problem in Chapter 1). Other ways of evaluating behavior must be used. For example, administration of the serotonin precursor, L-tryptophan, decreases motor activity in rats (Taylor, 1976). Gage and Springer (1981) injected serotonin directly into the hippocampus of rats. The animals became lethargic as a result, showing reduced reactivity and activity levels. In this study there was reduced reactivity to both non-noxious and noxious stimuli.

This behavioral result is interesting in view of the fact that noxious stimulation increases the firing rate of thalamic neurons. If the dorsal raphe serotonin neurons, which project to this part of the thalamus, are excited by this noxious stimulation, the firing rate of thalamic neurons is reduced. This indicates that serotonin activity (especially in limbic structures) has an important inhibitory effect on the responses to noxious stimuli. In this context, Llewelyn and colleagues (1983) have shown that serotonin, when applied directly to raphe neurons, excited those neurons and led to analgesia.

Recordings of activity of serotonin cells during behavior show highest activity during active waking. This activity gradually slows during the transition from waking through slow wave sleep. During rapid eye movement (REM) sleep there is a sharp drop in the activity of serotonin cells.

This seems almost paradoxical. How could serotonin activity decrease during sleep if injections of serotonin induce lethargy? One speculative explanation relates this evidence to the concept of a controlled system (see Chapter 1) in which serotonin could be active in a negative feedback mechanism throughout a behavioral hierarchy. Any behavioral activity—responses to noxious stimulation, well integrated aggressive behaviors, sex behavior—would require inhibitory feedback to decelerate the behavior even as it is initiated. This would provide behavioral smoothness and fine control. As activity levels decreased during sleep, requiring less negative feedback, serotonin feedback systems would consequently be less active.

Serotonin systems are well distributed hierarchically to act as this feedback mechanism, with bulbospinal serotonin systems inhibiting lower-level spinal reflex responses and rostral serotonin projections inhibiting more integrated behavior. Given that serotonin has a high turnover during stressful situations (which involve reactions from the entire behavioral hierarchy), it is easy to see how serotonin might be involved in the integrated behavioral life of the organism. Though this concept currently exists as speculation, the notion that dietary changes in serotonin activity can be a profound influence on behavior is well-grounded.

Diet

Milk, eggs, and beans contain relatively high amounts of tryptophan. Little tryptophan is found in bone or corn proteins, giving rise to the practice in several cultures of adding beans to corn-based diets to prevent deficiencies.

The key concept in considering the tryptophan/serotonin relationship to dietary behavior is that tryptophan is an essential amino acid. No biosynthetic pathway can manufacture tryptophan; it must be consumed in the diet along with other essential amino acids if the organism is to survive.

This strict requirement presents the forager with an exacting behavioral problem. Foods contain differing amounts of nutrients. Somehow, the forager must sense the consequences of nutrient intake and act to keep this intake adjusted to some reference condition (see Chapter 1). It is not clear just how the reference condition may be specified or even whether it can be specified. The important point, however, is that mechanisms have been elucidated that explain how foragers might be able to acquire these essential nutrients.

The first is the acquisition of nutrients. Predatory aggression is one way in which organisms acquire essential nutrients. Tryptophan is found in small amounts (about 1%) in the proteins of prey items. Gibbons and colleagues (1979) have shown that if tryptophan is excluded from the diet of rats who will not kill mice spontaneously, these animals turn into killer rats. Mouse killing is also facilitated in those rats who do kill mice spontaneously. This aggression abated when the diets were again supplemented with tryptophan. Given that manipulations lowering serotonin levels result in heightened aggression, and that the deficient diets lowered brain serotonin, it is reasonable to suppose that lower tryptophan levels result in heightened predation because of the lowered levels of serotonin. It would be interesting to determine in those animals showing more ritualized forms of predation (and who require tryptophan) whether lowered tryptophan levels heighten these behaviors.

It is a simplification to say that this predation mechanism regulates nutrient intake by enabling a predator to acquire essential amino acids from its prey. For one thing, essential amino acids do not present themselves as separately regulated entities in any complex system. Indeed, there is competition among tryptophan and other large neutral amino acids—tyrosine, phenylalanine, leucine, isoleucine, and valine—for the uptake carrier into the brain from the bloodstream. Also, amino acids such as tryptophan may participate in the regulation of the intake of "unrelated" nutrients.

Anderson and Ashley (1977) have shown that the plasma ratio of tryptophan to other neutral amino acids is highly correlated with protein intake, but the association is a negative one. Although absolute levels of tryptophan may rise in the plasma, proteins introduce an influx of the other neutral amino acids. Greater amounts of protein intake are thus associated with lower tryptophan ratios.

This presents a problem for the predation mechanism discussed above. If the tryptophan/serotonin axis regulates predation, intake of a prey item might be expected to shut off subsequent predation by elevating tryptophan/serotonin levels. But this is not the case, because intake of proteins tends to lower tryptophan ratios. This reasoning also does not take into account the element of time; subsequent predation might be shut off by satiety mechanisms operating immediately after a meal so that the tryptophan/serotonin axis may have little to do with the acquisition of protein by predation.

The amount of carbohydrate in the diet is also a strong determinant of plasma tryptophan ratios (and hence brain serotonin levels). One of the essential physiological features of carbohydrate intake is the consequent release of insulin. Insulin has little effect on plasma tryptophan levels directly, primarily because plasma tryptophan is bound to albumin. Insulin facilitates the entry into muscle of other unbound competing amino acids. Tryptophan ratios rise because of the reduced competition. Because of tryptophan's intimate relationship with serotonin synthesis, it has been argued that serotonin neurons may thus be variable ratio sensors for the carbohydrate content of the diet.

To determine whether this might be the case, Wurtman and Wurtman (1979) injected rats with drugs known to enhance serotonin neurotransmission (fenfluramine or fluoxetine). If serotonin neurons are detectors for carbohydrate intake, increased amounts of serotonin transmission (endogenously produced as a result of insulin's action to raise tryptophan levels) should shut off subsequent carbohydrate intake. That is exactly what happened. The drug injections caused the animals to reduce their selection of carbohydrates without affecting their selection of proteins. This effect was independent of whether the carbohydrate had a sweet taste.

The entire behavioral loop can be summarized as follows. Carbohydrate ingestion releases insulin, thereby elevating tryptophan ratios. The consequent increase in serotonin synthesis decreases the animal's self-selection of carbohydrates.

It should be kept in mind that the term *carbohydrate* does not denote a homogeneous substance. Recently, researchers have shown that complex carbohydrates (such as starch in potatoes) give a dramatic rise in blood glucose and therefore blood insulin. Sucrose, however, has only a moderate effect on blood glucose levels. More attention should therefore be given to the role of different carbohydrates in animals' self-selection behaviors for carbohydrates.

Evidence has accrued in Judith Wurtman's (1984) lab that the carbohydrate/serotonin behavioral loop may be involved in excessive carbohydrate snacking by obese carbohydrate cravers. In her study, obese subjects were not permitted to choose foods at meals. The outlay was predetermined to meet nutritional needs, except that the caloric content was below usual intake. The subjects were thus encouraged to snack freely from 10 isocaloric protein- and carbohydrate-rich snack foods, including potato chips, bagels and cream cheese, salami and cheese, and chocolate cupcakes.

Most of the subjects ate the carbohydrate-rich foods exclusively, showing that most snacking is for carbohydrates. The subjects received a dose of fenfluramine, tryptophan, or a placebo. The placebo had no effect. The subjects receiving fenfluramine reduced their carbohydrate snack intake. Half the subjects receiving tryptophan reduced their carbohydrate snack intake. Because these treatments elevate serotonin neurotransmission, Wurtman suggested that carbohydrate snacking occurs because of a "need" for elevated serotonin transmission that is fulfilled by the serotonin elevation inherent in the carbohydrate/serotonin behavior loop.

Insight into the central site of action of serotonin's effects on food intake and diet selection comes from pharmacologic and behavioral studies of its actions within the medial hypothalamus. In particular, the paraventricular nucleus (PVN) appears to be especially sensitive to serotonin's suppression of feeding behavior and carbohydrate intake. Drugs that increase the synthesis of serotonin, or that act presynaptically to release serotonin, are quite active in low doses in the PVN to suppress feeding.

The literature is not uniform with regard to the notion of diet selection being dependent on serotonin levels. Peters and colleagues (1984) showed that injections of tryptophan failed to alter food intake or protein or carbohydrate selection in rats. Failure to alter dietary behavior was found despite increases of 50% in brain concentrations of serotonin and its principal metabolite. Other studies have shown that the electrical activity of serotonin neurons in cats is unresponsive to diets containing varying proportions of tryptophan, though the diets produced significant changes in brain serotonin. However, it should be mentioned that various laboratories have had difficulty replicating this latter work (Wurtman, personal communication).

This is not to argue that the concept is wrong; other mechanisms of serotonin activation may serve to control diet selection. Also, the measurements of serotonin concentrations in these studies in no way indicate the activity of receptors that may be critical in the behavioral control. Moreover, treatments that increase serotonin neurotransmission tend to be effective only when the animal is intending to eat carbohydrates. However, these studies lead one to caution against uncritical acceptance of the idea.

The species specificity should also be kept in mind. Apparently, insulin administration in normal humans does not elevate plasma tryptophan. Patients with a major depressive disorder, however, show a *drop* in free plasma tryptophan levels for the first 30 minutes following insulin administration, and then an elevation of tryptophan levels 30-60 minutes thereafter. The underlying biochemical mechanism for these differences in depressed patients is unclear, but tryptophan levels, and perhaps brain serotonin levels, can be altered in humans by diet.

Within this context of species specificity, it is also interesting to consider that a tryptophan-free diet has an effect on tonic immobility. Tonic immobility is presumably a fear reaction to predation brought on by manual restraint. Animals (chickens, lizards, frogs) brought under this reaction remain immobile, and their muscle tone is characterized by waxy flexibility. Diets free of tryptophan, or manipulations that lower serotonin, tend to diminish tonic immobility. These data agree with pharmacologic data showing that serotonin is involved in tonic immobility.

So far, in the context of nutrient regulation, we have considered only the selection of macronutrients. What about a behavioral regulation for tryptophan itself? After all, humans and rodents can taste differences in single amino acids. Even if amino acids are acquired as constitutents of proteins, and it might seem that behavioral regulation for amino acids is beside the point, proteins are not uniform in quality. They contain varying proportions of the essential amino acids. It would behoove any forager to be able to select among proteins that might satisfy particular nutrient needs.

The mantled howling monkeys in Glander's (1981) observations appear to be capable of some amount of selection among proteins (see Chapter 1). Unpublished observations from my laboratory indicate also that rats can regulate intake of the single amino acid tryptophan. In this study, animals were housed in operant chambers in which they had to press a lever for a single pellet of food. We systematically manipulated the quality of food in the food hopper from 100% normal pellets to 100% tryptophan-free pellets.

The graph in Figure 3.6 shows that as we began to cut the normal food with tryptophan-free food, the animals began to respond with a demand for more food. This occurred despite a normal tendency in rats toward neophobia. Responses tended to increase each time we cut the food quality and to decrease each time the food quality was improved. At 0% tryptophan there appeared to be a regulatory breakdown; the animals became anorexic. During the subsequent 33% period, it appeared that the animals were taking in so little food (and still only getting 33% normal food) that there was little op-

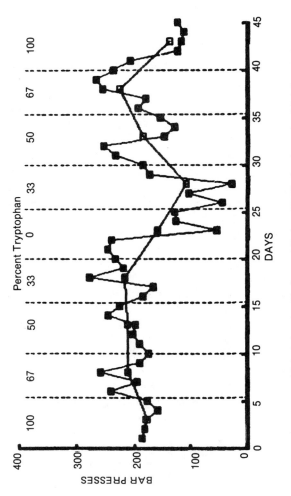

Figure 3.6 Unpublished data by Chafetz and Duhon (1983) showing animals' daily acquisition of food in an operant chamber as the level of tryptophan in the food was systematically manipulated. The daily means of 3 animals are represented by darkened squares. The mean of each tryptophan manipulation is represented by open squares.

portunity until the end of this period for them to determine that the food now contained some tryptophan. This work needs to be expanded to determine whether serotoninergic systems play a part in this regulation.

Now consider other behaviors. After a heavy meal rich in carbohydrates there is a tendency for the eater to become sleepy. A heavy carbohydrate-rich meal presumably elevates brain serotonin levels as does the administration of tryptophan. Researchers have found that tryptophan administration reduces sleep latency in rats and humans and, in some human studies, increased total sleep time. Conversely, tryptophan deficiencies elevate activity levels. Spring et al. (1982) has shown that a carbohydrate meal produces greater calmness than a protein meal in male subjects and greater sleepiness in female subjects.

In fact, food selections vary as a result of natural diurnal rhythms that could reflect natural variation in serotonin activity. Rats vary in their choice of protein intake during light and dark periods of a diurnal rhythm. Latham and Blundell (1979) have shown that injections of tryptophan in rats reduce food intake over a 24 hour period, and that the reduction occurs during the dark, and not the light, interval of the period.

Tryptophan deficiency also has an effect on sensory reactivity. Rats maintained on low-tryptophan diets show increases in sensitivity to pain, as well as increases in startle responses. This heightened reactivity is reduced by injections of tryptophan. These nutrient effects on pain and startle parallel those that occur when serotonin is directly manipulated in the brain. (At least some of aspirin's ability to relieve pain may be due to its displacement of tryptophan from binding proteins, thereby freeing up more tryptophan for serotonin synthesis.)

Developmental Effects

Adequate development of brain and behavior is dependent upon early dietary integrity with regard to serotonin systems. Low dietary tryptophan intake in several species early in life alters the ratio of tryptophan to the sum of neutral amino acids, thereby diminishing central serotonin activity. As expected, this has behavioral consequences. Lytle and colleagues (1975) have shown that rats fed corn diets poor in tryptophan grow up to have increased responsiveness to electric shock. This effect can be reversed by feeding the animals adequate amounts of tryptophan. Newly weaned female rats fed diets severely deficient in tryptophan also show a delay in reproductive aging, giving birth long after normal control animals are no longer able to.

It is particularly interesting that the dietary effect on the development of serotonin systems and behavior need not be restricted to a specific manipulation of tryptophan. Rats malnourished in protein from birth show significant elevations of brain tryptophan and serotonin levels long into adulthood. This is no doubt due to the elevated ratio of tryptophan to its competing neutral amino acids, and to the diminished amount of tryptophan bound to albumin. This effect on serotonin has its consequences in behavior. Protein malnutrition during development in rats results in a shift of REM sleep behavior from the light to the dark phases of the diurnal cycle.

Behavioral Pathology

As a way of establishing that tryptophan deprivation (usually in rats) is having its desired effect, experimenters often report clinical observations of anorexia during the deprivation phase of the experiment. Assuming that the deprivation in most cases results in diminished CNS serotonin levels, the anorexia seems paradoxical. After all, the "anorexic" drugs fenfluramine and fluoxetine act to increase CNS serotonin neurotransmission.

Biologically, it is interesting that deprivation of many essential nutrients (such as tryptophan) results in anorexia (see Figure 3.6 and Chapters 9 & 10). Animals often develop conditioned aversions to foods deficient in an essential nutrient. The taste of the food that produces a malaise becomes associated with the unpleasant feeling, thereby becoming a cue that elicits the food rejection response. Chafetz (1984) has argued that anorexia may be linked to a CNS error of metabolism in which the brain "feels" the error as the lack of a nutrient. Under these conditions, animals might develop conditioned aversions to foods generally, because all food would be perceived as lacking a nutrient. In this context, it would be interesting to determine whether tryptophan repletion supports a conditioned preference, which is the converse of the conditioned aversion. It would also be interesting to determine whether tryptophan deficiency results in an altered pattern of nutrient intake, not just a decrease in a composite lab chow.

From the perspective of changes in neural systems, it would also be necessary to determine other neural changes that accompany both the administration of anorexic drugs and the deprivation of essential nutrients. The fact that manipulations resulting in opposite neural effects lead to the same behavior—anorexia—should not go unchallenged.

With regard to other forms of pathologic change, there is considerable clinical evidence for altered indoleamine metabolism in depression. One dietary aspect of this altered metabolism is that plasma tryptophan levels fall within 30 minutes and then rise from 30 to 60 minutes thereafter following insulin administration to depressed patients (Menna-Perper et al., 1983). These sequelae of insulin do not occur in normal individuals, which suggests that depressed persons are perhaps more sensitive to the serotonergic consequences of carbohydrate consumption. The interpretation of different dietary patterns in depressed individuals would also be supported by these data. To this end, it is interesting that improvement in depressive symptoms is correlated with plasma increases in the ratio of tryptophan to five competitor amino acids: valine, leucine, isoleucine, phenylalanine, and tyrosine (Dunlop et al., 1983). Moreover, there has been some success, albeit controversial, in the treatment of depression with L-tryptophan, and Rosenthal et al. (1986) have shown that a carbohydrate lunch reduces depression to a greater degree than an isocaloric protein lunch.

Summary

Serotonin is widely distributed throughout the nervous system. As such, it has influences on almost every aspect of behavior. The synthesis of serotonin can be altered by changes in levels of tryptophan, its amino acid starting material. Levels of tryptophan are influenced by both protein and carbohydrate intake. Protein intake lowers tryptophan uptake into the brain by introducing other amino acids that compete with tryptophan for the uptake carrier. Carbohydrate intake elevates tryptophan by eliciting a release of insulin, which diminishes the levels of competing amino acids.

Experimentally, manipulation of tryptophan levels alter activity, reactivity, aggression, food and nutrient intake, and sleep. The relationship between tryptophan and brain serotonin has been implicated in the carbohydrate snacking by obese individuals, as well as in the changes in eating habits by depressed persons. Manipulation of the diet may be considered as a factor in the treatment of depression, both as a direct treatment and in avoidance of interaction with drugs.

References

Andersen, E., & Dafny, N. An ascending serotonergic pain modulation pathway from the dorsal raphe nucleus to the parafascicularis nucleus of the thalamus. *Brain Research, 269*, 1983, 57–67.

Anderson, G.H., & Ashley, D.V.M. Correlation of the plasma tyrosine to phenylalanine ratio with energy intake in self-selecting weanling rats. *Life Sciences, 21*, 1977, 1227–1234.

Ashley, D.V.M., Coscina, D.V., & Anderson, G.H. Selective decrease in protein intake following brain serotonin depletion. *Life Sciences, 24*, 1979, 973–984.

Azmitia, E.C. The serotonin-producing neurons of the midbrain median and dorsal raphe nuclei. In L.L. Iversen, S.D. Iversen, & S.H. Snyder (Eds.), *Chemical pathways in the brain, Handbook of psychopharmacology* (Vol. 9). New York: Plenum Press, 1978, pp. 233–314.

Beaudet, A., & Descarries, L. Radioautographic characterization of a serotonin-accumulating nerve cell group in adult rat hypothalamus. *Brain Research, 160*, 1979, 231–243.

Blundell, J.E. & Leshem, M.B. Dissociation of the anorexic effects of amphetamine and fenfluramine following intrahypothalamic injection. *British Journal of Pharmacology, 47,* 1973, 81–88.

Chafetz, M.D. Anorexia: A micronutrient model. *The Southern Psychologist, 2,* 1984, 39–47.

Cooper, J.R., Bloom, F.E., & Roth, R.H. *The biochemical basis of neuropharmacology* (4th ed.). New York: Oxford University Press, 1982.

Dahlstrom, A., & Fuxe, K. Evidence for the existence of monoamine neurons in the central nervous system. II. Experimentally induced changes in the intraneuronal amine levels of bulbospinal neuron system. *Acta Physiologica Scandinavica, 64* (247), 1965, 1–36.

Dunlop, S.R., Hendrie, H.C., Shea, P.A., & Brittain, H.M. Ratio of plasma tryptophan to five other amino acids in depressed subjects: A follow-up. *Archives of General Psychiatry, 40,* 1983, 1033–1034.

Ellison. G.D. Animal models of psychopathology. The low-norepinephrine and low-serotonin rat. *American Psychologist, 32,* 1977, 1036–1045.

Gage, F.H., & Springer, J.S. Behavioral assessment of norepinephrine and serotonin function and interaction in the hippocampal formation. *Pharmacology, Biochemistry, and Behavior, 14,* 1981, 815–821.

Geyer, M.A., Puerto, A., Menkes, D.B., Segal, D.S., & Mandell, A.J. Behavioral studies following lesions of the mesolimbic and mesostriatal serotonergic pathways. *Brain Research, 106,* 1976, 257–270.

Gibbons, J.L., Barr, G.A., Bridger, W.H., & Leibowitz, S.F. Manipulations of dietary tryptophan: Effects on mouse killing and brain serotonin in the rat. *Brain Research, 169,* 1979, 139–153.

Glander, K.E. Feeding patterns in mantled howling monkeys. In A.C. Kamil & T.D. Sargent (Eds.), *Foraging behavior: Ecological, ethological, and psychological approaches.* New York: Garland Press, 1981, pp. 231–258.

Hole, K., Johnson, G.E., & Berge, O.G. 5,7-Dihydroxytryptamine lesions of the ascending 5-hydroxytryptamine pathways: Habituation, motor activity and agonistic behavior. *Pharmacology, Biochemistry, & Behavior, 7,* 1977, 205–210.

Latham, C.J. & Blundell, J.E. Evidence for the effect of tryptophan on the pattern of food consumption in free-feeding and food deprived rats. *Life Sciences, 24,* 1979, 1971–1978.

Leibowitz, S.F., & Stanley, B.G. Neurochemical controls of appetite. In R. Ritter, S. Ritter, & C.D. Barnes (Eds.), *Feeding behavior: Neural and humoral controls,* New York: Academic Press, 1986, pp. 191–233.

Llewelyn, M.B., Azami, J., & Roberts, M.H.T. Effects of 5-hydroxytryptamine applied into nucleus raphe magnus on nociceptive thresholds and neuronal firing rate. *Brain Research, 258,* 1983, 59–68.

Lytle, L.D., Messing, R.B., Fisher, L., & Phebus, L. Effects of long term corn consumption on brain serotonin and the response to electric shock. *Science, 190,* 1975, 692–694.

Menna-Perper, M., Swartzburg, M., Mueller, R.S., Rochford, J., & Manowitz, P. Free tryptophan response to intravenous insulin in depressed patients. *Biological Psychiatry, 18,* 1983, 771–780.

Peters, J.C., Bellissimo, D.B., & Harper, A.E. L-Tryptophan injection fails to alter nutrient selection by rats. *Physiology and Behavior, 32,* 1984, 253–259.

Rosenthal, N.E., Genhart, M., Cabellero, B., Jacobsen, F.M., Skwerer, R., Wurtman, J., & Spring, B. Carbohydrate craving in seasonal affective disorder. *American Psychological Association,* Washington, DC, 1986, reported in Spring et al. (1987).

Smith, R.F., Mediation of footshock sensitivity by serotonergic projection to hippocampus. *Pharmacology, Biochemistry, & Behavior, 10,* 1979, 381–388.

Spring, B., Maller, O., Wurtman, J., Digman, L., & Cozolino, L. Effects of protein and carbohydrate meals on mood and performance: Interactions with sex and age. *Journal of Psychiatric Research, 17,* 1982-83, 155–167.

Taylor, M. Effects of L-tryptophan and L-methionine on activity in the rat. *British Journal of Pharmacology, 58,* 1976, 117–119.

Waldbillig, R.J. The role of the dorsal and median raphe in the inhibition of muricide. *Brain Research, 160,* 1979, 341–346.

Wurtman, J.J. The involvement of brain serotonin in excessive carbohydrate snacking by obese carbohydrate cravers. *Journal of the American Dietetic Association, 84,* 1984, 1004–1007.

Wurtman, J.J., & Wurtman, R.J. Drugs that enhance central serotoninergic transmission diminish elective carbohydrate consumption by rats. *Life Sciences, 24,* 1979, 895–904.

*S*uggested Readings

Ashley, D.V.M. & Curzon, G. Effects of long-term low dietary tryptophan intake on determinants of 5-hydroxytryptamine metabolism in the brains of young rats. *Journal of Neurochemistry, 37,* 1981, 1385–1393.

Blundell, J.E. Problems and processes underlying the control of food selection and nutrient intake. In R.J. Wurtman, & J.J. Wurtman (Eds.), *Nutrition and the Brain* (Vol. 6). New York: Raven Press, pp. 163–221.

Cooper, A.J. Tryptophan antidepressant "physiological sedative": Fact or fancy? *Psychopharmacology, 61,* 1979, 97–102.

Curzon, G. Relationships between plasma, CSF, and Brain tryptophan. *Journal of Neural Transmission, 15,* 1979, 81–82.

Dorner, G., Bewer, G., & Lubs, H. Changes of the plasma tryptophan to neutral amino acids ratio in formula-fed infants: Possible effects on brain development. *Experimental Clinical Endocrinology, 82,* 1983, 368–371.

Essman, W.B. (Ed.) *Serotonin in health and Disease. Availability, localization, and disposition* (Vol. 1). New York: SP Medical and Scientific Books, 1978.

Forbes, W.B., Tracy, C.A., Resnick, O., & Morgane, P.J. Effect of protein malnutrition during development on sleep behavior of rats. *Experimental Neurology, 57,* 1977, 440–450.

Gallup, G.G., Jr., Wallnau, L.B., Boren, J.L., Gagliardi, G.J., Maser, J.D, & Edson, P.H. Tryptophan and tonic immobility in chickens: Effects of dietary and systemic manipulations. *Journal of Comparative and Physiological Psychology, 91,* 1977, 642–648.

Geyer, M.A., Flicker, C.E., & Lee, E.H.Y. Effects of tactile startle on serotonin content of midbrain raphe neurons in rats. *Behavioural Brain Research, 4,* 1982, 369–376.

Hartmann, E., Lindsley, J.G., & Spinweber, C. Chronic insomnia: Effects of tryptophan, flurazepam, secobarbital, and placebo. *Psychopharmacology, 80,* 1983, 138–142.

Heym, J., Steinfels, G.F., & Jacobs, B.L. Activity of serotonin-containing neurons in the nucleus raphe pallidus of freely moving cats. *Brain Research, 251,* 1982, 259–276.

Iwasaki, K., & Sato, M. Taste preferences for amino acids in the house musk shrew, *Suncus murinus*. *Physiology and Behavior, 28*, 1982, 829–833.

Jenkins, D.J., Taylor, R.H., & Wolever, T.M. The diabetic diet, dietary carbohydrate and differences in digestibility. *Diabetologia, 23*, 1982, 477–484.

Kantak, K.M., Hegstrand, L.R., & Eichelman, B. Dietary tryptophan reversal of septal lesion and 5,7-DHT lesion elicited shock-induced fighting. *Pharmacology, Biochemistry, & Behavior, 15*, 1981, 343–350.

Leibowitz, S.F. Brain neurotransmitters and appetite regulation. *Psychopharmacology Bulletin, 21*, 1985, 412–418.

Malmnas, C.O., & Meyerson, B.J. p-Chlorophenylalanine and copulatory behaviour in the male rat. *Nature, 232*, 1971, 398–400.

Messing, R.B., Pettibone, D.J., Kaufman, N., & Lytle, L.D. Behavioral effects of serotonin neurotoxins: An overview. *Annals of the New York Academy of Sciences, 305*, 1978, 480–496.

Miller, M., Leay, J.P., Stern, W.C., Morgane, P.J., & Resnick, O. Tryptophan availability: Relation to elevated brain serotonin in developmentally protein-malnourished rats. *Experimental Neurology, 57*, 1977, 142–157.

Morgane, P.J. & Jacobs, M.S. Raphe projections to the locus coeruleus in the rat. *Brain Research Bulletin, 4*, 1979, 519–534.

Reinhard, J.F., Jr., Liebmann, J.E., Schlosberg, A.J., & Moskowitz, M.A. Serotonin neurons project to small blood vessels in the brain. *Science, 206*, 1979, 85–86.

Reinis, S., & Goldman, J.M. *The chemistry of behavior*. New York: Plenum Press, 1982.

Salis, P.J., & Dewsbury, D.A. p-Chlorophenylalanine facilitates copulatory behavior in male rats. *Nature, 232*, 1971, 400–401.

Segal, P.E. & Timiras, P.S. Low tryptophan diets delay reproductive aging. *Mechanisms of Aging and Development, 23*, 1983, 245–252.

Spring, B., Chiodo, J., & Bowen, D.J. Carbohydrates, tryptophan, and behavior: A methodological review. *Psychological Bulletin, 102*, 1987, 234–256.

Stern, W.C., Miller, M., Forbes, W.B., Morgane, P.J., & Resnick, O. Ontogeny of the levels of biogenic amines in various parts of the brain and in peripheral tissues in normal and protein malnourished rats. *Experimental Neurology, 49*, 1975, 314–326.

Sved, A.F. Precursor control of the function of monoaminergic neurons. In R.J. Wurtman, & J.J. Wurtman (Eds.) *Nutrition and the brain* (Vol. 6). New York: Raven Press, 1983, pp. 223–275.

Trulson, M.E. Dietary tryptophan does not alter the function of brain serotonin neurons. *Life Sciences, 37*, 1985, 1067–1072.

Wilson, J.M. & Meier, J.H. Tryptophan feeding induces sensitivity to short daylengths in photorefractory hamsters. *Neuroendocrinology, 36*, 1983, 59–63.

Wurtman, R.J. Nutrients that modify brain function. *Scientific American, 246*, 1982, 50–59.

Wurtman, R.J. & Fernstrom, J.D. Control of brain monoamine synthesis by diet and plasma amino acids. *The American Journal of Clinical Nutrition, 28*, 1975, 638–647.

Chapter 4

Catecholamines and Behavioral Arousal

Catecholamine (CA) neurotransmission may not be altered as directly or with as much sensitivity by the diet as serotonin transmission, but virtually any change in CA activity could have widespread consequences, especially if the CA system has been activated already by other physiological means. Nutrients that can alter CA activity include protein and an amino acid found in the sweetener aspartame (NutraSweet®).

Catecholamines make up a class of related neurochemicals having in common a basic structure: a catechol nucleus (a benzene ring with two adjacent OH groups attached) and a nitrogen (NH_2) group. In the central and peripheral nervous systems CAs act as neurotransmitters or modulators of other physiological systems. The synaptic actions of CAs can be either inhibitory or excitatory, the action depending largely on the target structure innervated and the relative proportion of various receptors present in that structure.

The "typical" CA nerve cell utilizes dopamine (DA), norepinephrine (NE), or epinephrine (EP) as the CA transmitter. Similarly to serotonin nerve cells, CA cells are "old" in evolution and are found in invertebrates. Although some fine differences in morphology exist, central nervous system CA fibers are thin and varicose (like serotonin fibers). Central NE fibers are also highly branched; some evidence even suggests that axons from NE cells may innervate structures as far apart as the forebrain and the cerebellum. Peripheral, sympathetic NE fibers, which have a widespread distribution throughout the body, are coarser in appearance than the central fibers.

Any change in the levels of the principal dietary precursor, tyrosine, or in other dietary substances that affect CA neurons or receptors, has the potential for altering the status of both central and peripheral neural function. Dietary events that can affect CA activity in this way are important in that they can have profound effects on behavior.

Biochemistry

The synthesis of CA is usually considered to begin with tyrosine, which is acquired from dietary protein at the normal human consumption rate of 3-4 g/day. Note, however, that additional tyrosine can be synthesized from dietary phenylalanine, another amino acid acquired from proteins, at the rate of 2-3 g/day. Phenylalanine hydroxylase, found primarily in the liver, is responsible for the conversion of phenylalanine to tyrosine. Because tyrosine is the branch point for several biosynthetic reactions, it is usually considered to be the primary synthetic starting source for CA.

The rate-limiting step for production of CA (Figure 4.1) is the conversion of tyrosine to dihydroxyphenylalanine (DOPA). ("Rate-limiting" means that

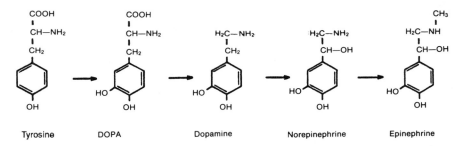

| Tyrosine | DOPA | Dopamine | Norepinephrine | Epinephrine |

Figure 4.1   Synthesis of catecholamines. The enzymes used in each step are described in the text.

the activity of the conversion enzyme is the lowest in the sequence.) The final production of CA occurs very quickly, usually dependent on the prior production of DOPA. The enzyme participating in this first step is tyrosine hydroxylase. This enzyme requires dietary iron, which may be a factor in this initial conversion step (see Chapters 9 and 10 on trace metals and vitamins).

Because this step is rate-limiting, it is crucial to examine whether dietary alterations in tyrosine or phenylalanine affect production of DOPA. Sved (1983) has provided a detailed review of the regulation of CA synthesis by tyrosine availability.

First, it is necessary that tyrosine hydroxylase not be fully saturated with its substrate tyrosine. This requirement is important so that dietary fluctuations can affect transmitter production, but it has not quite been met. The K_m for conversion of tyrosine to DOPA is about 1/10 to 1/5 of normal physiological concentrations of tyrosine. When Sved substituted the K_m and tyrosine concentrations into the appropriate kinetic equation, he calculated that conversion of tyrosine to DOPA would proceed at 88% of the maximal rate. If, under these conditions, you increased tyrosine intake (or, more to the point, plasma tyrosine levels) by 100%, you could expect only a small increase (14%) in CA synthesis. Indeed, it has been repeatedly shown that central CA levels are not reliably affected by injections of tyrosine, although administration of tyrosine does result in proportional increases in NE turnover.

Contrary findings, however, can be found. A report by Benedict and coworkers (1983) shows that, in humans, oral tyrosine intake significantly *decreases* levels of NE in plasma. They speculate that this reduction in peripheral NE comes about via a central *increase* in CA produced by the increased tyrosine. The increased central adrenergic activity has its action by decreasing peripheral sympathetic tone.

The kinetic values do indicate, however, that dietary *reduction* in tyrosine could have a large effect on CA synthesis. Injections of large neutral amino acids, which serve to reduce brain tyrosine levels, clearly reduce CA synthesis. On the other hand, given the highly branched terminal structure and extensive distribution of CA neurons, a 14% elevation could be functionally amplified throughout the nervous system. In other words, the numbers by themselves say nothing about the physiological value of any change, and CA levels per se certainly do not represent the synthesis, release, or physiological activity of CA neurons.

To illustrate this last point, Sved presented data to show that tyrosine injection alters CA synthesis primarily in "activated" CA systems. This is a reasonable idea given that the conversion activity of tyrosine hydroxylase is elevated in "activated" systems. For example, intracerebral injection of prolactin selectively activates hypothalamic DA neurons. Tyrosine injections increase the synthesis of DA in the median eminence, one of the (activated) projection sites. These injections, however, do not affect the unactivated striatum, indicating that fluctuations of tyrosine availability may thus have rather selective effects depending upon the current state of activation of any particular CA system. Furthermore, the striatum is not refractory to administration of tyrosine. Striatal DA synthesis can be affected by tyrosine when treatments that activate these particular neurons are applied.

Sved further supported this argument with reports of data on the peripheral nervous system. In one of these experiments, when rats are placed in a cold environment to enhance sympathetic nervous system activity, tyrosine administration dramatically elevates urinary CA levels. This result once again invokes the idea that tyrosine administration elevates CA levels primarily when the particular system is activated.

This result should be contrasted with Benedict's finding in humans that tyrosine decreases plasma CA levels. Aside from obvious species differences, the possibility remains that plasma levels of CA could fall while accumulated urinary levels rise. Another, more intriguing, possibility is that an early increase in sympathetic activity or tyrosine availability could have recruited central CA activity. A feedback system would be necessary to regulate this central nervous system arousal. Increases in bulbar NE activity can thus lead to a decrease in peripheral sympathetic tone. In other words, the Benedict study could have measured the decreased sympathetic activity on the "feedback inhibition" side of tyrosine ingestion.

The next step in CA biosynthesis is the decarboxylation of DOPA to DA (Figure 4.1). This step is catalyzed by a general L-aromatic amino acid decarboxylase, which also works on histidine, tyrosine, tryptophan, phenylalanine, and 5-hydroxytryptophan. This is the last (synthetic) step in DA neurons. In NE neurons another step is required.

The conversion from DA to NE is catalyzed by the enzyme dopamine beta-hydroxylase. This enzyme attaches an OH group to the ethylamine portion of DA. There is the potential for other nutrients in foods to affect this conversion. Dietary copper (see Chapter 9) is an integral component of this enzyme. Additionally, ascorbic acid (vitamin C) is a cofactor for this enzymatic step (see Chapter 10). These enzymatic steps converting DOPA to DA and DA to NE proceed quite rapidly under normal conditions. Neurotransmitter formation is primarily dependent upon the conditions affecting the initial step from tyrosine to DOPA.

In EP neurons (or in adrenal medulla) another enzyme is needed to convert NE to EP. This is phenylethanolamine-N-methyl-transferase (PNMT), which transfers a methyl (CH_3) group to the nitrogen atom.

The principal enzymes important in the breakdown of CA are monoamine oxidase and catechol-O-methyl-transferase. The first converts CA molecules to their corresponding aldehydes, which are then usually oxidized to the corresponding acids. The second enzyme catalyzes the attachment of a methyl group to one of the catechol OH groups.

Although it appears that primary dietary effects of tyrosine ingestion are focused on "classic" CA neurotransmitters, it is worthwhile to consider that tyramine and octopamine, both of which have neurotransmitter activity, are also formed initially from tyrosine. In fact, investigators have shown that conversion of tyrosine to tyramine is a major route of tyrosine metabolism. Moreover, Edwards (1982) has suggested that the antidepressant effects of tyrosine may be due in part to formation of tyramine and octopamine following tyrosine administration.

*A*natomy

Catecholamine Cells

At least 15 groups of cells that contain CA have been identified in the rat central nervous system. In accordance with the nomenclature that originated with the papers by Dahlstrom and Fuxe (1965), these cellular masses are named A1-A15 (Figure 4.2). (See Lindvall and Bjorklund (1978) for more detail.)

The most caudal of these cells (A1 and A3) have been found in the medulla at about the level where the pyramidal tracts decussate (cross). These cells are located ventrally and laterally in this area. Cells in the rostral part of this grouping contain PNMT, the enzyme that converts NE into EP, and thus might utilize EP as a neurotransmitter.

Cells at this caudal level (A2) also appear in a dorsal and medial location, primarily located in the nucleus of the solitary tract and in the dorsal motor nucleus of the vagus. These cells utilize DA, NE, or EP as neurotransmitters.

The cell groups A4-A7 are best explained with reference to the locus ceruleus (A6). The locus ceruleus is the largest CNS group of cells that contain NE (Figure 4.3). It is located in the dorsal pons around the lateral edge of the fourth ventricle, primarily at the level of the trigeminal nerve. The A4 group lies more caudally on the lateral roof of the fourth ventricle. The A5 and A7 cells, like the A1 and A3 cells, are located laterally, and A7 cells are rostral to A6.

The cells labeled A8, containing DA, can be found in the midbrain caudal, ventral, and lateral to the red nucleus, but the A9 DA nucleus has claimed the most research attention. A9 cells are located in the compact zone of the substantia nigra. These are the cells that send massive DA projections to the basal ganglia. The DA cells lying medial to this band of cells are designated A10.

Surrounding the aqueduct where it joins with the third ventricle are the A11 cells, most of which contain DA. These periventricular and periaqueductal cells appear to project within ventricular regions and are therefore quite distinct from the previously mentioned DA cells.

As we move forward into hypothalamus, we find DA cells that project

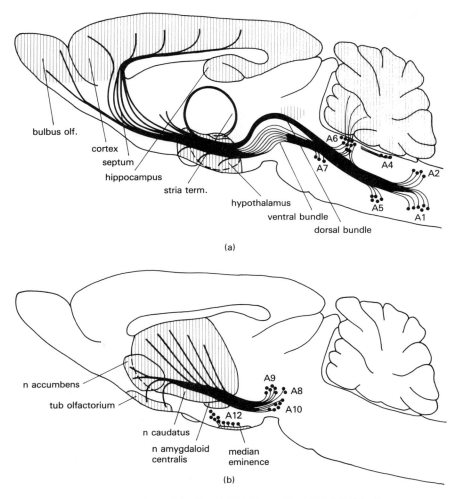

Figure 4.2 Catecholamine cell bodies (A13-A15 not shown). (a) Cell bodies containing norepinephrine. (b) Cell bodies containing dopamine. [(a) From U. Ungerstedt, *Acta Physiol. Scand.*, 62, Suppl. 232:1 (1971); (b) From U. Ungerstedt, *Acta Physiol. Scand.*, Suppl. 367:1 (1971).]

within the hypothalamus. These form the incertohypothalamic system and the tuberohypophyseal system (A12-A14). The latter system has cells located in the hypothalamic arcuate nucleus that interact directly with the pituitary. Some of the axons from these cells terminate in the median eminence, while others project to the intermediate lobe of the pituitary.

Other DA systems seem to have distinctly sensory functions. The so-called A15 DA neurons are periglomular cells in the olfactory bulb. There are also DA interneurons in the retina, where DA is probably released when light strikes the retina.

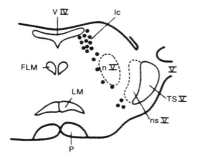

Figure 4.3 Cross-section of the brain stem (pontine level) showing location of the locus coeruleus (lc), which is the principal site of norepinephrine cells. Abbreviations: V IV = 4th ventricle; n V = principal trigeminal nucleus; V = trigeminal nerve; TS V = spinal tract of trigeminal nerve; ns V = spinal trigeminal nucleus; FLM = medial longitudinal fasciculus; LM = medial lemniscus; P = pyramidal tract. (From Lindvall and Bjorklund, 1978.)

This does not exhaust the available discussion of CA cells. There are numerous CA cells in the periphery, many of which participate in sympathetic nervous system function (Chapter 2). Virtually all the cells in the chain of sympathetic ganglia contain NE. Also, some small cells in sympathetic ganglia contain DA. Cells in the adrenal medulla, a sympathetically innervated structure, secrete EP.

Catecholamine Cell Projections

The principal NE projection systems arise from cells in the locus ceruleus (LC). This major cell group gives rise to axons that innervate virtually the entire central nervous system. Even more remarkable is the fact that the number of cells in each LC cluster (in the rat) is only about 1500, so that you might suppose these axons to have a highly branched pattern of distribution. Indeed, many of these axons initially bifurcate with a characteristic T-shaped pattern to send one projection into the brain and one into the spinal cord.

Descending CA fibers from the LC and from A1 and A2 groups run in anterior and lateral portions of the spinal cord to terminate in ventral horn motor cell areas. A smaller system descends in a lateral and dorsal manner to innervate dorsal horn sensory areas and the sympathetic lateral column. This projection onto preganglionic sympathetic areas may provide physiological antagonism to serotonin projections in this area.

The locus ceruleus also gives rise to a bundle of fibers that ascends in the superior cerebellar peduncle to innervate the cerebellum. Many of these fibers may in fact arise from primary branches of LC axons otherwise destined to ascend toward the forebrain. This means that single LC cells may give rise to a projection system that innervates areas as far apart as the cerebellum and forebrain.

The ascending LC systems are confined largely to two main tracts: central tegmental tract (CTT) and dorsal periventricular system (DPS). Figure 4.4 describes these ascending pathways. The sites of innervation will be described according to the contributions of different NE systems, after Lindvall and Bjorklund.

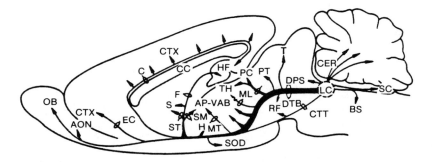

Figure 4.4 Principal norepinephrine pathways originating from cells in the locus coeruleus. Abbreviations: AON, anterior olfactory nucleus; AP-VAB, ansa peduncularis-ventral amygdaloid bundle system; BS, brainstem nuclei; C, cingulum; CC, corpus callosum; CER, cerebellum; CTT, central tegmental tract; CTX, cerebral neocortex; DPS, dorsal periventricular system; DTB, dorsal catecholamine bundle; EC, external capsule; F, fornix; H, hypothalamus; HF, hippocampal formation; LC, locus ceruleus; ML, medial lemniscus; MT, mammillothalamic tract; OB, olfactory bulb; PC, posterior commissure; PT, pretectal area; RF, reticular formation; S, septal area; SC, spinal cord; SM, stria medullaris; SOD, supraoptic decussations; ST, stria terminalis; T, tectum; TH, thalamus. (Diagram compiled by R. Y. Moore. From the observations of Lindvall and Björklund, 1974b; Jones and Moore, 1977.)

As NE fibers ascend from pontine areas into the midbrain, they give rise to tectal projections innervating the superior and inferior colliculi. The periventricular system, as its name implies, gives rise to NE fibers that innervate nuclei in the thalamus and hypothalamus surrounding the midline ventricles.

The predominant ascending bundle for the central tegmental tract is through the medial forebrain bundle. Fibers are contributed to this bundle after turning ventrally as they ascend from the midbrain. As these fibers begin to turn ventrally, some branch off to join the fasciculus retroflexus to innervate the habenula. Others branch off to innervate the ventral thalamus. From the medial forebrain bundle, fibers branch off to innervate the piriform lobe and to join the supraoptic decussations. NE fibers branch off dorsally from this bundle to join the fornix. These curve dorsally and caudally under the corpus callosum to innervate the hippocampal formation. Many of the fibers continue further rostrally and extend into olfactory nuclei. Others branch off dorsally to loop around the genu of the corpus callosum. These fibers initially run in the cingulum bundle and provide much of the innervation of the cerebral cortex. Some of these fibers continue in the cingulum above the corpus callosum and eventually pass down behind the splenium to join the hippocampus.

Figure 4.5 illustrates DA pathways. One of the principal DA pathways is the nigrostriatal system, so named because it originates in the substantia nigra (compact portion, A9) and terminates primarily in neostriatum, where it is involved in the control of motor behavior. This pathway also receives projections from A8 and A10 DA cell groups.

DA fiber systems also course through the medial forebrain bundle. As these fibers ascend almost to the level of the optic chiasm, one group leaves

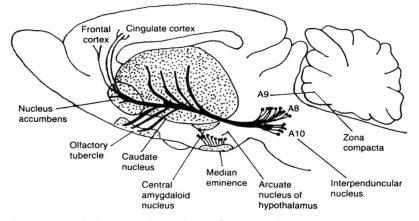

Figure 4.5 Principal dopamine pathways. [Modified after U. Ungerstedt. *Acta Physiol. Scand.* (1971) Suppl. 367.]

the bundle laterally to innervate amygdala, piriform cortex, and entorhinal cortex. Other fibers fan out ventrally and rostrally to innervate the olfactory tubercle. These are the mesolimbic DA projections. The DA fibers that continue forward, rising at the rostral septal area to branch into frontal and cingulate cortices, are called collectively the mesocortical DA system.

As previously mentioned, shorter DA projection systems in the arcuate and periventricular hypothalamic nuclei innervate median eminence and the posterior pituitary. The DA system (incertohypothalamic) originating in dorsal and caudal hypothalamus extends forward to innervate anterior and preoptic regions of the hypothalamus.

There are also EP projections to the hypothalamus and brain stem. The cell bodies of origin of these fibers are located in the caudal brainstem.

In the periphery, the sympathetic nervous system contributes EP and (primarily) NE projections to virtually all organs and regions of the body (Chapter 2). Arterioles have a dense innervation by sympathetic fibers throughout the body. Because these terminals have first access to available tyrosine as a precursor to NE, this system would probably be the first altered by dietary changes in tyrosine supply.

*B*ehavior

Catecholamine Systems

Recalling Gaylord Ellison's work cited in Chapter 3, we note that it was based on a concept of behavioral roles of NE and serotonin that originated in the late 1950s. At that time, Brodie and Shore (1957) proposed that the two transmitters act antagonistically. Serotonin and NE were considered to activate parasympathetic and sympathetic systems, respectively. If you administered a drug that blocked the action of serotonin, NE sympathetic actions would prevail (Figure 4.6). These investigators compared this concept for the

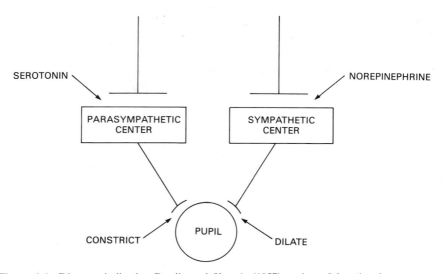

Figure 4.6 Diagram indicating Brodie and Shore's (1957) notion of functional antagonism between norepinephrine and serotonin systems.

central nervous system to the (peripheral) antagonism observed for pupillary dilation: drugs will dilate the pupil if they enhance sympathetic activity or if they block parasympathetic activity.

Keeping in mind the mutual antagonism of the transmitters, Ellison analyzed his experimental results in terms of a NE/serotonin balance. He viewed the results as reflective of either low-NE/high-serotonin or high-NE/low-serotonin brain states. For convenience, we will refer to these states as low-NE and high-NE.

Low-NE rats exhibited typical clinical signs of inactivity and depression. These animals remained in their burrows more than normal and were lethargic and inactive, though they provoked more fights when they came out of their burrows. By contrast, the high-NE rats stayed out of their burrows and in the open more than any other group. These animals were hyperactive and exploratory.

Converging results are found when rats are treated neonatally with 6-hydroxydopamine (or 6-hydroxydopa) to destroy developing NE systems. McLean and co-workers (1976) found that when these animals are tested as adults, they show hypophagia, reduced activity, and increased emotionality and aggression.

These data converge nicely with the findings of Gage and Springer (1981), who injected NE directly into the hippocampus of rats. Shortly after the injection these animals were hyperactive in the open field, and hyperreactive to somatosensory stimuli. Flicker and Geyer (1982) also infused NE into the hippocampus of rats. Their animals did not increase locomotor activity per se but showed more diverse exploration.

It is not easy to reconcile the two different sets of data that show increased hyperreactivity (also called hyperemotionality) with such radically different methods: by injecting NE or by removing its influence with the use of a specific neurotoxin. A developing receptor supersensitivity to remaining NE is a phenomenon that could be invoked to "explain" the hyperreactivity in lesioned animals, but it is best to let further research resolve the discrepancy.

The activity of locus ceruleus NE-containing cells can be correlated directly with behavior. Recordings show that firing of these cells increases in response to various external stimuli in freely moving rats. A progressive decline in firing rate occurs as the animal's state of arousal recedes from wakefulness through slow-wave sleep to paradoxical sleep. Recordings from substantia nigra in cats show that the highest discharge of DA cells also occurs during active waking. This rate of activity is about 20% higher than that during quiet waking, though there is no further diminishing of cellular activity as the animal progresses through sleep stages. There is also no change in the activity of these DA neurons at any time during feeding or immediately following satiety, though these neurons are active during orienting responses.

Although these data are generally consistent with a role for CA in behavioral arousal, such a generalization is not immediately warranted. After all, serotonin neurons show a similar progressive decline in activity as the animal recedes from behavioral arousal. The question then is whether the activity of monoamine neurons follows or leads to arousal. This question can be answered only by means of direct converging evidence.

Evidence so far suggests that activity of serotonin cells follows behavioral arousal. Because serotonin administration seems to depress behavioral arousal, it could be argued that the activity of serotonin cells occurs as a feedback response to behavioral arousal. Conversely, NE administration seems to heighten behavioral arousal. A similar line of argument would therefore suggest that NE activity leads to behavioral arousal. Accordingly, elevations in NE activity would tend to arouse the organism, leading to a feedback response in serotonin systems. But what of dopamine?

Carey (1983) compared the differential effects of limbic and striatal DA loss on motor functions. He injected the neurotoxin 6-hydroxydopamine into the ventral tegmental area to remove the (limbic) DA projections to the nucleus accumbens-olfactory tubercle area. The same neurotoxin was injected into the substantia nigra (compact region) to remove striatal DA projections. He then injected a drug (apomorphine) that activates DA receptors. An important point to keep in mind in this experiment is that there are more DA receptors in a target site (accumbens or striatum) that has been deprived of DA input.

The drug enhanced spontaneous locomotor activity only in those animals deprived of limbic DA. In the animals deprived of striatal DA, there was no effect of the drug on spontaneous locomotor activity, but there was a persistent augmentation of motor rigidity. These results suggest that limbic DA normally mediates locomotor activity and that striatal DA normally mediates other forms of motor behavior. Parkinsonian patients who show motor rigidity typically have destruction of the substantia nigra projection system. Administration of L-DOPA, the immediate precursor to DA, is helpful in alleviating these symptoms.

More recent work confirms these roles for DA, and extends our knowledge of the activation of different DA receptors in different brain areas. When a D_1 agonist of DA is administered to the accumbens of rats treated with neurotoxin, there is a dose-related increase in locomotor activity. Administration of the D_1 agonist into the caudate of similarly lesioned rats produces little locomotion, but does induce stereotypy. A D_2 agonist also induces stereotypic behavior when injected into the caudate, but does little to affect locomotion in the accumbens.

Of course, any consideration of CA mediation of behavior must take into account the sympathetic nervous system (Chapter 2). Activation of this (primarily) noradrenergic system leads to peripheral organ changes that mediate behavioral arousal. Cardiac and respiratory systems increase in activity, and EP is released into the bloodstream from the adrenal medulla, further increasing sympathetic arousal. Peripheral vasoconstriction occurs, thereby maintaining internal body temperature against heat dissipation. On the other hand, relaxation of this system, as when people are taught a specific relaxation technique, reduces sympathetic responsiveness, thereby lessening arousal.

Superior cervical ganglionic (sympathetic) fibers innervate cerebral blood vessels. (Locus ceruleus projections also innervate cerebral blood vessels.) Activity by these fibers usually results in constriction, thereby reducing cerebral blood flow. This action alone does not permit one to make a direct inference about behavior, because reduced blood flow to a behaviorally inhibitory region could result in arousal. It is also clear that there is no uniform cerebral vasoconstriction and that regional vasoconstriction may be mediated by regional brain activity. There is also evidence that locus ceruleus NE is necessary for the recovery of oxidative metabolism after regional activity in cortex.

To summarize the CA mediation of behavior, it is helpful to consider the separate contributions of different catecholamines as well as of different nervous systems. The participation of DA in behavioral functions appears to be more specific than that of NE, which generally seems to mediate behavioral arousal, both centrally and peripherally. The architecture of central NE projections is not unlike that of serotonin projections, so it is tempting to ascribe an antagonistic (compared to serotonin) arousal function to NE at every hierarchical level of the nervous system. However, caution is advised, especially because of local differences in transmitter function. For example, locus ceruleus projections decrease somatosensory communication by inhibiting transmission in spinal cord and in spinal trigeminal nucleus.

Diet

For a discussion of dietary effects, it will be helpful to focus on the arousal properties of CA, and on the particular relationship between NE and feeding behavior. This makes sense in the context of widespread distribution of peripheral and central NE systems, and of the well-researched relationship between NE and hypothalamic areas that control feeding.

The administration of the amino acid tyrosine has arousal effects compatible with the general arousal properties of CA, but these occur primarily when CA systems are first activated. For example, Conlay and colleagues (1981) found that a dose-related effect of tyrosine was to increase systolic blood pressure in hypotensive animals. This is in contrast to tyrosine's effect of decreasing blood pressure in hypertensive animals.

In hypertensive animals, brainstem NE neurons probably fire frequently, thereby diminishing sympathetic outflow. Under these conditions, tyrosine administration probably accelerates NE synthesis in the more active NE neurons: the brainstem neurons. Because NE activity in the brainstem reduces activity in the sympathetic nervous system, blood pressure falls after tyrosine administration. Conversely, the sympathetic nervous system is quite active in hypotensive animals. Under these conditions, tyrosine administration probably enhances the release of NE from sympathetic neurons and EP from the adrenal medulla, thereby increasing systolic blood pressure.

Under conditions of uncontrolled stress, turnover in central NE neurons increases. This kind of stress can decrease locomotor and exploratory behavior, presumably by depleting NE neurons of available transmitter. Data from the Wurtman (Reinstein et al., 1984) laboratory show that if tyrosine is given before the administration of a stressor (shock) uncontrolled by the rats, the animals display neither NE depletion nor decrements in locomotion.

If you have consumed any products containing the artificial sweetener Nutra-Sweet® (Figure 4.7), you have almost certainly affected activity in your own NE systems (depending of course on the relative state of activity in these systems). The essential ingredient in Nutra-Sweet® is aspartame (1-methyl-N-L-α aspartyl-L-phenylalanine), a dipeptide that liberates its phenylalanine when digested.

The Wurtman laboratory (1983) studied the effects of aspartame in rats at doses consistent with the amount a thirsty 8 year old child might consume during a hot afternoon (three soft drinks plus an additional 100 mg in other foods). The aspartame administration doubled levels of phenylalanine in the rat brains. The effect doubled again when the rats consumed high amounts of carbohydrates, presumably because of the reduced competition with other branched chain amino acids. The aspartame-carbohydrate combination increased tyrosine levels by 344% and reduced by 50% the increase in tryptophan that normally occurs after carbohydrate consumption. Aspartame can thus also prevent the rise in serotonin that occurs after carbohydrate ingestion.

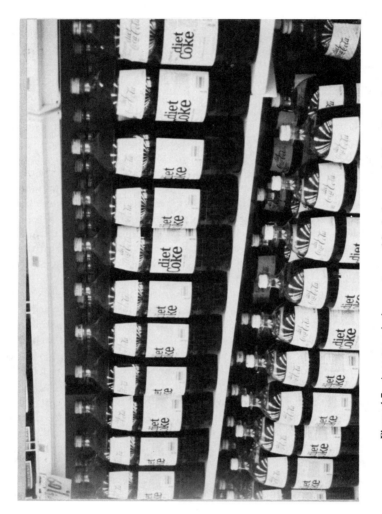

Figure 4.7 Aspartame is the sweetener of foods that contain Nutra-Sweet.®

In other studies, it was shown that oral or injected aspartame—in high doses that correspond to 40-50 mg/kg for a human consuming the sweetener with a carbohydrate snack—reduced blood pressure in spontaneously hypertensive rats. Aspartame also elevated brain levels of tyrosine and NE. The finding is therefore consistent with the data showing that tyrosine administration reduces blood pressure in hypertensive animals.

Elevated intake of foods sweetened with aspartame has been implicated in increased susceptibility to seizures. Wurtman (1985) has reported case studies in which persons who consume high levels of aspartame undergo seizures. When all aspartame is removed from the diet, the seizures cease. Recent news accounts of research presentations by Paul Spiers indicate that aspartame may be a factor in decreased cognitive function in normal individuals. Spiers gave subjects aspartame capsules containing the FDA's maximum allowable limit (50 mg/kg) daily for 12 days. When he tested these people on "Think Fast," a demanding and self-paced computer test, he found that subjects on aspartame failed to improve and often worsened in their performance. These findings are consistent with the record of impairment of mental function by increased phenylalanine and may reflect interference with NE involvement in memory consolidation.

Torii and colleagues (1986) have shown that consumption of meals with protein along with aspartame may lessen some of its effects. They found that animals receiving large doses of aspartame with their 25% casein (high-protein) diet have no change in brain monoamines.

Blundell and Hill (1986) have reported paradoxical effects of aspartame on appetite in humans. They showed that ratings of pleasantness of sucrose decline in humans after aspartame consumption, though not as much as when glucose is consumed. However, whereas glucose causes a decline in rated motivation to eat and an increase in the ratings of fullness, aspartame does just the reverse: it increases rated motivation to eat and decreases ratings of fullness. These findings probably reflect NE's ability to stimulate feeding. Aspartame thus has stimulatory effects on appetite and can lead to disordered patterns of eating and loss of control over appetite.

Several conflicting reports of the effects of tyrosine or phenylalanine on food intake have been published. The Anderson group (1977) in Toronto has shown that the plasma tyrosine/phenylalanine ratio correlates positively with energy intake (the tryptophan/neutral amino acid ratio correlates negatively with protein intake). Møller (1983) showed that in humans the plasma tyrosine/neutral amino acid (NAA) and tryptophan/NAA ratios were related to the choice of between-meal snacks in the forenoon. Subjects who had high ratios of these amino acids consistently preferred snacks with low proportions of protein to carbohydrate (high-carbohydrate).

These two studies seem to be in close agreement until you consider that protein preferences did not change in the Møller study; the ratios were related primarily to carbohydrate preferences. This study therefore did not confirm that tryptophan ratios are negatively related to protein intake. Moreover, elevations in serotonin levels usually decrease carbohydrate intake; the correlation between tryptophan ratios and increased preference for carbohydrates is not compatible with previous findings on serotonin. However, tyrosine ratios *are* associated with carbohydrate preferences. This finding is compatible with data showing tyrosine ratios correlated positively with energy intake.

Unless an extended extrapolation is made, neither of these findings seem especially related to a behavioral (total organismic) regulation for tyrosine or phenylalanine. One possible extrapolation is that many foods with a high carbohydrate content (and therefore high energy) have low amounts of protein. If tyrosine ratios correlate positively with energy intake, high tyrosine levels would serve to reduce protein intake. But this extrapolation is probably not warranted because of the findings that tyrosine ratios seem unrelated to protein intake, and that protein intake can be divorced from energy intake.

The notion of phenylalanine or tyrosine regulation becomes somewhat more substantiated when the central nervous system is examined more directly. Injection of amino acids directly into the hypothalamus reduces food intake, and consequently intake of these amino acids. On the other hand, Mauron and colleagues (1980) have also shown that administration of low doses of clonidine, a NE alpha$_2$ agonist, increases total food and protein intake in rats. Consistent with these findings are the results showing that chickens intubated with tyrosine increase their food intake.

Work from the Leibowitz laboratory (Leibowitz et al., 1985; Leibowitz and Stanley, 1986) (see also Chapter 8) provides more direct evidence of CA regulation of food intake, especially of carbohydrates, though little attention has been given to specific regulation of tyrosine or phenylalanine. Administration of NE directly into the paraventricular nucleus (PVN) of the hypothalamus selectively stimulates carbohydrate intake. This effect occurs in the absence or presence of a change in total calorie intake, indicating a potential dissociation of the mechanisms controlling nutrient and total energy intake. Receptors in the PVN responsible for this effect are likely the alpha$_2$-adrenoceptors, because administration of alpha$_2$ agonists such as clonidine also result in specific carbohydrate ingestion. Furthermore, selective alpha$_2$ antagonists attenuate feeding responses induced by NE and clonidine. Moreover, circadian increases in NE activity in this area of the hypothalamus are greatest at the onset of the dark period, during which time rats increase their preference for carbohydrates (Jhanwar-Uniyal et al., 1986).

The relative state of activity of NE systems before and after a meal may therefore more closely determine food intake, especially of carbohydrates, than the ingestion of phenylalanine or tyrosine. Intake of these essential amino acids could well bias the specific selection of foods.

Developmental Effects

Rats whose mothers were fed a low-protein diet the last week of pregnancy and during nursing, and who were fed a low-protein diet until they were 50 days old, have an enhanced rate of brain CA turnover, even when fed a balanced lab chow for 90 days before they were sacrificed (Keller et al., 1982). This enhanced turnover is reflected in a significant increase in the rate-limiting enzyme for CA production (tyrosine hydroxylase). Moreover, these animals have a reduction in NE receptor binding (alpha and beta), probably as a result of the increased turnover. Stern and colleagues (1975) have shown that early protein malnourishment elevates brain CA levels at most ages from birth through 300 days of age.

These adult consequences of early protein deprivation also reflect altered brain function. Leahy and colleagues (1978) have shown that early protein deprivation diminishes the ability of apomorphine to produce stereotyped behavior.

Behavioral Pathology

The mode of action of tricyclic antidepressant drugs has been controversial. One immediate action of many of these drugs is to decrease uptake of NE, thereby elevating its action at the synapse. This mechanism fits nicely with the notions of NE and behavioral arousal, but the major problem is one of time. Clinically depressed patients who take these drugs do not get better within the short time frame of this action of the drug. It has more recently been shown that another action of these drugs is to alter production of beta-adrenergic receptors ("up-" or "down-regulation"). This action takes considerably longer than uptake inhibition and has about the same time frame as the clinical improvement, indicating that altered action at NE receptors could still elevate depressed behavior. The major problem with this argument, however, is that these drugs tend to diminish the responsiveness of central beta receptors.

A study by Gelenberg and others (1980) has suggested that administration of tyrosine to increase NE turnover may also be an effective means of treating depression. In their case study, a therapist who did not know the order of administration of tyrosine or placebo rated the symptoms of depression in the patient. Whenever tyrosine was administered, clinical ratings improved. These included judgments as to mood, self-esteem, sleep, energy level, anxiety, and somatic complaints. Depressive signs worsened whenever the placebo was administered. Blood samples were taken in this study, and it was clear that plasma tyrosine levels rose only after the administration of tyrosine; that is, plasma tyrosine levels were associated with improvement in the clinical picture.

In the history of the treatment of depression there is also a case of food-related tragedy. Before the present use of tricyclic antidepressants, monoamine oxidase inhibitors were used frequently. These drugs tend to elevate monoamines (including NE) by inhibiting the first enzymatic step in degredative metabolism. Some patients who were using these drugs died of hypertensive crises during treatment, and it later became clear that these patients had eaten sharp cheeses or other fermented foods. These foods have an especially high level of tyramine, the decarboxylated product of tyrosine. Tyramine, like NE, is a sympathomimetic and would therefore tend to enhance sympathetic tone. Because the drugs were inhibiting the breakdown of NE and of tyramine, the enhanced sympathetic activity produced an increased risk of cardiac arrhythmias in these patients. The ingestion of foods (such as cheese) with a high tyramine content (or a high caffeine content) is now contraindicated for patients using these drugs.

Summary

Catecholamines have widespread effects on brain and behavior. NE especially is distributed throughout the CNS and is the principal transmitter of the sympathetic nervous system. Increased activity of NE is associated with behavioral arousal. Animals with experimentally elevated brain NE levels are typically more active and reactive, and they consume more food, especially carbohydrates.

Although changes in tyrosine levels do not have as much potential for affecting CA systems as tryptophan does for serotonin systems, the potential for any change to have widespread effects has been established. This is particularly important in light of the evidence that consumption of NutraSweet can contribute relatively high amounts of phenylalanine to the synthesis of catecholamines.

Catecholamines are also important in the etiology of depression. Evidence exists that oral tyrosine administration may be a factor in the treatment of depression by virtue of its ability to enhance catecholamine synthesis.

References

Anderson, G.H., & Ashley, D.V.M. Correlation of the plasma tyrosine to phenylalanine ratio with energy intake in self-selecting weanling rats. *Life Science*, *21*, 1977, 1227–1234.

Benedict, C.R., Anderson, G.H., & Sole, M.J. The influence of oral tyrosine and tryptophan feeding on plasma catecholamines in man. *The American Journal of Clinical Nutrition, 38*, 1983, 429–435.

Blundell, J.F. & Hill, A.J. Paradoxical effects of an intense sweetener (aspartame) on appetite. *The Lancet, 1*, 1986, 1092–1093.

Brodie, B.B., & Shore, P.A. A concept for a role of serotonin and norepinephrine as chemical mediators in the brain. *Annals of the New York Academy of Sciences, 66*, 1957, 631–642.

Carey, R.J. Differential effects of limbic versus striatal dopamine loss on motoric function. *Behavioural Brain Research, 7*, 1983, 283–296.

Conlay, L.A., Maher, T.J., & Wurtman, R.J. Tyrosine increases blood pressure in hypotensive rats, *Science, 212*, 1981, 559–560.

Dahlstrom, A. & Fuxe, K. Evidence for the existence of monoamine neurons in the central nervous system. II. Experimentally induced changes in the intraneuronal amine levels of bulbospinal neuron systems. *Acta Physiologica Scandinavica, 64* (247), 1965, 1–36.

Edwards, D.J. Possible role of octopamine and tyramine in the antihypertensive and antidepressant effects of tyrosine. *Life Sciences, 30*, 1982, 1427–1434.

Ellison, G.D. Animal models of psychopathology: The low-norepinephrine and low-serotonin rat. *American Psychologist, 32*, 1977, 1036–1045.

Flicker, C., & Geyer, M.A. Behavior during hippocampal microinfusion. I. Norepinephrine and diversive exploration. *Brain Research Reviews, 4*, 1982, 79–103.

Gage, F.H., & Springer, J.S. Behavioral assessment of norepinephrine and serotonin function and interaction in the hippocampal formation. *Pharmacology, Biochemistry, and Behavior, 14*, 1981, 815–821.

Gelenberg, A.J., Wojcik, J.D., Growdon, J.H., Sved, A.F., & Wurtman, R.J. Tyrosine for the treatment of depression. *American Journal of Psychiatry, 137*, 1980, 622–623.

Jhanwar-Uniyal, M., Roland, C.R., & Leibowitz, S.F. Diurnal rhythm of α_2-noradrenergic receptors in the paraventricular nucleus: Relation to circulating corticosterone and feeding behavior. *Life Sciences, 38*, 1986, 473–482.

Keller, E.A., Munaro, N.I., & Orsingher, O.A. Perinatal undernutrition reduces alpha and beta adrenergic receptor binding in adult rat brain. *Science, 215*, 1982, 1269–1270.

Leahy, J.P., Stern, W.C., Resnick, O., & Morgane, P.J. A neuropharmacological analysis of central nervous system catecholamine systems in developmental protein malnutrition. *Developmental Psychobiology, 11*, 1978, 361–370.

Leibowitz, S.F., Brown, O., Tretter, J.R., & Kirschgessner, A. Norepinephrine, clonidine, and tricyclic antidepressants selectively stimulate carbohydrate ingestion through noradrenergic system of the paraventricular nucleus. *Pharmacology, Biochemistry, & Behavior, 23*, 1985, 541–550.

Leibowitz, S.F., & Stanley, B.G. Neurochemical controls of appetite. In R. Ritter, S. Ritter, & C.D. Barnes (Eds.), *Feeding behavior: Neural and humoral controls*, NY: Academic Press, 1986, pp. 191–233.

Lindvall, O., & Bjorklund, A. Organization of catecholamine neurons in the rat central nervous system. In L.L. Iversen, S.D. Iversen, & S.H. Snyder (Eds.), *Chemical pathways in the brain* (Vol. 9). *Handbook of psychopharmacology*. New York: Plenum Press, 1978, pp. 139–232.

Mauron, C., Wurtman, J.J., & Wurtman, R.J. Clonidine increases food and protein consumption in rats. *Life Sciences, 27*, 1980, 781–791.

McLean, J.H., Kostrzewa, R.M., & May, J.G. Behavioral and biochemical effects of neonatal treatment of rats with 6-hydroxydopa. *Pharmacology, Biochemistry, and Behavior, 4*, 1976, 601–607.

Møller, S.E. Tryptophan and tyrosine availability: Relation to food choice and sleeping habits: A preliminary study. *Human Neurobiology, 2*, 1983, 45–48.

Reinstein, D.K., Lehnert, H., Scott, N.A., & Wurtman, R.J. Tyrosine prevents behavioral and neurochemical correlates of an acute stress in rats. *Life Sciences, 34*, 1984, 2225–2231.

Stern, W.C., Miller, M., Forbes, W.B., Morgane, P.J., & Resnick, O. Ontogeny of the levels of biogenic amines in various parts of the brain and in peripheral tissues in normal and protein malnourished rats. *Experimental Neurology, 49*, 1975, 314–326.

Sved, A.F. Precursor control of the function of monoaminergic neurons. In R.J. Wurtman, & J.J. Wurtman (Eds.), *Nutrition and the brain* (Vol. 6). New York: Raven Press, 1983, pp. 223–275.

Torii, K., Mimura, T., Takasaki, Y., & Ichimura, M. Effect of mealing on plasma and brain monoamine in rats after oral aspartame. *Physiology and Behavior, 36*, 1986, 759–764.

Wurtman, R.J. Aspartame: Possible effect on seizure susceptibility. *The Lancet, 2*, 1985, 1060.

Wurtman, R.J. Neurochemical changes following high-dose aspartame with dietary carbohydrates. *New England Journal of Medicine, 309*, 1983, 429–430.

Suggested Readings

Altman, H.J., & Quartermain, D. Facilitation of memory retrieval by centrally administered catecholamine stimulating agents. *Behavioural Brain Research, 7*, 1983, 51–63.

Aston-Jones, G., Ennis, M., Pieribone, V.A., Nickell, W.T., & Shipley, M.T. The brain nucleus locus coeruleus: Restricted afferent control of a broad efferent network. *Science, 234*, 1986, 734–737.

Blundell, J.E. Problems and processes underlying the control of food selection and nutrient intake. In R.J. Wurtman, & J.J. Wurtman (Eds.), *Nutrition and the brain* (Vol. 6). New York: Raven Press, 1983, pp. 163–221.

Breese, G.R., Duncan, G.E., Napier, T.C., Bondy, S.C., Iorio, L.C., & Mueller, R.A. 6-Hydroxydopamine treatments enhance behavioral responses to intracerebral microinjection of D_1- and D_2-dopamine agonists into nucleus accumbens and striatum without changing dopamine antagonist binding. *The Journal of Pharmacology and Experimental Therapeutics, 240*, 1987, 167–76.

Cooper, J.R., Bloom, F.E., & Roth, R.H. *The biochemical basis of neuropharmacology* (4th ed.). New York: Oxford University Press, 1982.

David, J-C., Dairman, W., & Udenfriend, S. Decarboxylation to tyramine: A major route of tyrosine metabolism in mammals. *Proceedings of the National Academy of Sciences, USA, 71*, 1974, 1771–1775.

Gibson, C.J., & Wurtman, R.J. Physiological control of brain norepinephrine synthesis by brain tyrosine concentration. *Life Sciences, 22*, 1978, 1399–1406.

Goldman, C., Marino, L. & Leibowitz, S.F. Postsynaptic α_2-noradrenergic receptor in the paraventricular nucleus mediate feeding inducted by norepinephrine and clonidine. *European Journal of Pharmacology, 115*, 1985, 11–19.

Gordon, F.J., Brody, M.J., Fink, G.D., Buggy, J., & Johnson, A.K. Role of central catecholamines in the control of blood pressure and drinking behavior. *Brain Research, 178*, 1979, 161–173.

Harik, S.I., LaManna, J.C., Light, A.I., & Rosenthal, M. Cerebral norepinephrine: Influence on cortical oxidative metabolism *in situ*. *Science, 206*, 1979, 69–71.

Hoffman, J.W., Benson, H., Arns, P.A., Stainbrook, G.L., Landsberg, L., Young, J.B., & Gill, A. Reduced sympathetic nervous system responsivity associated with the relaxation response. *Science, 215*, 1982, 190–192.

Lacy, M.P., Van Krey, H.P., Denbow, D.M., Siegel, P.B., & Cherry, J.A. Amino acid regulation of food intake in domestic fowl. *Nutrition and Behavior, 1*, 1982, 65–74.

Maher, T.J., & Wurtman, R.J. High doses of aspartame reduce blood pressure in spontaneously hypertensive rats. *New England Journal of Medicine, 309*, 1983, 1125.

Marcus, M.L., & Heistad, D.D. Effects of sympathetic nerves on cerebral blood flow in awake dogs. *American Journal of Physiology, 236*, 1979, H549-H553.

McNaughton, N., & Mason, S.T. The neuropsychology and neuropharmacology of the dorsal ascending noradrenergic bundle—A review. *Progress in Neurobiology, 14*, 1980, 157–219.

Panksepp, J., & Booth, D.A. Decreased feeding after injections of amino acids into the hypothalamus, *Nature, 233*, 1971, 341–342.

Rovner, S. NutraSweet: The debate continues. *The Washington Post*, quoted in: *The Times-Picayune*, New Orleans, LA, May 26, 1987.

Shor-Posner, G., Grinker, J.A., Marinescu, C., & Leibowitz, S.F. Role of hypothalamic norepinephrine in control of meal patterns. *Physiology & Behavior, 35*, 1985, 209–214.

Steinfels, G.F., Heym, J., Strecker, R.E., & Jacobs, B.L. Behavioral correlates of dopaminergic unit activity in freely moving cats. *Brain Research, 258*, 1983, 217–228.

Woodward, D.J., Moises, H.C., Waterhouse, B.D., Hoffer, B.J., & Freedman, R. Modulatory actions of norepinephrine in the central nervous system. *Federal Proceedings, 38*, 1979, 2109–2116.

Yokogoshi, H. & Wurtman, R.J. Acute effects of oral or parenteral aspartame on catecholamine metabolism in various regions of rat brain. *Journal of Nutrition, 116*, 1986, 356–364.

Zornetzer, S.F., & Gold, M.S. The locus coeruleus: Its possible role in memory consolidation. *Physiology and Behavior, 16*, 1976, 331–336.

Chapter **5**

Acetylcholine: Diet Affects Memory and Movement

The richest sources of choline in the diet usually supply choline in the form of lecithin, which can elevate levels of brain choline and acetylcholine (ACh). Given ACh's involvement in memory and motor function, dietary changes in lecithin and choline have a large potential for influencing brain function.

ACh was recognized as a neurotransmitter several years before serotonin and the catecholamines were identified as chemical transmitters, but the tracing of its pathways lagged far behind that of the monoamines. Until recently, the problem was the lack of availability of a technique with which to visualize ACh directly in neurons. With the development of immunocytochemical detection of ACh, the historical problems of uncertainty about the indirect methods of determining location are being overcome.

The best techniques available for ACh have historically involved a staining procedure for the primary enzymes of ACh degradation (first discovered) or synthesis (most recently discovered). These methods assume that ACh neurons are indeed those staining for degradative or synthetic enzymes. This assumption has not always been borne out by the evidence, though the synthetic enzyme staining is considered to be far more reliable. This staining shows the relative proportion of presumptive ACh neurons to be small and diffusely grouped throughout the CNS. Some of them have longer projection systems, but others are clearly short projecting interneurons. In the periphery, parasympathetic ganglia also use ACh as their primary transmitter. Classic cholinergic neurons are the motor cells of the ventral (anterior) horn of the spinal cord.

*B*iochemistry

Acetylcholine is synthesized directly by the joining of an (activated) acetate group from the donor acetyl-coenzyme A (acetyl-CoA) to a choline group derived in part from the circulating blood (Figure 5.1). The acetate group is derived from the breakdown of glucose (see Chapter 8). Carbohydrate metabolism thus has the potential for affecting ACh synthesis.

Because of the evidence that acetyl-CoA is a rate-limiting step in ACh synthesis, the conversion of pyruvate to acetyl-CoA takes on special importance. Factors that affect this conversion—the presence of pyruvate, calcium, and magnesium—may affect the synthesis of ACh. Calcium is also important for the transfer of mitochondrial acetyl-CoA into the cholinergic nerve ending, where it can be used for the conversion to ACh.

Choline can be synthesized in the brain, but it is also transported to the

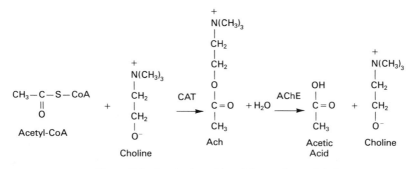

Figure 5.1 Synthesis and breakdown of acetylcholine.

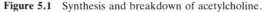

brain from the bloodstream. The transport occurs in both free and lipid (phosphatidylcholine) form. These forms of choline are derived from endogenous synthesis in the liver and from exogenous sources: eggs and meats supply a fair amount. Choline for ACh synthesis is also conserved upon breakdown of ACh; approximately half of the liberated choline is reused to make new ACh.

Choline has two uptake systems: low- and high-affinity. The low-affinity system is present in nonneural tissue and is thought to function in the formation of phospholipids. The high-affinity system is found primarily in (acetylcholine) nerve terminals, where the choline transported by this process is used for ACh synthesis. In some areas of the brain (primarily the septohippocampal pathway), an increase in the flow of neural activity increases the amount of choline transported. Moreover, exogenous choline enhances the synthesis of ACh only under conditions—usually drug treatments—that increase the neuronal activity of ACh cells. Dietary choline supplements also prevent the depletion of ACh in the brain by drug treatments that increase the firing of ACh neurons. The situation for ACh synthesis may thus be somewhat like that for catecholamines: an increase in nerve activity may accelerate the utilization of the precursor. The transport of choline, however, is also regulated by the amount of ACh in nerve tissue. The relative balance of these regulatory processes probably depends on the specific ACh system being studied.

Choline easily crosses the blood-brain barrier. Its passage is bidirectional, and its carrier is normally unsaturated. Dietary choline supplements increase the transport velocity of choline across the blood-brain barrier. However, this effect appears to be a compensation for an endogenous serum inhibitor that is elevated during choline supplementation, and it may explain why ACh cannot be elevated directly by dietary supplementation of choline, as compared with exogenous choline treatments. The direction of choline flow is usually from brain to blood, except when the concentration in blood has been elevated.

Choline acetyltransferase (CAT) is the enzyme responsible for the joining of the choline and acetyl groups. Kinetic values for half-maximal activity of this enzyme (0.4-1.0 mM for choline and 10-20 uM for acetyl-CoA) are higher than the physiological concentrations of its substrates, choline (30 uM) and acetyl CoA (2-20 uM). Treatments or diets that elevate either substrate therefore have the potential for accelerating ACh synthesis.

Blusztajn and Wurtman (1983) have shown in rats that whole brain ACh levels were reliably elevated by 22% after a single intraperitoneal dose of choline chloride, but work in other laboratories has contradicted these findings. Although this result is confounded by the fact that the chloride ion activates CAT, ACh synthesis is also elevated upon administration of phosphatidylcholine (no chloride ion) as lecithin alone, or as a dietary component. By contrast, choline deficient diets have not been found to diminish brain

choline levels to a significant degree, though they do diminish brain phos-
phocholine. This could be due to liberation of choline from membrane phospholipids when necessary.

Wecker (1986) has shown that dietary supplements of choline do not
directly elevate brain ACh. Her evidence supports the concept that choline
is supplied to ACh from a bound source and that this process is initiated and
enhanced in the brain when the activity of ACh neurons increases.

Acetyl-CoA concentrations in the brain can also be reduced by the induction of thiamine deficiency, and injections of a thiamine derivative increase
high-affinity uptake of choline (see Chapter 10), indicating interaction with
other dietary components.

The action of ACh is effectively terminated by cholinesterases. The most
effective of these is acetylcholinesterase (AChE), but other esterases serve
to hydrolyze ACh, breaking it down into choline and acetate. Although about
half of the choline thus released is taken back up by the presynaptic neuron
to be reformed into ACh, not all of the remaining ACh released at the synapse
is hydrolyzed. Some of the neurotransmitter is actively taken up by the postsynaptic neuron for yet unknown functions.

Choline also has biochemical effects on other transmitter systems that
receive inputs from cholinergic neurons. For example, choline administered
to rats will increase the activity of tyrosine hydroxylase in the adrenal medulla
and in dopamine nerve endings in the caudate nucleus.

*A*natomy

Acetylcholine Cells

Our description of the mapping of cholinergic cells derives from work
principally by the McGeer laboratory (1984) and from Cuello and Sofroniew
(1984) on the synthetic enzyme, choline acetyltransferase (CAT).

The McGeer laboratory has classified at least four major cholinergic systems in the brain, and claim a high probability that a fifth exists. These authors,
as do others, also list several minor cholinergic systems in the brain (Figure 5.2).

The first major cholinergic system described is the *medial forebrain complex*. This relatively continuous stream of giant cholinergic cells occupies
anterior positions on the medial surface of the cortex and extends in a cau-
dolateral direction. These cholinergic cells maintain their basic position close
to the medial and ventral surfaces of the brain, terminating toward the caudal
aspect of the lentiform nucleus (putamen and globus pallidus). One can identify various distinct subregions along this rostral-caudal stream of cells: the
medial septal nucleus, the nuclei of the diagonal band of Broca, and the

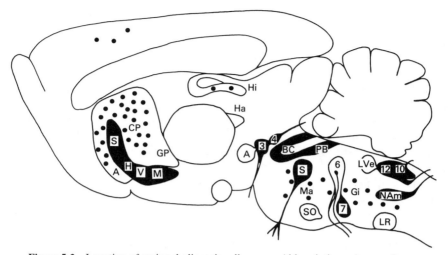

Figure 5.2 Location of major cholinergic cell groups. Abbreviations: A = nucleus accumbens; Am = Amygdala; BC = brachium conjunctivum; CP = caudate-putamen; Gi = gigantocellular aspect, reticular formation; GP = globus pallidus; H = horizontal limb, diagonal band; Ha = habenula; Hi = hippocampus; IC = inferior colliculus; IP = interpeduncular nucleus; LR = lateral reticular nucleus; LVe = lateral vestibular nucleus; M = nucleus basalis of Meynert; Ma = mag-nocellular aspect, reticular formation; NAm = Nucleus ambiguus; PB = para-brachial complex; R = red nucleus; S = medial septum; SN = substantia nigra; SO = superior olive; V = vertical limb, diagonal band. (From McGeer et al., 1984.)

nucleus basalis of Meynert. One distinctive component of the diagonal band nuclei is the preoptic area, where cholinergic cells are thought to play a part in hypothalamic functions.

In the rat, the rim of large cholinergic neurons bordering the globus pallidus is considered the rodent equivalent of the primate nucleus basalis. In the primate, the nucleus basalis is located in a more ventral position, close to the anterior commissure.

The second major cholinergic system so labeled in the McGeer lab involves the *striatal interneurons*. The CAT and AChE levels of the caudate, putamen, and accumbens are high, yet the giant cholinergic neurons represent no more than 1% of the neuronal population of the striatum. Smaller cholinergic cells have also been reported in the striatum.

The third major system consists of the *motor nuclei of cranial nerves*. Cholinergic cells exist in cranial nerve nuclei 3-7 and 9-12 as the innervation source of efferent fibers to skeletal muscle and autonomic ganglia. Their counterparts in the ventral and lateral horns of the spinal cord also stain positively for CAT. The principal source of parasympathetic outflow is cho-linergic (Chapter 2).

The fourth major system, the *parabrachial nuclei*, makes up the most concentrated cholinergic cell group in the brainstem. These cells surround the brachium conjunctivum, initially in the most rostral aspect of the pons and then following the direction of the brachium in a caudodorsal manner. The most commonly described nucleus in this system is the pedunculopontine tegmental nucleus in the lateral aspect of the most rostral region.

The fifth system considered as "probably major" is the scattered collection of cells throughout the gigantocellular and magnocellular tegmental fields of the *reticular formation*. Caudally, these cells gradually aggregate in a medial direction toward the raphe nuclei and in a ventral direction to the area near the inferior olivary nucleus. These cells thus extend as a column from the pons into the medulla.

Several so-called minor central cholinergic systems exist. Evidence indicates magnocellular cholinergic neurons in the red nucleus. These neurons concentrate labeled choline by retrograde flow, suggesting that dietary choline is utilized by them. The lateral reticular, superior olivary, and vestibular nuclei also stain positively for CAT.

Growing evidence indicates that some small bipolar neocortical interneurons are cholinergic. Similar CAT-positive interneurons have been found in hippocampus. CAT-positive cells have also been found in olfactory tubercle and in amygdala, as well as in medial habenula and interpenducular nucleus.

Acetylcholine Pathways

On the basis of cholinesterase staining and lesion technique, Lewis and Shute (1967) identified a septohippocampal cholinergic system. Recent confirmation has shown fibers from cholinergic cells in medial septum and diagonal band entering into fimbria-fornix. These cells also project to the cingulate gyrus and dorsomedial frontal lobe. The relative contribution of septal versus other cholinergic projections to the fornix, however, is not clear. These fibers distribute to dendritic fields of both granule and pyramidal cells in the hippocampus. Figure 5.3 shows this cholinergic projection, as well as the other major central cholinergic pathways.

The more caudal cells in this column, principally in the horizontal limb of the diagonal band and in nucleus basalis, project primarily to the remainder of frontal, parietal, and occipital lobes. Workers in the McGeer laboratory have also shown a heavy cholinergic projection from the basal forebrain to the amygdala and to the temporal lobe.

The interpeduncular nucleus receives a dense distribution of cholinergic fibers from at least two sources. One source, via stria medullaris, comes from the mediobasal forebrain complex. These fibers descend from the dorsal diencephalic regions into interpeduncular nucleus via fasciculus retroflexus, but this is not the only source of cholinergic fibers in this fascicle. The second source likely descends from the medial habenula.

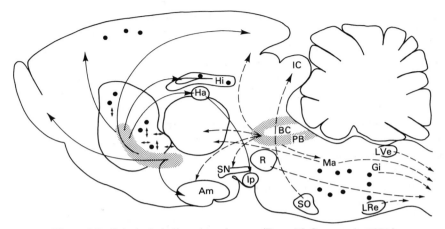

Figure 5.3   Principal cholinergic pathways. (From McGeer et al., 1984.)

The pedunculopontine nucleus projects to medial thalamic nuclei, subthalamus, and substantia nigra. Other projections from these nuclei have been described to ventral basal thalamic nuclei, hypothalamus, and amygdala. This pontine region can thus be described as a major supplier of cholinergic fibers to the diencephalon and limbic system.

Other principal brainstem cholinergic nuclei are the likely suppliers of descending cholinergic fibers. For example, the magnocellular division of the red nucleus is the primary source of the rubrospinal tract. Lateral reticular nucleus projects to cerebellum as well as to spinal cord. Much work remains to be done on the characterization of descending cholinergic projections.

The parasympathetic division of the autonomic nervous system is primarily cholinergic. Cholinergic cells in the lateral horn of the spinal cord innervate the sympathetic ganglionic chain as well as the celiac and mesentary ganglia. Vagal nuclei (N. X) supply cholinergic innervation to the heart, lungs and bronchi, liver, spleen, kidney, and gastrointestinal tract.

Skeletal muscle is supplied by cholinergic fibers originating segmentally in the ventral horn of the spinal cord. Chapter 2 provides a brief description of the organization of this cholinergic innervation.

*B*ehavior

Acetylcholine

To provide a general understanding of the influence of ACh on behavior, it might be helpful to contrast the organization of ACh systems with that of monoamine systems. You will recall that monoamine cell bodies are concentrated principally in the brainstem, from which they project diffusely throughout the brain and spinal cord. ACh cells appear to have a more discrete organization.

For example, ACh cells in brainstem project to diencephalon, as do monoamine cells located in the brainstem. Unlike monoamine neurons, however, these cholinergic neurons do not branch out further to innervate neocortical areas. Another group of rostral, telencephalic ACh neurons have principal innervation sites throughout the cortex. It is not surprising, therefore, that investigations into the behavioral activity of ACh have focused on particular "higher" cortical motor, sensory, and memory functions, as opposed to the general "behavioral tone" modulation supplied by monoamines.

Consistent with the involvement of hippocampal and thalamic systems in behavioral reactivity to somatosensory stimuli, ACh plays a role in reactions to somatosensory stimulation. Hemicholinium-3, which decreases ACh synthesis, or septal lesions, which destroy ACh cells and projections to the hippocampus, increase reactivity to environmental stimuli. The administration of deanol, a direct precursor of ACh in the brain, is associated with hyporeactivity. These findings are consistent with the results showing increased reactivity following administration of the ACh neurotoxin, ethylcholine mustard aziridinium ion (AF64A).

Given the presence of ACh in striatum, you would expect it to be involved in motor behavior. Drugs that increase ACh activity by mimicking its effect at central muscarinic receptors or by decreasing its rate of breakdown depress motor behavior. Lesions that destroy medial septal cholinergic neurons result in hyperactivity, which is attenuated by ACh agonists and augmented by antagonists. Systemic administration or localized application of agonists to the caudate nucleus produces tremor. Administration of AF64A into the lateral ventricles, which destroys cholinergic neurons, results in an increase in motor activity.

To the extent that cholinomimetic drugs decrease sensory reactivity and motor activity, the suggestion that ACh might be involved in preparing the organism for sleep is justified. Indeed, sleep is a prominent effect following injection of cholinomimetic drugs into the vertebral artery of dogs. The sleep is natural, and the animals can be readily awakened.

ACh also has a role in mediating effects of light on reproduction. Short day photoperiods inhibit testicular function, thus preparing animals for hibernation. These inhibitory effects are prevented by nighttime, but not daytime, administration of carbachol, a cholinergic agonist, in the cerebral ventricles. ACh therefore likely plays a role in the mechanism through which information about the light-dark environment is transferred to the hypothalamic-pituitary-gonadal axis. These results suggest that alterations in dietary choline could have different effects on the organism depending upon diurnal and seasonal variation.

ACh's heavy presence in hippocampus and neocortex, taken together with early pharmacologic work by Deutsch (1971), has long implicated its involvement in processes of learning and memory. For a variety of anatomic, physiologic, and behavioral reasons, much of the work has focused on septohippocampal connections. To give an idea of why the rationale is so strong, consider that the position of the fimbria-fornix affords a simple opportunity for surgically severing the septum's cholinergic contribution to the hippocampus. Physiologic effects on hippocampal theta and behavioral correlates on learning, memory, and motor activity can be easily studied. Furthermore, the hippocampus retains its gross structural integrity after such an operation, which allows investigators to study histochemical and biochemical correlates of the ensuing behavioral changes.

David Olton, working at The Johns Hopkins University, has been one of the major contributors to this body of knowledge (see Olton & Samuelson, 1976). He pioneered the use of the radial eight-arm maze (Figure 5.4) to study memory processes in rodents. The maze has a center platform, with eight arms radiating from it like spokes from the hub. The maze is typically elevated, with only a short ridge at the edges, so the animals can see clearly through the room. A single animal is placed on the center platform and allowed to choose freely for a small food or water reward at the end of each

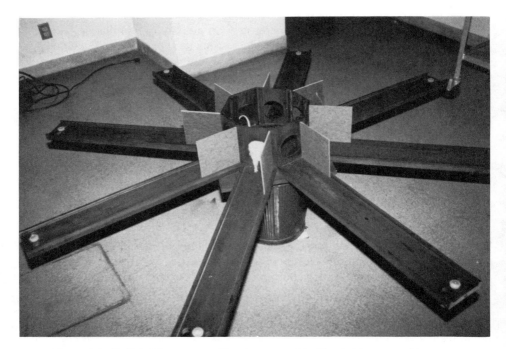

Figure 5.4 Radial eight-arm maze like the one used in Olton's laboratory. (From Olton & Samuelson, 1976.)

of the arms. The animal usually consumes the reward on the trip out to the end of the arm. Because this reward is not replenished after each visit, the animal's task is to remember the location of the visit, lest it not be able to retrieve all the rewards in eight attempts.

Through careful experimentation, Olton and his collaborators have been able to eliminate odor trails or algorithms as sources of adequate maze performance. It is clear from much of the work that animals develop memories of their previously visited locations using the sights available in the room. Two types of memories can be formed: *reference memories*, from the use of visual cues always present every time the animal is on the maze; and *working memories*, from the different sequence of arm entries the animal makes each new time it is given the particular choice. The differences between working and reference memories are not unlike the differences between new and old memories that are so often dissociated in human pathologic conditions.

Damage to hippocampus, or to fimbria-fornix, but not to frontal cortex, caudate, or amygdala results in a behavioral deficit on the 8-arm maze in rats. In particular, this deficit has been characterized primarily as an impairment of working, rather than reference, memory. Moreover, electrolytic or neurotoxic (AF64A) lesions that damage septal cholinergic nuclei normally projecting to hippocampus produce similar impairments.

The striatum may participate in memory formation as well. Cholinergic lesions of striatum through the use of AF64A produce significant impairments in acquisition and retention of a stepdown passive avoidance task. These cholinergic striatal lesions apparently produce no other impairment in spontaneous motor activity or sensitivity to electric shock.

Neurotoxic lesions of the nucleus basalis ACh cells, which distribute cholinergic projections widely throughout cerebral cortex, also impair acquisition of a one-way active avoidance, and produce severe deficits in retention of passive avoidance.

Prior to these advances in our understanding of the involvement of cholinergic systems in acquisition and retention of habits, Deutsch provided strong suggestions from pharmacologic studies about ACh's involvement in storage and retrieval of new information. He hypothesized that receptors on postsynaptic membranes at a specific set of synapses become more sensitive to transmitter. This sensitivity, he suggested, increases with time after learning and then declines, leading to forgetting. Anticholinesterase drugs, which by inhibiting ACh breakdown tend to increase available ACh at the synapse, generally were useful in enabling animals to retain memories when control animals were forgetting.

More recent pharmacologic research has focused Deutsch's suggestions. In humans, drugs that block central ACh receptors disrupt higher cognitive functions and induce transient amnesic states. For example, scopolamine, which blocks muscarinic receptors, produces selective deficits in recent memory and a profile on the Wexler Adult Inventory Scale resembling that seen in elderly drug-free individuals. Deficits produced by scopolamine can be partially, but reliably, reduced by physostigmine, a compound that prevents endogenous breakdown of ACh. Administration of physostigmine plus arecoline, which activates muscarinic receptors directly, tends to improve geriatric memory.

When rodents are studied on the 8-arm radial maze, their performance is significantly impaired by administration of scopolamine. Scopolamine appears to increase the number of errors on this task by enhancing the effect of stimuli interfering with storage of the visuospatial information. Intraventricular administration of CAT inhibitors also produces an impairment of passive avoidance learning in mice that is potentiated by addition of scopolamine. From these studies in humans, nonhuman primates, and rodents, it is clear that some aspects of memory and cognition are enhanced by drugs that activate cholinergic neurotransmission. Drugs that decrease cholinergic activity tend to produce the opposite effect: a tendency toward forgetting and an inability to produce new storage.

Diet

In reviewing sources of choline in our diets, Judith Wurtman (1981) concluded that almost all the choline we consume is derived from lecithin. Choline itself is found only in small amounts in food. Pure lecithin is phosphatidyl-choline (Figure 5.5), but "lecithin" found in commercially processed foods is really a mixture of phosphatides and other substances, although it does

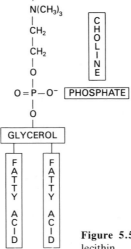

Figure 5.5 Chemical components of lecithin.

contain some "pure" lecithin. The richest sources of lecithin and other forms of choline in the diet are eggs, liver, soybeans, wheat germ, and peanuts, but other sources of animal protein also contain significant amounts. Oatmeal, pecans and rice contribute some lecithin to our diets. Fruit and vegetables contain little lecithin, but cauliflower and kale contain high amounts of choline. Torula yeast, which is added to foods as a flavor enhancer or emulsifier, is also a source of lecithin, containing about 2.5-3.0% lecithin.

Few studies deal with behavioral regulation of choline intake, perhaps because, unlike tryptophan or tyrosine, choline is not an essential nutrient. It can be manufactured in brain cells for use in assembling the ACh molecule. This does not really address the issue, however, because choline excess or deficiency has important physiological consequences. These consequences presuppose a mechanism for the regulation of dietary choline. It would therefore be important for behavioral physiologists to address this issue.

We do know that choline has important central and peripheral physiological effects. Consumption of a diet that includes choline chloride increases the concentration of serum choline, brain choline, and brain ACh in rats. In fact, a single meal containing lecithin granules elevates serum choline within 3 hours, and increases the ACh levels in the adrenal gland and the brain. In the adrenal gland, choline interacts directly with nicotinic receptors on chromaffin cells to induce catecholamine secretion.

Choline deficiency, by contrast, appears to increase the responsiveness of urinary bladders to ACh, while dietary choline excess leads to a drop in bladder responsiveness to ACh. Changes in dietary choline thus have important physiological effects involving central and peripheral cholinergic neurotransmission.

Bartus and coworkers (1980) have shown that mice raised on a diet deficient in choline have decrements in retention of a passive avoidance task. Mice raised on a diet enriched in choline show better retention on this task than mice raised on a control diet. Other investigators have shown that dietary choline can enhance memory in the simple cholinergic system of a mollusc. The increased choline elevates both plasma choline and cholinergic transmission at the neuromuscular junction.

So far we have discussed how dietary choline can alter neurotransmission, thereby presumably having an effect on behaviors involving ACh activity. But it is also interesting that behavior itself can alter the uptake of choline. Adequate behavior on radial and T mazes, and in active avoidance tasks, apparently depends upon activity in cholinergic systems. Participation in these tasks therefore is likely to involve increased flow of endogenous cholinergic activity in circuits critical for these responses. For example, behavioral experience on these tasks alters sodium dependent high affinity choline uptake in hippocampus, but not in frontal cortex. Furthermore, it takes a memory task to alter the choline uptake; activity on a treadmill has no effect. Apparently, at times during memory formation the system places increased demands on the available choline.

Choline During Development

There are at least three sources of choline present for infants in human milk: lecithin, sphingomyelin, and choline itself. This is an important finding; the mother's intake or deficiency of sources of choline could be reflected in the developing infant's metabolism and behavior.

In rats and mice, the cholinergic transmitter system attains functional maturity during the third week of life (about 15 to 20 days postnatally). It is not until that age that rodents respond to drugs that affect ACh systems. Smith and colleagues (1982), however, showed that scopolamine decreases rats' latency to escape in a spatial discrimination escape task in 7, 9, and 12 day old animals. Scopolamine disrupts the rate of acquisition of this response when the animals are 15 days old. The rather late development of cholinergic systems, including muscarinic receptors, suggests that dietary alterations in choline or lecithin can influence the development of behavior.

Behavioral Pathology

As might be expected from an analysis of the roles of ACh systems in motor activity and memory, the applications of cholinergic treatments and the influences of diet focus on disorders of motor behavior and memory. There is growing evidence that dietary treatments that influence cholinergic systems may be useful in alleviating symptoms associated with tardive dyskinesia, Huntington's chorea, and Alzheimer's disease.

Tardive dyskinesia is an iatrogenic choreiform motor disorder, commonly thought to result in psychotic patients from prolonged treatment with neuroleptic drugs. Symptoms usually involve buccal-lingual masticatory movements. Physostigmine is sometimes useful in treating this disorder. Double-blind crossover studies have also indicated that administration of choline suppresses these masticatory movements in about 45% of treated patients. This is interesting in view of the fact that choline may elevate ACh activity in areas of the striatum thought to be affected by neuroleptic drugs. Neuroleptics do not act on ACh systems per se, but are thought to affect dopamine projections to striatal cholinergic neurons. Thus choline does not directly antagonize effects of neuroleptics, but acts on one particular transmitter system affected as a net result.

There is, however, a problem with this mode of treatment. An intestinal bacterial enzyme synthesizes trimethylamine directly from choline. This substance imparts a marked fishy odor to any patient receiving choline treatment.

To avoid such problems, lecithin can be given instead of choline. This is advantageous, because lecithin does not have the bitter taste of choline, nor can it react with the gut bacteria. When patients with tardive dyskinesia are treated with lecithin, choreiform movements are also reduced.

Huntington's chorea is an autosomal genetic disorder that results in degeneration of striatal interneurons, most of them cholinergic. Biochemical studies of choreic brains have shown that the specific activity of CAT is decreased markedly in caudate nucleus. Coincident with the decrease in cholinergic enzyme activity is an elevation in muscarinic receptor binding. These biochemical markers are unchanged in cerebral cortex, indicating specificity to the movement disorder. Choline therapy has a spotty record in improving symptoms of this disorder. In many patients, it does not conclusively alter the involuntary movements. Trials with lecithin, however, have produced objective improvement in some patients with Huntington's chorea, as well as in some patients with another movement disorder known as Friedrich's ataxia.

Individuals with Alzheimer's disease that is not far advanced may be able to recall in considerable detail events from the distant past, but they can not seem to remember what occurred just minutes earlier. The onset of this disease can be seen much earlier than senile dementia, and for this reason it is often termed a presenile dementia. In Alzheimer's patients, higher cognitive functions deteriorate. There may be accompanying psychiatric symptoms of emotional lability, or even hallucinations, but there are no neurologic deficits (paralysis, sensory loss).

Alzheimer's patients have a marked loss of cholinergic cells in nucleus basalis (which distributes projections widely throughout cortex). Accompanying this loss, there is a decrease in CAT activity in cerebral cortex and hippocampus. Animal models have been somewhat successful in mimicking this disease state in that destruction of nucleus basalis cholinergic cells produces a similar loss in cholinergic activity, as well as a similar decrease in a working memory with less disruption of reference memory.

Choline and lecithin have been used to treat patients with Alzheimer's disease. Choline has had mixed success. In one patient, increased plasma levels of choline coincide with some improvement in a block designs test, but there was no clear improvement in other patients. Lecithin has also met with similar mixed success in the treatment of symptoms. At this writing, there is yet no information on whether treatment with combinations of lecithin and thiamine derivatives (see Chapter 10) may prove beneficial.

Another aspect of pathology potentially involves cholinergic function, but dietary treatments to elevate ACh activity may exacerbate this. In depression, it is possible that a relative ACh hyperactivity alters the neurochemical balance between NE and ACh. Treatments that elevate ACh or depress NE can potentially increase symptoms of depression. When oral choline is given for tardive dyskinesia, some patients experience severe depression, feelings of worthlessness, and suicidal thoughts. When choline treatment is stopped, these symptoms of depression show remission. It is not known whether self-treatment with lecithin from supplements purchased at health food stores produces similar symptoms in normal persons. It is also wise for depressed persons to curtail ingestion of eggs and other sources of lecithin and choline.

Summary

In contrast to the widespread distribution of NE and serotonin in the brain, ACh has a restricted distribution, suggesting a specific contribution to particular behaviors. In fact, ACh is important for the control of memory and motor behavior, and has been shown to be a factor in neurologic illnesses. Manipulation of ACh by drugs or diet has important effects on memory and motor behavior.

Dietary elevation of choline or lecithin increases levels of ACh in the brain. Choline deficiency also alters ACh neurotransmission. Clinicians have taken advantage of this ability of diet to alter the brain and have shown that oral lecithin or choline may be factors in the treatment of tardive dyskinesia, Huntington's chorea, and Alzheimer's disease. The neurochemical balance in depression indicates that depressed persons should refrain from ingestion of foods with high amounts of lecithin or choline.

References

Bartus, R.T, Dean, R.L., Goas, J.A., & Lippa, A.S. Age-related changes in passive avoidance retention: Modulation with dietary choline. *Science, 209,* 1980, 301–303.

Blusztajn, J.K. & Wurtman, R.J. Choline and cholinergic neurons. *Science, 221,* 1983, 614–620.

Cuello, A.C. & Sofroniew, M.V. The anatomy of the CNS cholinergic neurons. *Trends in Neurosciences,* March, 1984, 74–78.

Deutsch, J.A. The cholinergic synapse and the site of memory. *Science, 174,* 1971, 788–794.

Lewis, P.R. & Shute C.C.D. The cholinergic limbic system: Projections to hippocampal formation, medial cortex, nuclei of the ascending cholinergic reticular system, and the subfornical organ and supra-optic crest. *Brain, 90,* 1967, 521–543.

McGeer, P.L., McGeer, E.G., & Peng, J.H. Choline acetyltransferase: Purification and immunohistochemical localization. *Life Sciences, 34,* 1984, 2319–2338.

Olton, D.S. & Samuelson, R.J. Remembrance of places passed: Spatial memory in rats. *Journal of Experimental Psychology: Animal Behavior Processes, 2,* 1976, 97–116.

Smith, G.J., Spear, L.P., & Spear, N.E. Detection of cholinergic mediation of behavior in 7-, 9-, and 12-day old rat pups. *Pharmacology, Biochemistry, & Behavior, 16,* 1982, 805–809.

Wecker, L. Neurochemical effects of choline supplementation. *Canadian Journal of Physiology and Pharmacology, 64,* 1986, 329–333.

Wurtman, J.J. Sources of choline and lecithin in the diet. In Barbeau, A., Growdon, J.H., & Wurtman, R.J. (Eds.), *Nutrition and the brain* (Vol. 5). New York: Raven Press, 1981, pp. 73–81.

*S*uggested *R*eadings

Aquilonius, S.M. & Eckernas, S.A. Choline therapy in Huntington's chorea. *Neurology, 27,* 1977, 887–889.

Barbeau, A. Phosphatidylcholine (lecithin) in neurological disorders. *Neurology, 28,* 1978, 358.

Barbus, R.T. Physostigmine and recent memory: Effects in young and aged non-human primates. *Science, 206,* 1979, 1087–1089.

Bartus, R.T., Dean, R.L., Beer, B., & Lippa, A.S. The cholinergic hypothesis of geriatric memory function. *Science, 217,* 1982, 408–417.

Beatty, W.W. & Carbone, C.P. Septal lesions, intramaze cues, and spatial behavior in rats. *Physiology and Behavior, 24,* 1980, 675–678.

Becker, J.T., Walker, J.A., & Olton, D.S. Neuroanatomical bases of spatial memory. *Brain Research, 200,* 1980, 307–320.

Benjamin, A.M. & Quastel, J.H. Acetylcholine synthesis in synaptosomes: Mode of transfer of mitochondrial acetyl coenzyme A. *Science, 213,* 1981, 1495–1497.

Buresova, O. & Bures, J. Radial maze as a tool for assessing the effect of drugs on the working memory of rats. *Psychopharmacology, 77,* 1982, 268–271.

Butcher, L.L. Nature and mechanisms of cholinergic-monoaminergic interactions in the brain. *Life Sciences, 21,* 1977, 1207–1226.

Coyle, J.T., Price, D.L., & DeLong, M.R. Alzheimer's disease: A disorder of cortical cholinergic innervation. *Science, 219,* 1983, 1184–1190.

Davis, K.L., Berger, P.A., & Hollister, L.E. Choline for tardive dyskinesia. *New England Journal of Medicine, 293,* 1975, 152.

Drachman, D.A. Memory and cognitive function in man: Does the cholinergic system have a specific role? *Neurology, 27,* 1977, 783–790.

Earnest, D.J. & Turek, F.W. Role for acetylcholine in mediating effects of light on reproduction. *Science, 219,* 1983, 77–79.

Eckenstein, F. & Sofroniew, M.V. Identification of central cholinergic neurons containing both choline acetyltransferase and acetylcholinesterase and of central neurons containing only acetylcholinesterase. *The Journal of Neuroscience, 3,* 1983, 2286–2291.

Enna, S.J., Bird, E.D., Bennett, J.P., Bylund, D.B., Yamamura, H.I., Iversen, L.L., & Snyder, S.H. Huntington's chorea: Changes in neurotransmitter receptors in the brain. *New England Journal of Medicine, 294,* 1976, 1305–1309.

Etienne, P., Gauthier, S., Johnson, G., Collier, B., Mendis, T., Dastoor, D., Cole, M., and Muller, H.F. Clinical effects of choline in Alzheimer's disease. *Lancet, 1,* 1978, 508–509.

Fibiger, H.C. The organization and some projections of cholinergic neurons of the mammalian forebrain. *Brain Research Reviews, 4,* 1982, 327–388.

Flicker, C., Dean, R.L., Watkins, D.L., Fisher, S.K., & Bartus, R.T. Behavioral and neurochemical effects following neurotoxic lesions of a major cholinergic input to the cerebral cortex in the rat. *Pharmacology, Biochemistry, & Behavior, 18,* 1983, 973–981.

Geffard, M., McRae-Degueurce, A., & Souan, M.L. Immunocytochemical detection of acetylcholine in the rat central nervous system. *Science, 229,* 1985, 77–79.

Glick, S.D., Mittag, T.W., & Green, J.P. Central cholinergic correlates of impaired learning. *Neuropharmacology, 12*, 1973, 291–296.

Growdon, J.H., Gelenberg, A.J., Doller, J., Hirsch, M.J., & Wurtman, R.J. Lecithin can suppress tardive dyskinesia. *New England Journal of Medicine, 298*, 1978, 1029–30.

Haranath, P.S.R.K., Indira, G., & Krishnamurthy, A. Effects of cholinomimetic drugs and their antagonists injected into the vertebral artery of unanaesthetized dogs. *Pharmacology, Biochemistry, and Behavior, 6*, 1977, 259–263.

Hepler, D.J., Olton, D.S., Wenk, G.L., & Coyle, J.T. Lesions in nucleus basalis magnocellularis and medial septal area of rats produced qualitatively similar memory impairments. *The Journal of Neuroscience, 5*, 1985, 866–873.

Hirsch, M.J. & Wurtman, R.J. Lecithin consumption elevates ACh concentrations in rat brain and adrenal gland. *Science, 202*, 1978, 223–225.

Holz, R.W. & Senter, R.A. Choline stimulates nicotinic receptors on adrenal medullary chromaffin cells to induce catecholamine secretion. *Science, 214*, 466–468.

Jarrard, L.E., Levy, A., Meyerhoff, J.L., & Kant, G.J. Intracerebral injections of AF64A: An animal model of Alzheimer's disease? *Annals of the New York Academy of Sciences, 444*, 1985, 520–522.

Karczmar, A.G. Overview: cholinergic drugs and behavior—what effects may be expected from a "cholinergic diet." In A. Barbeau, J.H. Growdon, & R.J. Wurtman (Eds.), *Nutrition and the brain* (Vol. 5). New York: Raven Press, 1981, pp. 141–185.

Leathwood, P.D. & Schlosser, B. Phosphatidylcholine, choline, and cholinergic function. *International Journal for Vitamin and Nutrition Research*, Supplement 29, 1986, 49–67.

LoConte, G., Bartolini, L., Casamenti, F., Marconcini-Pepeu, I., & Pepeu, G. Lesions of cholinergic forebrain nuclei: Changes in avoidance behavior and scopolamine actions. *Pharmacology, Biochemistry, & Behavior, 17*, 1982, 933–937.

Nagai, T., Kimura, H., Maeda, T., McGeer, P.L., Peng, F., & McGeer, E.G. Cholinergic projections from the basal forebrain of the rat to the amygdala. *The Journal of Neuroscience, 2*, 1982, 513–520.

Price, D.L., Whitehouse, P.J., Struble, R.G., Clark, A.W., Coyle, J.T., Delong, M.R., & Hedreen, J.C. Basal forebrain cholinergic systems in Alzheimer's disease and related dementias. *Neuroscience Commentaries, 1*, 1982, 84–92.

Russell, R.W. & Jenden, D.J. Behavioral effects of deanol, of hemicholinium and of their interaction. *Pharmacology, Biochemistry, & Behavior, 15*, 1981, 285–288.

Russell, R.W. & Macri, J. Central cholinergic involvement in behavioral hyperreactivity. *Pharmacology, Biochemistry, and Behavior, 10*, 1979, 43–48.

Sahley, C.L., Barry, S.R., & Gelperin, A. Dietary choline augments associative memory function in *Limax maximus*. *Journal of Neurobiology, 17*, 1986, 113–120.

Sandberg, K., Sandberg, P.R., Hanin, I., Fisher, A., & Coyle, J.T. Cholinergic lesion of the striatum impairs acquisition and retention of a passive avoidance response. *Behavioral Neuroscience, 98*, 1984, 162–165.

Shute, C.C.D. & Lewis, P.R. The ascending cholinergic reticular system: Neocortical, olfactory, and subcortical projections. *Brain, 90*, 1967, 497–521.

Tamminga, C.A., Smith, R.C., Chang, S., Haraszti, J.S., & Davis, J.M. Depression with oral choline. *Lancet, 2*, 1976, 905.

Trommer, B.A., Schmidt, D.E., & Wecker, L. Exogenous choline enhances the synthesis of acetylcholine only under conditions of increased cholinergic neuronal activity. *Journal of Neurochemistry, 39*, 1982, 1704–1709.

Wallace, L.J., Kolta, M.G., Gerald, M.C., & Mervis, R.F. Dietary choline affects response to acetylcholine by isolated urinary bladder. *Life Sciences, 36*, 1985, 1377–1380.

Walsh, T.J., Tilson, H.A., DeHaven, D.L., Mailman, R.B., Fisher, A., & Hanin, I. AF64A, a cholinergic neurotoxin, selectively depletes ACh in hippocampus and cortex, and produces long term passive avoidance and radial arm maze deficits in the rat. *Brain Research, 321*, 1984, 91–102.

Wecker, L. & Trommer, B.A. Effects of chronic (dietary) choline availability on the transport of choline across the blood-brain barrier. *Journal of Neurochemistry, 43*, 1984, 1762–1765.

Wenk, G., Hepler, D., & Olton, D. Behavior alters the uptake of [3H]choline into acetylcholinergic neurons of the nucleus basalis magnocellularis and medial septal area. *Behavioural Brain Research, 13*, 1984, 129–138.

Whitehouse, P.J., Price, D.L., Struble, R.G., Clark, A.W., Coyle, J.T., & DeLong, M.R. Alzheimer's disease and senile dementia: Loss of neurons in the basal forebrain. *Science, 215*, 1982, 1237–1239.

Zeisel, S.H., Char, D., & Sheard, N.F. Choline, phosphatidylcholine, and sphingomyelin in human and bovine milk and infant formulas. *Journal of Nutrition, 116*, 1986, 50–58.

Chapter **6**

Excitatory Amino Acids and GABA

Glutamic acid is one of the most common amino acids found in nature. It is a constituent of virtually every protein, as well as being ubiquitous in its "free form." It is therefore consumed every day as a fundamental constituent of foodstuffs. It is also added as the salt (monosodium glutamate) to foods as a flavor enhancer. Controversy currently exists over the extent to which monosodium glutamate may influence behavior.

Unlike the essential neutral or basic amino acids, glutamate and aspartate (the acidic amino acids) can be synthesized by several metabolic pathways in brain cells. The synthesis of these compounds may occur at rates commensurate with the metabolic demands placed on them. Glutamate (GLU) and aspartate (ASP) lower the threshold and increase the firing rate of most neurons with which they come into contact.

Gamma-amino butyric acid (GABA), by contrast, raises the threshold and decreases the firing rate of most neurons. GABA is synthesized directly from GLU in neurons that contain the enzyme glutamate decarboxylase. In the brain, GABA is contained mostly in short projection interneurons, whereas GLU and ASP tend to project together in fibers that interconnect functional regions of the brain. Considerable evidence shows that GLU and ASP have the same uptake carrier and are therefore taken up as putative transmitters within the same nerve endings. Within some brain regions, the excitatory amino acids GLU and ASP balance the functional output with the inhibitory transmitter GABA. Increases in GLU or ASP, or decreases in GABA, are associated with epileptic convulsive states, and treatments for epilepsy involve drugs that stimulate the GABA system. Figure 6.1 shows the molecular structure of these three substances.

Biochemistry

As major amino acid constituents of dietary protein, GLU and ASP must be liberated from the protein module for uptake into plasma for distribution to other organs. Digestion of dietary protein is dependent upon hydrolysis by gastric pepsin, followed by proteolytic enzymes secreted by the pancreas and intestinal mucosa. Much of dietary protein is hydrolyzed to free amino acids prior to absorption, although it is now generally recognized that small peptides may play a role in the assimilation of dietary protein. These peptides may also undergo hydrolysis to free amino acids. As Figure 6.2 shows, a small proportion of dietary protein mixed with secreted proteins is excreted. Most of the dietary protein is hydrolyzed, and the free amino acids are absorbed from the mucosa for transport in plasma. Some transamination of amino acids (e.g., ASP and alpha-ketoglutarate to oxaloacetic acid and GLU) occurs within the intestinal mucosa.

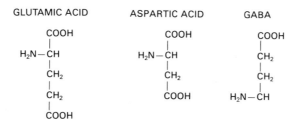

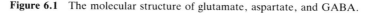

Figure 6.1   The molecular structure of glutamate, aspartate, and GABA.

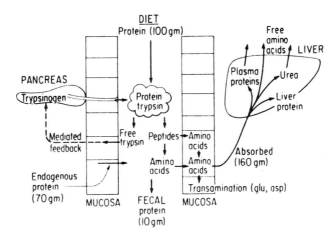

Figure 6.2   The digestion of dietary protein for the release and absorption of free amino acids. (From Crim and Munro, 1977.)

Figure 6.3 outlines glutamate metabolism in mammalian tissues. Reactions of the tricarboxylic acid cycle, also known as the citric acid cycle, produce alpha-ketoglutarate as an intermediate. Alpha-ketoglutarate can then be converted to GLU by GLU dehydrogenase (pathway 2 in the figure). Some authors question the active biosynthetic role for this enzyme in the regular production of GLU, because of its relatively low *in vivo* affinity for ammonia. This may simply reflect an ability for metabolic or dietary changes in ammonia to influence the production of GLU via this catabolic step (see Wurtman's requirements discussed in Chapter 1).

Alternatively, Meister (1979) has suggested that GLU dehydrogenase might be linked *in vivo* with an enzyme such as glutaminase (reaction 5) to make the amide nitrogen atom directly available for the synthesis of GLU and the formation of the alpha amino group of other amino acids.

Transamination reactions (such as described above for the intestinal mucosa) also serve to produce GLU. This is shown in pathway 3. GLU is also formed during the degradation of arginine, ornithine, proline, and histidine (reaction pathway 17). The glutaminase reaction to form GLU from glutamine, however, is probably the largest single contributor to GLU formation.

Once GLU is liberated from proteins or formed from any of its many catabolic reactions, several pathways contribute it to the formation of other compounds. The alpha carboxyl group of GLU, as well as ASP, is activated by a tRNA synthetase to be used directly for protein synthesis. GLU is also the precursor to two gamma-glutamyl compounds of major biochemical importance: glutamine and glutathione. Especially in brain, a significant pathway of GLU metabolism involves decarboxylation to GABA, an im-

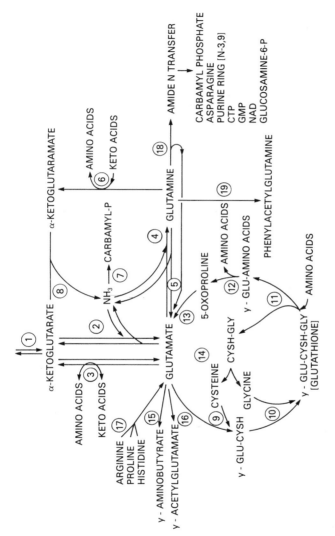

Figure 6.3 Schematic of GLU metabolism in mammalian tissues. 1, Reactions of the citric acid cycle; 2, glutamate dehydrogenase; 3, glutamate transaminases; 4, glutamine synthetase; 5, glutaminase; 6, glutamine transaminase; 7, carbamyl phosphate synthetase (liver); 8, α-keto acid w-amidase; 9, γ-glutamyl cysteine synthetase; 10, glutathione synthetase; 11, γ-glutamyl transpeptidase; 12, γ-glutamyl cyclotransferase; 13, 5-oxoprolinase; 14, cysteinylglycinase; 15, glutamate decarboxylase; 16, glutamate N-acylase; 17, various enzymes involved in the degradation of these amino acids; 18, glutamine amidotransferases known to occur in mammalian tissues; and 19, phenylacetyl glutamine synthetase (Acyl-CoA-L-glutamine N-acyltransferase). (From Meister, 1979.)

portant inhibitory neurotransmitter. The decarboxylase enzyme is a metal-loenzyme that incorporates dietary zinc in the molecule. As you will see in Chapter 9 on trace metals, changes in dietary zinc can alter the activity of this enzyme.

The catabolism of the neurotransmitter pool of GLU is thought to have its origins in both glucose and glutamine (Figure 6.4). Each molecule of glutamine may serve as a source of amino nitrogen for two molecules of GLU. The reaction is catalyzed by glutaminase. If this is correct, this pathway assumes that the carbon portion of GLU is supplied by glutamine and by alpha-ketoglutarate in equal amounts. The mechanism to produce the carbon skeleton in this case would be quite complex.

It is also likely that some of the transmitter GLU molecules have glucose as their metabolic origin, though recent evidence tends to discount this pathway as a major source. Energy metabolism is quite vigorous in the central nervous system. The synthesis of GLU from glucose precursors is therefore likely to be rapid. This reaction would occur via oxidative metabolism and transamination of the oxoglutarate. Nerve terminals, however, contain large quantities of glutaminase, indicating that the glutamine pathway is very important in the production of the transmitter pool of GLU. In Cotman's laboratory (1981), it has been shown that brain slices exposed to glutamine release far more GLU than slices incubated with glucose alone. Use of radioactive precursors can also show that more GLU is derived from glutamine than from glucose. It is therefore not likely that dietary influences on blood glucose levels have a significant influence on GLU formation or metabolism, though some influence is not ruled out.

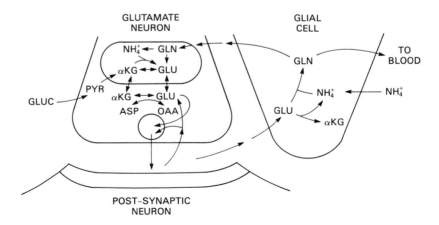

Figure 6.4 The neurotransmitter pool of GLU is thought to have its origins in both glucose and glutamine. (From Shank and Aprison, 1979.)

   Amino acids such as tryptophan cannot be synthesized in brain cells at all, much less at a rate commensurate with the metabolic demands for their use. By contrast, the acidic amino acids GLU and ASP can be synthesized at a rate that satisfies most of their metabolic demands. As a consequence, their rate of transport from the blood to the brain is much lower than that for the neutral or basic amino acids. The GLU carrier for uptake of GLU into the brain has a K_m of only about 25% of the normal plasma GLU level. This indicates that the carrier is virtually saturated by the normal physiological levels of GLU. Indeed, GLU leaves the brain faster than any of the basic or neutral amino acids.

   Changes in cerebral blood flow to various areas of the brain are indicative of the relative activity of those areas. Areas that are more active typically have increased blood flow, and consequently an increased flow and uptake of nutrients. Because the GLU uptake carriers are mostly saturated with GLU, increased activity and blood flow do not normally influence the brain's uptake of GLU or ASP. Areas of the brain surrounding the ventricles (Figure 6.5), however, lack an effective blood brain barrier. In these areas increased blood flow (perhaps from epileptic seizure activity) may accelerate the uptake of GLU and ASP. Dietary or metabolic changes in the levels of these com-

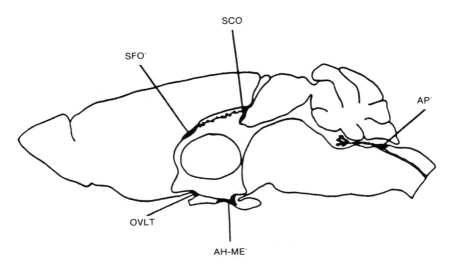

Figure 6.5 Drawing of a mid-sagittal section of a rat brain showing the location of the circumventricular organs that lack an effective blood-brain-barrier. Neurons in or near these areas are subject to changes in plasma levels of excitatory amino acids. Abbreviations: SCO—subcommissural organ; SFO—subfornical organ; OVLT—organum vasculosum lamina terminalis; AH-ME—anterior hypothalamus-median eminence. (From Olney, 1979.)

pounds may thus influence neural activity in certain areas of the brain, and changes in neural activity in these areas may also conversely influence the uptake of acidic amino acids.

Anatomy

The concept of the CNS anatomy of cells and fibers containing acidic amino acids or GABA neurotransmitters is considerably different from that for the biogenic amines. We conceive of serotonin and norepinephrine central projections as having an "ascending" anatomy, with small groups of nerve cells in the brainstem sending widely branching fiber projections through the central neuraxis. Though many of these fibers branch to descend into the spinal cord, their origin is still at "low levels" in the brain. Dopamine is considerably more restricted, but its principal system is also an ascending one. Acetylcholine differs from these monoaminergic systems in having a hierarchically "higher" distribution of nuclei, but its projections are still considered to ascend, whether from the reticular formation up into the thalamus, or from the basal forebrain up into the neo- and allocortex.

By contrast, GLU and ASP have largely "descending" systems or systems that interconnect functional regions of the CNS. Virtually every suborgan of the brain has GLU or ASP cells that send fibers to descending systems or to other suborgans. GABA cells are primarily local-acting neurons, often called interneurons. They are usually interspersed within the same suborgans that contain GLU or ASP fibers, often counteracting the excitatory effects of GLU or ASP. Even though GABA is synthesized from GLU, the amount of GLU in various brain regions bears no resemblance to the amount of GABA in those regions, indicating that the transmitter function of GLU can be differentiated from its role as precursor.

High-affinity GLU uptake is not considered to be a specific marker for "GLU-using" as opposed to "ASP-using" neurons. In fact, GLU and ASP share the same high-affinity uptake process, which suggests that the same uptake sites are present on neurons that utilize either amino acid as a neurotransmitter. Some findings show high affinity uptake of these amino acids in glial preparations. Nevertheless, several pathways in the nervous system show a reduction of GLU/ASP uptake after various treatments or lesions that destroy their source of GLU/ASP fiber projections. The use of other converging techniques has strengthened the likelihood that these pathways use GLU/ASP as neurotransmitters.

Beginning from the "top down," we note the laminar pattern of uptake of ASP into cortical slices that corresponds to the different cortical layers. In somatosensory cortex, the greatest amount of ASP appears in the molecular layer, or layer I. In layer IV an extensive labelling corresponds to the barrel pattern characteristic of sensory function in this region of cortex. Within the cortex, groups of neurons transport GABA and are therefore likely to use GABA as a neurotransmitter. These neurons form an inhibitory, bidirectional system of connections that joins cells in superficial and deep layers of functional cortical columns.

GLU and ASP cells in the cerebral cortex project to other areas of cortex, as well as subcortically to innervate regions of the striatum and the thalamus. In olfactory cortex, the highest uptake of GLU/ASP occurs in the deep part of the plexiform layer, which receives a dense cortical input, and GLU neurons have been identified in the lateral olfactory tract. If frontal cortex or the entire hemicortex is ablated, a considerable loss of GLU uptake is seen in the whole rostrocaudal extent of the neostriatum, and several converging techniques show GLU as the transmitter of the corticostriatal pathway.

Figure 6.6 shows the scheme of GLU and GABA interactions in the striatum. As noted, the primary cortical projections to the striatum utilize GLU as a neurotransmitter. GLU fibers synapse upon GABA interneurons as well as upon other local striatal neurons. Two types of GABA neurons apparently exist in the striatum: classic GABA interneurons, and GABA neurons that project to dopamine cells in the substantia nigra.

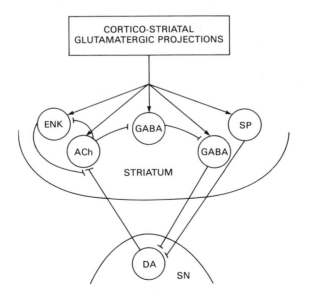

Figure 6.6 Scheme of GLU and GABA interactions in the striatum. (From Costa et al., 1979.)

At least two sources of GLU fibers project to nucleus accumbens. The ipsilateral frontal neocortex supplies about 18-25% of the GLU innervation to accumbens. Most of the accumbens GLU innervation, however, is derived from the subiculum of the hippocampal formation; transection of the fimbria-fornix results in a 50% drop in GLU uptake.

The cortex supplies GLU innervation to other areas of the extrapyramidal motor system. Anatomic studies show evidence for cortical GLU projections to the substantia nigra. Moreover, ablation of frontal cortex is accompanied by a loss of 20-50% GLU uptake in substantia nigra. Pharmacologic studies support these findings.

The cortical projections to the thalamus are unilateral and reciprocal to thalamocortical projections. Hemidecortication is accompanied by a large reduction (up to 70%) in ASP uptake on the ipsilateral side of the thalamus. A large part of this reduction can be obtained by removal of the pyriform cortex alone. The specific projections from cortex to thalamus can be described according to classic functional anatomy. For example, ablation of the visual cortex leads to a 75% drop in GLU uptake and a 30% drop in endogenous GLU in the lateral geniculate body. The concept that GLU cells provide the "effector" projections of cortex is further supported by the finding that ablation of visual cortex also reduces GLU uptake by 50% and endogenous GLU by 30% in superior colliculus. Direct GABA immunocytochemistry reveals that intrinsic thalamic nuclei contain 27-33% GABA neurons. This evidence strengthens the concept of local GABA inhibition acting to counter GLU or ASP excitation.

The amygdala is a recipient of cortical GLU fibers, receiving projections from mediofrontal, pyriform, and entorhinal cortex. Lesions of pyriform cortex, which also interrupt entorhinal fibers, reduce GLU uptake by greater than 50% in amygdala. The origin and distribution of cortical GLU fibers are shown in Figure 6.7.

GLU projections in allocortex form a circuit of critical importance for the study of epilepsy. The primary GLU and ASP input to the hippocampal region is derived from cells in the entorhinal cortex, the projections of which traverse the perforant path to terminate on the outer two-thirds of dendrites in the dentate molecular layer. Activity in this pathway excites the dentate granule cells, whose mossy fiber projections carry the excitation to hippocampal pyramidal cells in the CA_3 region and to modified pyramidal cells in the CA_4 region. The excitatory targets of these pyramidal cells are the basilar and apical dendrites in the CA_1 and CA_2 region of both ipsilateral and contralateral hippocampus. The contralateral projections are the commissural fibers; the ipsilateral projections are identified as the Schaeffer collaterals. These pathways utilize both GLU and ASP as neurotransmitters.

Intrinsic basket cells in the hippocampus contain GABA, thereby providing an inhibitory counterpoint to the loop of excitation carried in the hip-

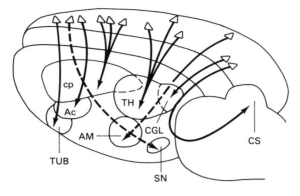

Figure 6.7 Schematic of the origin and distribution of GLU fibers from neocortex. Ac, nucleus accumbens; cp, neostriatum; TH, thalamus; CGL, lateral geniculate body; CS, colliculus superior; SN, substantia nigra; AM, amygdala; TUB, olfactory tubercle. (From Fonnum et al., 1981.)

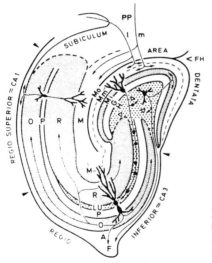

Figure 6.8 Diagram of a hippocampal slice showing the loop of excitation brought about by GLU and ASP fibers. (From Storm-Mathisen, 1981.)

pocampal circuit. These GABA cells are distributed in a laminar fashion in the hippocampal strata. The hippocampal slice in Figure 6.8 shows the loop of excitation brought about by GLU and ASP fibers.

Hippocampal output is also regarded as excitatory and is at least partially carried by GLU fibers. Pyramidal cells in the CA_3 region project bilaterally through the fimbria-fornix to the lateral, but not the medial, part of the septum. When these CA_3 cells are destroyed by the selective application of kainic acid, GLU uptake is reduced in the lateral (but not the medial) septum. Evidence from electrical stimulation of slices also indicates an evoked release of ASP from septal terminals. The concept that GABA provides *local* inhibition was further supported when this work failed to show an evoked GABA release under similar conditions. There is also evidence that GLU fibers project from the hippocampal formation to other projection areas of the fimbria-fornix. The distribution of these hippocampal projections is shown in Figure 6.9.

In the pituitary and hypothalamus, there is considerably more GLU than GABA, which indicates that GLU and GABA may have separate functions apart from a simple precursor relationship. In fact, the absence of the GLU decarboxylase in the anterior pituitary indicates another biosynthetic source of GABA in the organ. It has been suggested that in several hypothalamic nuclei GABA nerve terminals arise from cell bodies located outside the hypothalamus. Some findings indicate that GABA neurons in the posterior hypothalamus may project to the neocortex. These findings show that the distribution and projections of GABA cells are not limited to the classic concept of interneurons, though there is also evidence for intrinsic GABA neurons within the hypothalamus.

Other areas of the central nervous system that utilize GLU as a neurotransmitter include the cerebellum, the cochlear nucleus, and the spinal cord. There are high concentrations of GLU in the cerebellum, consistent with the presence of GLU as a neurotransmitter in the parallel fibers originating from the granule cells. High-affinity uptake of GLU in the cerebellum is reduced upon damage to this system. GLU and ASP may be transmitters for the auditory nerve in the cochlear nucleus. When kainic acid, a neurotoxin for neurons with GLU input, is injected into the brainstem, a selective pattern of degeneration occurs in the cochlear nucleus

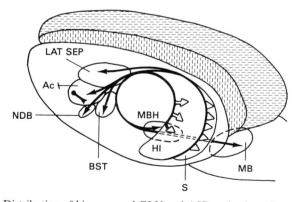

Figure 6.9 Distribution of hippocampal GLU and ASP projections. Lat sep, lateral septum; Ac, nucleus accumbens; NDB, nucleus of diagonal band; MBH, mediobasal hypothalamus; MB, mammillary body; S, subiculum; HI, hippocampus. The fibers to lat sep and NDB come mainly from hippocampus, whereas the other fibers come mainly from subiculum. (From Fonnum et al., 1981.)

corresponding to the distribution of primary auditory fibers. In the spinal cord, iontophoresis of ASP and GLU excites neurons in the superficial dorsal horn (Rexed's laminae I & II), correlating with the distribution of GLU fibers there.

*B*ehavior

Neurotransmitter Systems

No one concept of behavior for GLU, ASP, or GABA systems exists, although generally GLU and GABA tend to have antagonistic effects. To some extent, the participation of these transmitters in behavioral control depends on the functional aspects of the circuit in which they are used. For example, because GLU appears to be the primary transmitter of the auditory nerve, there is little doubt about its function in audition. Similarly, GLU afferents to the striatum appear to be involved in motor control; intrastriatal injection of GLU analogs into the awake, unrestrained animal produces relatively immediate motor effects, and injection of muscimol into the striatum inhibits the display of non-stimulus directed behavior. In the hippocampus, long-term potentiation has been suggested as a mechanism of memory; it is associated with an increase in calcium-dependent release of GLU in the commissural pathways.

In the somatosensory cortex, GLU and GABA may be involved in shaping the receptive fields of cortical neurons. GLU lowers the threshold for activation by cutaneous stimuli but does not enlarge the receptive field. Bicuculline, however, does enlarge the receptive field size of neurons, but GABA has no effect on receptive field size.

The hypothalamus, containing large amounts of GABA and receiving GLU projections, has functional contributions from these substances. Microinjection of GLU in the posterior hypothalamus produces hypertension and tachycardia. These cardiovascular responses are accompanied by signs of behavioral arousal: increased searching, rearing, and sniffing. Agonists of GABA also reduce sexual behavior in male rats that is not dependent upon the reduced activity produced by GABA stimulants.

With regard to hypothalamic function, there is also considerable evidence for GABA's mediation of feeding, though its effect depends upon the particular feeding system studied. For example, injection of a GABA agonist into medial hypothalamic areas elicits feeding in satiated rats, but injection into lateral areas suppresses feeding in deprived rats.

Another way of viewing the functional participation of GABA is to examine the effects of benzodiazepines (e.g., Valium). Benzodiazepine binding sites are physically associated with post-synaptic GABA receptors. In fact, the presence of GABA increases the affinity of benzodiazepine receptors, and vice versa: the presence of benzodiazepines increases the affinity of GABA receptors. Benzodiazepines are administered for their anxiolytic, sedative, muscle-relaxant, and anticonvulsant effects. Growing evidence indicates that GABA may be involved in these effects, depending upon the site of activity (i.e., the particular receptor involved). For example, in decorticate, unanesthetized cats displaying sequences of stereotyped locomotor movements in response to electrical stimulation of the footpad, local injections of either GABA or diazepam into the mesencephalic locomotor region completely suppress the movements.

Diet

Sources of dietary protein for the "average American" in this century have increasingly emphasized animal foods over cereal sources (see Appendix). Nevertheless, the daily protein intake of 100 g has not changed appreciably. Examination of the intake of individual amino acids shows that the eight essential amino acids account for 38% of this daily protein amount. Of the remaining 62% of nonessential amino acids, the total intake of GLU is about 20% and that of ASP about 8%. Of these amino acids, approximately half of the intakes are likely to be in the form of the corresponding amide.

Free GLU and ASP are present in animal and plant tissues. A large amount of GLU is found in muscle. Brain has slightly over a third of the GLU present in muscle. Kidneys, liver, and plasma all have free GLU, but in smaller amounts than in muscle or brain. In beets, apples, apricots, and avocados, as well as in other fruits and vegetables, ASP is present in higher concentrations than GLU. Wheat gluten and wheat flour have 37.4% and 34.2% GLU as a percentage of the total nitrogen, respectively.

GLU is also present naturally in the diet in the form of its salt, monosodium glutamate (MSG). Natural sources of MSG include tomatoes, and parmesan and Roquefort cheeses. In Japanese cuisine, dried bonito, black mushroom, and the seaweed sea tangle are used extensively as condiments to impart a "savory" taste. The sea tangle contains MSG and other salts of GLU. Bonito contains the histidine salt of inosinic acid, whereas the black mushroom contains guanosine monophosphate (GMP). A powerful taste synergism exists with mixtures of these compounds: the taste intensity of the mixture is described as much greater than the intensity of each of the substances alone. Research with catfish, which have taste buds distributed all over their bodies, shows that the addition of GMP to the binding medium causes a marked increase in the binding of GLU to receptors in taste tissue, but not in non-taste epithelium.

Psychometric studies on the taste of MSG show that the addition of

MSG to beef consomme has no effect on perceived aroma, but it increases the overall taste intensity. Saltiness, sweetness, sourness, and bit-
terness are not significantly enhanced, but the addition of MSG does increase some of the aspects of flavor. More specifically, continuity, mouth-
fulness, impact, mildness, and thickness are perceived to be enhanced.
MSG also increases the "meaty" flavor and overall preference for consomme.

When given a choice, animals are able to select nutrients according to
their physiological needs. Often this happens by an association of the sensory
quality of the food with its postingestional consequences. Because GLU is
such a ubiquitous constituent of the diet and has so many biosynthetic sources,
you would not expect much of a behavioral control for its intake. Indeed, in
a two-choice situation, rats will not select high concentrations of MSG, but
will select low concentrations when the sensory characteristics of MSG are
apparent to them. This selection is not dependent upon sodium or pH factors.
There is no selection for MSG when the "taste" is disguised in solid foods,
indicating that rats prefer the sensory enhancement of the compound; no
significant postingestional consequences exist.

Tews (1981, 1984, 1986) have amassed considerable data on the dietary
regulation of GABA, indicating either that GABA supplies a general satiety
signal or that there is a specific element to the food regulation effect of GABA.
In either case, the avoidance of diets that contain GABA is quite strong and
is not overcome by the addition of an acceptable flavoring agent or by the
forced association of the amino acid with a palatable food. Because GABA
has opposite effects on food intake in different brain regions, it is not known
whether this dietary effect on food intake is mediated centrally or by some
peripheral action.

When added to a low protein diet that contains the appropriate amounts
of the essential amino acids, GABA (4.5%) can strongly reduce food intake
and the growth of rats and other animals. In contrast, the addition of serine,
alanine, or glycine in equimolar amounts to the same low-protein diet does
not depress food intake and growth. When rats are allowed to choose between
a diet containing 2.5% or 4.5% GABA and a diet inadequate in other nutrients, the GABA diet is avoided in favor of the inadequate diet. Odor does
not appear to be critical to this effect: bulbectomized rats still avoid diets that
contain GABA. This deleterious effect of GABA on food intake occurs
despite the fact that the amino acid is rapidly cleared from the body by
excretion in the urine and by metabolism to CO_2. GABA also depresses food
intake in genetically obese mice (*ob/ob*), but not as much as in normal, lean
controls.

Related to the issue of whether GABA might alter the transport of amino
acids into brain and thereby alter food intake, Tews and colleagues (1984)
studied the dietary effects of GABA on cats, who require greater dietary
levels of protein for growth and maintenance than do other mammals. The
question was whether kittens normally consuming relatively higher amounts

of protein would reduce their food intake and growth when fed GABA. GABA at 5%, but not 3%, of a low-protein diet depressed the food intake of kittens, but adaptation to a high-protein diet prevented these effects, suggesting some possible interaction of GABA and the transport of other amino acids into brain.

Pathology

Because GLU is a ubiquitous neurotransmitter that increases the firing rate of neurons on which it is released, it is the first suspect as cause of the neurologic signs collectively known as Chinese restaurant syndrome. These symptoms include numbness and tingling in the extremities and lips, and backaches that do not feel muscular in origin. Many attribute these neurologic signs to the addition of MSG to oriental foods. Several studies in nonhuman species show that peripherally administered MSG can result in retinopathy and hypothalamic damage, and can produce neurologic signs.

However, several studies also show that the risks of consumption of MSG as an additive have been somewhat overstated. Questionnaire surveys that led to the 30-50% "findings" of incidence of the syndrome were considerably biased by demand and population characteristics. When these are controlled in a "neutral," or more objective, questionnaire, the incidence of the syndrome drops to 1-2%.

Moreover, although hypothalamic lesions are induced in a variety of rodent species with massive doses of MSG or by routes of administration that bypass the normal peripheral metabolism, little or no evidence exists for induced pathologic change in feeding studies. Diets containing 4% MSG for the rat and up to 10% for the dog have not been associated with any clinical or histopathologic evidence of CNS damage for up to 2 years of feeding. MSG given with the meal results in only slight increase in plasma GLU in rodents. In humans, plasma GLU increases proportionally to the dose of MSG added to consomme, except when the meal contains carbohydrates; then there is little effect on plasma GLU. An oriental rice dish may therefore allow little opportunity for the added MSG to elevate plasma GLU levels.

The situation, however, in young rodents is different. Forced meals containing 5% GLU double the plasma GLU and lead to a 60% increase in plasma alanine. Also, studies in humans show that MSG dissolved in tomato juice (150 mg/kg) results in a marked increase in plasma GLU compared to a similar amount of sodium chloride as control. Although there are several biochemical and nervous system controls on the intake and uptake of MSG, some percentage of the population may be susceptible to the slight amounts used as a flavor enhancer, and this percentage could vary depending upon the other constituents of the diet to which MSG has been added.

In this context, we should mention that one of the original criticisms of the dipeptide sweetener, aspartame (see also Chapter 4), was that increased consumption could potentially release significant amounts of ASP into the bloodstream (see Figure 6.10 for chemical diagram of aspartame). In fact, aspartame administration to infant mice in large doses results in neuronal destruction in the hypothalamus. But high doses given to infant primates do not destroy hypothalamic neurons even though plasma ASP and GLU levels are elevated. Moreover, the addition of aspartame to meals containing MSG does not further increase plasma GLU or ASP levels above values induced by MSG alone. These data do not support the suggestion that the addition of aspartame to a meal produces a dangerous rise in plasma GLU or ASP.

Because of their organization and distribution, GLU and GABA may act in excitatory/inhibitory balance. Epileptic convulsions may result from either an increase in GLU or a decrease in GABA activity. After intraperitoneal injections of large doses of MSG, rats become somnolent and then develop seizures. Injections of kainic acid, an analogue of GLU that binds with higher affinity to GLU receptors than does GLU, produces seizure activity and, at least initially, wet-dog shakes—a convulsive shudder in rats and dogs. Kainic acid applied to the amygdala or to the septal region produces "remote" destruction of hippocampal cells thought to result from increased excitation of GLU afferents to these neurons and a consequent increase in the number of GLU binding sites. Repeated intraventricular injection of GLU or ASP for one hour produces morphologic changes in the hippocampus similar to the pathologic changes seen in brains of human epileptics, and in experimental animals in which hippocampal seizure activity is induced by kainic acid or by electrical stimulation of the perforant path.

Impairment of GABA inhibition is also associated with convulsions. Nitsch (1978) has shown that convulsions produced by vitamin B_6 deficiency can be mimicked by the administration of a pyridoxine analogue, methoxypyridoxine. This treatment diminishes the activity of the GABA synthetic enzyme, GLU decarboxylase, so that the synthesis of GABA decreases as a consequence. Similarly, GABA nerve terminals have been shown to be reduced at the sites of focal epilepsy. Other studies have suggested that the site mediating the GABA inhibition of convulsions is the substantia nigra, which not only receives GABA projections from the striatum but also sends dopamine

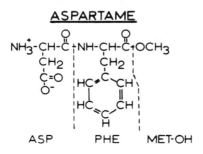

Figure 6.10 Diagram of aspartame showing how ASP is incorporated.

projections to the striatum. An effective recommendation for persons prone to epileptic seizure activity might therefore not only include abstinence from MSG and aspartame (see Chapter 4), but increased GABA in the diet. Indeed, evidence in mice shows that phosphatidylserine enhances the anticonvulsant effect of GABA and can be used to lower the doses of GABA needed to protect against seizures.

Huntington's chorea is another disorder that may involve an impaired balance between GLU and GABA. Choreic patients show a large loss of neurons in the striatum that contain GABA and its synthesizing enzyme GLU decarboxylase. In fact, to produce a model of the disorder, investigators have injected kainic acid into the striatum of experimental animals. This treatment results in a large and permanent decrease in the activity of GLU decarboxylase and choline acetyltransferase because of the loss of intrinsic striatal cells. Treated animals show motor disorders and impairment of cognitive functioning that resemble those of choreic patients. At the present time, there is no information of the use of dietary GABA as a treatment for this condition.

Summary

The excitatory amino acids, GLU and ASP, are often consumed in natural dietary sources and when added as a flavor enhancer: MSG. These amino acids act predominantly as excitatory neurotransmitters in the brain. GABA, which acts as an inhibitory transmitter usually in local interneurons, opposes the brain actions of GLU and ASP.

The addition of MSG to foods alters the flavor without adding its own taste. The change in flavor occurs mostly in taste intensity. Subtle tastes in foods are "brought out," and subjects often describe these tastes in more intense ways. When GABA is added to foods, it creates a strong aversion to them. It is not known whether this aversion is centrally or peripherally mediated.

MSG is the primary suspect in the Chinese restaurant syndrome, although many aspects of this syndrome have been overstated. Epileptic convulsions may result from a shift in the balance of excitatory amino acids and GABA such that excitation prevails in the circuits. Huntington's chorea is another disorder that may involve an impaired balance between excitatory amino acids and the inhibition from GABA. Whereas epilepsy often involves limbic circuits, Huntington's chorea involves the striatum.

References

Costa, E., Guidotti, A., Moroni, F., & Peralta, E. Glutamic acid as a transmitter precursor and as a transmitter. In Filer, L.J. et al. (Eds.), *Glutamic acid: Advances in biochemistry and physiology*, New York: Raven Press, 1979, pp. 151–161.

Cotman, G.W., Foster, A., & Lanthorn, T. An overview of glutamate as a neurotransmitter. In DiChiara, G. & Gessa, G. L. (Eds.), *Glutamate as a neurotransmitter* (Vol 27). New York: Raven Press, 1981, pp. 1–27.

Crim, M.C. & Munro, H.N. Protein and amino acid requirements and metabolism in relation to defined formula diets. In Shils, M.E. (Ed.), *Defined formula diets for medical purposes*, AMA: Chicago, 1977, pp. 5–15.

Fonnum, F., Soreide, A., Kvale, I., Walker, J., & Walaas, I. Glutamate in cortical fibers. In DiChiara, G. & Gessa, G.L. (Eds.), *Glutamate as a neurotransmitter* (Vol 27). New York: Raven Press, 1981, pp. 29–41.

Meister, A. Biochemistry of glutamate: Glutamine and glutathione. In Filer, L.J. et al. (Eds.), *Glutamic Acid: Advances in biochemistry and physiology*, New York: Raven Press, 1979, pp. 69–84.

Nitsch, C. Role of hippocampus in convulsions caused by a critical GABA decrease. *Advances in Epileptology, Proceedings, 13*, 1978, 151–154.

Olney, J.W. Excitotoxic amino acids: Research applications and safety implications. In Filer, L.J. et al. (Eds.), *Glutamic acid: Advances in biochemistry and physiology*, New York: Raven Press, 1979, pp. 287–319.

Shank, R.P. & Aprison, M.H. Biochemical aspects of the neurotransmitter function of glutamate. In Filer, L.J. et al. (Eds.), *Glutamic acid: Advances in biochemistry and physiology*, New York: Raven Press, 1979, pp. 139–150.

Storm-Mathisen, J. Glutamate in hippocampal pathways. In DiChiara, G. & Gessa G.L. (Eds.), *Glutamate as a neurotransmitter* (Vol. 27). New York: Raven Press, 1981 pp. 43–55.

Tews, J.K. Dietary GABA decreases body weight of genetically obese mice. *Life Sciences, 29*, 1981, 2535–2542.

Tews, J.K., Repa, J.J., & Harper, A.E. Dietary GABA and food selection by rats (42229). *Proceedings of the Society for Experimental Biology and Medicine, 181*, 1986, 98–103.

Tews, J.K., Rogers, Q.R., Morris, J.G., & Harper, A.E. Effect of dietary protein and GABA on food intake, growth and tissue amino acids in cats. *Physiology and Behavior, 32*, 1984, 301–308.

*S*uggested Readings

Agmo, A. & Paredes, R. GABAergic drugs and sexual behavior in the male rat. *European Journal of Pharmacology, 112*, 1985, 371–378.

Bhagavan, H.N., Coursin, D.B., & Stewart, C.N. Monosodium glutamate induces convulsive disorders in rats. *Nature, 232*, 1971, 275–276.

Bird, S.J., Gulley, R.L., Wenthold, R.J., & Fex, J. Kainic acid injections result in degeneration of cochlear nucleus cells innervated by the auditory nerve. *Science, 202*, 1978, 1087–1089.

Ben-Ari, Y., Tremblay, E., Ottersen, O.P., & Meldrum, B.S. The role of epileptic activity in hippocampal and 'remote' cerebral lesions induced by kainic acid. *Brain Research, 191*, 1980, 79–97.

Cagan, R.H., Torii, K., & Kare, M.R. Biochemical studies of glutamate taste receptors: The synergistic effect of L-glutamate and 5'-ribonucleotides. In Filer, L.J. et al. (Eds.), *Glutamic acid: Advances in biochemistry and physiology*. New York: Raven Press, 1979. pp. 1–9.

DeFelipe, J. & Jones, E.G. Vertical organization of gamma-aminobutyric acid-accumulating intrinsic neuronal systems in monkey cerebral cortex. *The Journal of Neuroscience, 5*, 1985, 3246–3260.

Dykes, R.W., Landry, P., Metherate, R., & Hicks, T.P. Functional role of GABA in cat primary somatosensory cortex: Shaping receptive fields of cortical neurons. *Journal of Neurophysiology, 52*, 1984, 1066–1093.

Feasey, K.J., Lynch, M.A., & Bliss, T.V.P. Long-term potentiation is associated with an increase in calcium-dependent, potassium stimulated release of [^{14}C]glutamate from hippocampal slices: An *ex vivo* study in the rat. *Brain Research, 364,* 1986, 39–44.

Filer, L.J., Baker, G.L., & Stegink, L.D. The effect of aspartame loading on plasma and erythrocyte free amino acid concentrations in one year old infants. *Journal of Nutrition, 113*, 1983, 1591–1599.

Filer, L.J., Garattini, S., Kare, M.R., Reynolds, W.A., & Wurtman, R.J. (Eds.), *Glutamic acid: Advances in biochemistry and physiology.* New York: Raven Press, 1979.

Fonnum, F. Glutamate: A neurotransmitter in mammalian brain. *Journal of Neurochemistry, 42,* 1984, 1–11.

Gamrani, H., Onteniente, B., Seguela, P., Geffard, M., & Calas, A. Gamma-aminobutyric acid-immunoreactivity in the rat hippocampus. A light and electron microscopic study with anti-GABA antibodies. *Brain Research, 364,* 1986, 30–38.

Giacometti, T. Free and bound glutamate in natural products. In Filer, L.J. et al. (Eds.), *Glutamic acid: Advances in biochemistry and physiology*, New York: Raven Press, 1979, pp. 25–34.

Grandison, L. & Guidotti, A. Stimulation of food intake by muscimol and beta endorphin. *Neuropharmacology, 16,* 1977, 533–536.

Heywood, R. & Worden, A.N. Glutamate toxicity in laboratory animals. In Filer, L.J. et al. (Eds.), *Glutamic acid: Advances in biochemistry and physiology*, New York: Raven Press, 1979, pp. 203–215.

Iadarola, M.J. & Gale, K. Substantia nigra: Site of anticonvulsant activity mediated by gamma-aminobutyric acid. *Science, 218,* 1982, 1237–1240.

Kelly, J. & Grossman, S.P. GABA and hypothalamic feeding systems: A comparison of GABA, glycine, and acetylcholine agonists and their antagonists. *Pharmacology, Biochemistry, and Behavior, 11,* 1979, 649–652.

Kerr, G.R., Wu-Lee, M., El-Lozy, M., McGandy, R., & Stare, F.J. In Filer, L.J. et al. (Eds.), *Glutamic Acid: Advances in Biochemistry and Physiology*, New York: Raven Press, 1979, pp. 375–387.

Kessler, M. Baudry, M., Cummins, J.T., Way, S., & Lynch, G. Induction of glutamate binding sites in hippocampal membranes by transient exposure to high concentrations of glutamate or glutamate analogs. *The Journal of Neuroscience, 6,* 1986, 355–363.

Lanthorn, T. & Isaacson, R.L. Studies of kainate-induced wet-dog shakes in the rat. *Life Sciences, 22,* 1978, 171–178.

Madarasz, M., Somogyi, G., Somogyi, J., & Hamori, J. Numerical estimation of gamma-aminobutyric acid (GABA)-containing neurons in three thalamic nuclei of the cat: Direct GABA immunocytochemistry. *Neuroscience Letters, 61,* 1985, 73–78.

Meldrum, B. GABA-agonists as anti-epileptic agents. In Costa, E., DiChiara, G., & Gessa, G.L. (Eds.), *GABA and benzodiazepine receptors* (Vol 26). New York: Raven Press, 1981, pp. 207–217.

Munro, H.N. Factors in the regulation of glutamate metabolism. In Filer, L.J. et al. (Eds.), *Glutamic Acid: Advances in biochemistry and physiology*, New York: Raven Press, 1979, pp. 55–68.

Naim, M. Self-selection of food and water flavored with monosodium glutamate. In

Filer, L.J. et al. (Eds.), *Glutamic acid: Advances in biochemistry and physiology*, New York: Raven Press, 1979, pp. 11–23.

Ohta, H., Nakamura, S., Watanabe, S., & Ueki, S. Effect of L-glutamate, injected into the posterior hypothalamus, on blood pressure and heart rate in unanesthetized and unrestrained rats. *Neuropharmacology, 24*, 1985, 445–451.

Oldendorf, W.M. Brain uptake of radiolabelled amino acids, amines, and hexoses after arterial injection. *American Journal of Physiology, 221*, 1971, 1629–1639.

Pardridge, W.M. Regulation of amino acid availability to brain: Selective control mechanisms for glutamate. In Filer, L.J. et al. (Eds.), *Glutamic acid: Advances in biochemistry and physiology*, New York: Raven Press, 1979, pp. 125–137.

Peng, Y., Gubin, J., Harper, A.E., Vavich, M.G., & Kemmerer, A.R. Food intake regulation: Amino acid toxicity and changes in rat brain and plasma amino acids. *Journal of Nutrition, 103*, 1973, 608–617.

Pointis, D. & Borenstein, P. The mesencephalic locomotor region in cat: Effects of local application of diazepam and gamma-aminobutyric acid. *Neuroscience Letters, 53*, 1985, 297–302.

Racagni, G., Apud, J.A., Civati, C., Cocchi, D., Casanueva, F., Locatelli, V., Nistico, G., & Muller, E.E. Neurochemical aspects of GABA and glutamate in the hypothalamo-pituitary system. In Costa, E., DiChiara, G., & Gessa, G.L. (Eds.), *GABA and benzodiazepine receptors* (Vol. 26). New York: Raven Press, 1981, pp. 207–217.

Ribak, C.E., Hunt, C.A., Bakay, R.A.E., & Oertel, W.H. A decrease in the number of GABAergic somata is associated with the preferential loss of GABAergic terminals at epileptic foci. *Brain Research, 363*, 1986, 78–90.

Sanberg, P.R., Lehmann, J., & Fibiger, H.C. Impaired learning and memory after kainic acid lesions of the striatum: A behavioral model of Huntington's disease. *Brain Research, 149*, 1978, 546–551.

Sanger, D.J. GABA and the behavioral effects of anxiolytic drugs. *Life Sciences, 36*, 1985, 1503–1513.

Schneider, S.P. & Perl, E.R. Selective excitation of neurons in the mammalian spinal dorsal horn by aspartate and glutamate in vitro: Correlation with location and excitatory input. *Brain Research, 360*, 1985, 339–343.

Sloviter, R.S. & Dempster, D.W. "Epileptic" brain damage is replicated qualitatively in the rat hippocampus by central injection of glutamate or aspartate but not by GABA or acetylcholine. *Brain Research Bulletin, 15*, 1985, 39–60.

Stegink, L.D., Filer, L.J., & Baker, G.L. Plasma amino acid concentrations in normal adults fed meals with added monosodium L-glutamate and aspartame. *Journal of Nutrition, 113*, 1983, 1851–1860.

Stegink, L.D., Filer, L.J., & Baker, G.L. Plasma glutamate concentrations in adult subjects ingesting monosodium L-glutamate in consomme. *The American Journal of Clinical Nutrition, 42*, 1985, 220–225.

Taxt, T. & Storm-Mathisen, J. Uptake of D-aspartate and L-glutamate in excitatory axon terminals in hippocampus: Auto-radiographic and biochemical comparison with gamma-aminobutyrate and other amino acids in normal rats and rats with lesions. *Neuroscience, 11*, 1984, 79–100.

Toffano, G., Mazzari, S., Zanotti, A., & Bruni, A. Synergistic effect of phosphatidylserine with gamma-aminobutyric acid in antagonizing the isoniazid-induced convulsions in mice. *Neurochemical Research, 9*, 1984, 1065–1073.

Vincent, S.R., Hokfelt, T., Skirboll, L.R., & Wu, J-Y. Hypothalamic gamma-aminobutyric acid neurons project to the neocortex. *Science, 220*, 1983, 1309–1310.

Vrijmoed-DeVries, M.C., & Cools, A.R. Differential effects of striatal injections of dopaminergic, cholinergic and GABAergic drugs upon swimming behavior of rats. *Brain Research, 364*, 1986, 77–90.

Waddington, J.L. & Cross, A.J. Neurochemical changes following kainic acid lesions of the nucleus accumbens: Implications for a GABAergic accumbal-ventral tegmental pathway. *Life Sciences, 22*, 1978, 1011–1014.

Yamaguchi, S. & Kimizuka, A. Psychometric studies on the taste of monosodium glutamate. In Filer, L.J. et al. (Eds.), *Glutamic acid: Advances in biochemistry and physiology*, New York: Raven Press, 1979, pp. 35–54.

Part III

Macronutrients

Chapter *7*
Salty Behavior

T he importance of salt in economic and dietary history is underscored in numerous biblical and semantic references. Its economic value can be seen in the word "salary," which in the Latin denotes money given to Roman soldiers to buy salt. "Salubrious" and "salutary" both derive from the same root, as salt is beneficial to health and well-being. Job asks "Can that which is unsavory be eaten without salt?" Matthew calls the most respectable element of mankind "the salt of the earth." In salt scarce areas of the world, the mineral was traded for gold, and salt is still used as a major currency in isolated areas in Nepal and in the Andes (Hollenberg, 1980).

Every cell in the body utilizes sodium, and in nerve cells it is the major currency of an action potential. The appetite for salt encompasses several aspects of behavior. Individuals have a liking for salt beyond that required to maintain health, and will ingest salt to maintain a total body concentration well above critical homeostatic levels. Different hungers for salt also exist. One is dependent upon a deficiency in sodium intake and its hormonal consequences. Another is elicited by hormones of the reproductive system, and yet another is evoked by the hormonal response to stress.

Considerable species variation exists in the gustatory responses of mammals to chemical stimulation of the tongue. Carnivores have a higher sensitivity to potassium or ammonium, whereas herbivores generally respond better to sodium or lithium. Rats, with omnivorous habits, are salt gluttons.

Tracing of the gustatory pathways from the cranial nerves to the first and second level responsive areas of the brainstem, to the ventral posterior thalamus, and to cortical areas has supported the concept of a hierarchy of gustatory regulation, from responses to simple taste stimuli up to more complex learned behaviors. A close complementary relationship exists between sodium appetite and thirst; examination of the renin-angiotensin system has revealed some of the interactions with the CNS that regulate blood pressure, drinking, and electrolyte balance. The recent discovery of atrial natriuretic peptide and examination of its physiology has shown that it counteracts the aldosterone system in the regulation of sodium balance.

Because sodium regulatory systems participate in the maintenance of blood pressure, there is intense research into their involvement in the pathology of hypertension. The notion that mineral appetites manifest themselves in the exploration of potential nutrient sources has led to research on mineral deficiencies in pica, which is a perversion of appetite.

*B*iochemistry and Physiology

In general, we do not maintain a body sodium content at a homeostatic "set point." Instead, we operate at a level well above the controlled value. As Hollenberg (1980) has pointed out, we have prophylactic reasons for doing so in a world in which physical trauma, pregnancy, lactation, and losses in sweat or gastrointestinal disease all contribute to a profound sodium loss and could lead to a critical sodium deficit. According to Hollenberg, we should drop the notion that a "normal" individual, in the absence of extrarenal losses, is sodium replete only when ingesting salt and depleted when deprived of salt.

For example, a person given a diuretic along with a diet low in sodium so that a much larger amount of sodium is excreted on the first day, reduces his or her sodium content to minimal levels on the second day, when the direct influence of the diuretic on the kidney has dissipated. Also, a person who is in balance on a low sodium diet, when given even a trace amount of sodium will promptly excrete it. The data suggest that the controlled value, or "set point," around which sodium is regulated in the "normal" person is that amount of sodium chloride at which a person is in balance on a no-salt intake. This concept may also be viewed, as Denton (1984) has discussed, as the situation in which small obligatory losses in the urine, feces, and skin are balanced by dietary sodium intake, approximately 1-2 mmol/day.

The afferent and efferent limbs of the control of sodium have come under intense scrutiny. As Figure 7.1 shows, sodium loss is regulated by a number of hormones. The synthesis of the mineralocorticoid aldosterone, secreted by the adrenal cortex, is controlled by corticotropin released from the anterior pituitary. Alterations in body sodium, toward excess or deficiency, result in compensatory changes in the morphology and cytochemistry of the adrenal glomerulosa. Mild to moderate sodium depletion results in a 20-25 fold increase in aldosterone secretion. Repletion of sodium restores baseline levels of aldosterone. During sodium deficiency, increased aldosterone is associated

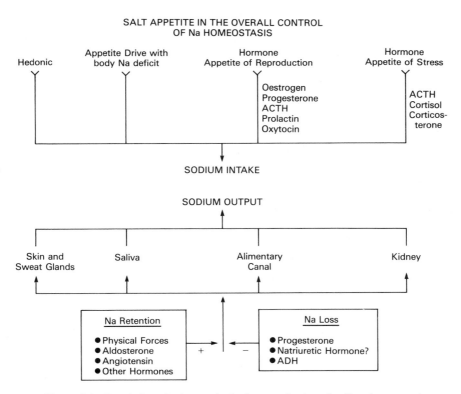

Figure 7.1 Regulation of salt appetite in the organization of sodium homeostasis. (From Denton, 1984.)

with enhanced sodium retention in target organs. Sodium levels fall, for example, in sweat and saliva, reflecting binding of aldosterone to its receptor, and the subsequent intranuclear transport of the complex.

Adrenalectomy rapidly permits sodium to be excreted in the various aldosterone target organs. Over 50 years ago, Richter (1936) wondered whether the resulting salt needs of adrenalectomized rats were accompanied by an increased salt appetite. He found that indeed adrenalectomized animals showed increased survival if they were allowed to consume salt-containing solutions. These animals also showed normal increases in body weight. Richter extended these observations to suggest that increased appetite was a typical consequence of removing the regulating gland. For example, parathyroidectomized rats given a diet as free of calcium as possible show a reliable increase in intake of calcium lactate. The amount of calcium taken spontaneously by these animals agrees with an empirically derived calculation of their calcium needs.

Subcutaneous injections of long-acting adrenocorticotropic hormone (ACTH) in rats result in a mineral appetite specific for sodium; other minerals such as calcium, magnesium, and potassium are unaffected. The resulting sodium intake is so large that the rats turn over daily an amount approximating their total body sodium. ACTH is ineffective in adrenalectomized rats, which indicates that sodium appetite is dependent upon adrenal hormones. However, this finding may be species-specific: ACTH produces a four-fold increase in NaCl intake in adrenalectomized wild rabbits. In these animals, injections of cortisol or corticosterone produce a significant stimulation of sodium appetite that is also synergistic with the action of ACTH. Moreover, in these animals, increases in sodium appetite produced by these hormones are independent of treatments producing a body sodium deficit. The stress-induced release of ACTH may therefore participate in producing a sodium appetite.

Adrenalectomized rats have a biphasic salt ingestion response to treatment with aldosterone. Low doses of mineralocorticoid reduce sodium appetite by reducing sodium loss. High doses reinstate appetite, as if by signaling the brain that a prolonged state of sodium depletion exists. Mineralocorticoids, though sufficient as stimuli for sodium appetite in rats, need not, however, have a vital role in the salt ingestion response. The threshold for sodium appetite in adrenalectomized rats is associated with the same small sodium deficits that are effective in stimulating salt appetite in intact rats. Neither intact nor adrenalectomized rats adjust sodium intake with precision. It is clear that other mechanisms of control exist.

One of these control mechanisms is the renin-angiotensin system (RAS). The RAS was originally linked to the kidney, as its name implies, to mechanisms of renal hypertension, and to sodium and volume regulation. It was subsequently shown, however, that renin is found at even higher concentrations in the uterus, salivary glands, brain, and various other tissues, and in tumors. In the brain, initial results suggested that renin-like activity was due to nonspecific action of acid proteases, but subsequent efforts clearly showed a distinct renin.

The system begins with the release of renin. This step is typically the rate-limiting one in the system. Angiotensinogen, which peripherally is manufactured primarily in the liver, is secreted into the blood. Renin then cleaves angiotensinogen to form the decapeptide angiotensin I. Angiotensin I is converted to the octapeptide angiotensin II by a carboxypeptidase converting enzyme. Angiotensin II is the primary active peptide of the system. Additional evidence, however, shows a further conversion to angiotensin III, which is also biologically active.

Stimulation of angiotensin II receptors in the arteries and adrenal gland produces vasoconstriction and secretion of mineralocorticoid hormones, respectively, which in turn leads to increased arterial blood pressure, and to salt and water retention. Considerable evidence shows that angiotensin II also elevates blood pressure by stimulating sites in the brain, presumably in the area postrema and the nucleus solitarius. Several differences between the peripheral and central effects of angiotensin II, however, suggest that mediation of blood pressure occurs by actions on different receptors. For example, stimulation of the area postrema via the vertebral artery increases heart rate, while the effect of angiotensin II in this area is to increase blood pressure without affecting heart rate.

These differences suggest the existence of two RAS functions, which probably interact via the circumventricular organs: the kidney-plasma RAS, which controls vasoconstriction and aldosterone release, and the brain RAS, which regulates vasopressin release, sympathetic tone, and drinking. The brain RAS and the plasma RAS are coupled: high plasma levels of angiotensin II suppress the brain RAS. In fact, it has been suggested by Ganten and Speck (1978) that the choroid plexus may act as a "miniature kidney," with its high concentration of renin and converting enzyme, presumably to control water and electrolyte balance in the cerebrospinal fluid.

Despite the differences between peripheral and central RAS effects, a number of CNS interactions suggest the existence of a single physiological system rather than a coupling of two systems. For example, electrical stimulation of particular regions in the mesencephalon, pons, medulla, and hypothalamus increases the rate of renin section by the kidneys, thereby helping to determine the rate at which angiotensin II is generated. This effect appears to result from activation of the sympathetic nervous system, because it is accompanied by increased arterial pressure, and abolished by renal denervation. The complementary inhibition of renal secretion can be achieved by stimulating areas of the hypothalamus that inhibit sympathetic activity.

Angiotensin II acts on the brain to produce a variety of interrelated effects, including elevation of blood pressure, stimulation of drinking, and increased secretion of vasopressin, and corticotropin (ACTH). These effects primarily involve circulating angiotensin, though there is growing evidence for a coordination by local angiotensin II formation in the brain. Angiotensin II also acts peripherally to release aldosterone. Vasopressin, however, inhibits renin secretion by direct action on renin-secreting cells, thereby providing feedback control for the physiological loop. The system can be "set into motion" by alterations in the sodium chloride concentration in the cerebrospinal fluid, causing reciprocal changes in the rate of renin secretion. For example, low sodium chloride content tends to elevate the amount of renin secreted.

Consider the physiological "layering" in the control of sodium intake: The elevated renin secretion produced by low sodium content would, of course, increase the production of angiotensin. In the normal rat, this would tend to elevate the production of vasopressin and the secretion of aldosterone, which help to conserve sodium. In the adrenalectomized rat, increased angiotensin produces a significant increase in salt appetite, thereby ruling out aldosterone as the sole mediator of the behavior. In fact, with mineralocorticoid doses that suppress salt appetite maximally in the adrenalectomized rat, addition of angiotensin stimulates salt appetite, indicating that angiotensin is the prime stimulus for the regulatory behavior.

Mineralocorticoid excess or absence, however, are two physiological states that rarely occur in nature. Epstein (1982) has shown that salt appetite is probably the sum of the actions of physiological amounts of aldosterone and angiotensin, which are likely to occur prior to significant central changes in sodium.

The stimulation of salt appetite by angiotensin can be further seen in studies in which angiotensin II is infused into the third ventricle of intact rats. Long-term infusions produce large and sustained increases in the intake of sodium and water, but carbachol has no such effect. The sodium appetite is specific; rats offered a choice of sodium and potassium take only sodium. Furthermore, the sodium appetite is not secondary to increased water intake, since it occurs even when a solution of 2.7% sodium is the only available fluid. The increased sodium appetite is also not secondary to natriuresis: rats stimulated with angiotensin develop a positive sodium balance; intracranial injections of renin do not cause sodium excretion in rats loaded with sodium; and rats with diminished urinary excretion also show a sodium appetite in response to renin.

In a physiological control system such as this one, you might expect at least one substance to counteract all the forces of sodium retention to balance the system with sodium excretion. Atrial natriuretic factor (ANF) is such a substance. This peptide is produced in myocytes of mammalian atria and exerts potent natriuretic and diuretic actions in the kidney, as well as a variety of other effects coordinated to balance extracellular fluid volume. As with many other peptides found in peripheral organs, ANF is also found in the brain. Recent immunocytochemical findings suggest that ANF exists in the hypothalamus, septum, and pontine nuclei.

Considerable evidence has accrued for central actions of ANF in the regulation of sodium balance. Intraventricular injection of ANF inhibits the increased water drinking produced by central administration of angiotensin. ANF also inhibits saline intake when infused into the third ventricle of conscious, salt-depleted rats, which effect is dose-dependent and long-lasting.

Both peripherally and centrally, ANF tends to oppose actions of angiotensin. In the heart, ANF is released in response to atrial stretching caused by increased venous return; the elevated blood pressure caused by actions of the RAS is thereby regulated by vasorelaxant actions of ANF. The central action of the peptide to reduce salt intake is matched peripherally by enhanced sodium and water excretion in the kidney. Moreover, direct actions of ANF inhibit aldosterone, renin, angiotensin, and vasopressin. More work remains to be done to determine whether ANF's action on sodium intake is direct or a consequence of its inhibition of the positive sodium balance hormones.

There have been a number of studies on the cravings of pregnant women. Richter (1955) reviewed a report published in 1691 by Christiani of Frankfurt of a woman who ate over 1,400 salted herrings during her pregnancy. Pregnant women commonly crave fruit, or strongly flavored or savory foods.

Our knowledge of specific appetites during pregnancy remained meager, however, until Richter and Barelare (1938) produced what are regarded as the first empirical studies. They offered rats a cafeteria of pure or relatively pure nutrients. During pregnancy, the appetite for protein and fat showed a definite increase, whereas that for carbohydrate showed a small decrease. The appetites for sodium chloride, sodium phosphate, and calcium lactate showed a marked increase, but there was no such increase for potassium chloride. There was also an increased appetite for yeast, but no change in appetite for wheat germ oil or cod liver oil.

Later studies of the hormonal factors influencing salt appetite during pregnancy revealed that sodium ingestion increases from the 11th to 25th day after initiation of pseudopregnancy and during treatment with estradiol. Daily treatment with progesterone only has no influence, but when given together with estradiol it enhances the latter's stimulation of salt intake. There may be species differences; these findings are not reproduced in sheep. During lactation, a large increase in salt appetite also occurs, and it has been shown that both prolactin and oxytocin stimulate salt ingestion. In rabbits, ACTH induces lactogenesis, and it is of course effective in stimulating salt appetite.

*A*natomy

Pathways Mediating Gustation and Salt Appetite

Ralph Norgren, who has done much of the gustatory mapping of the rat brain, has provided us with a synopsis of gustatory pathways shown in Figure 7.2. Peripheral gustatory afferents reach the brain via the facial (VII), glosso-

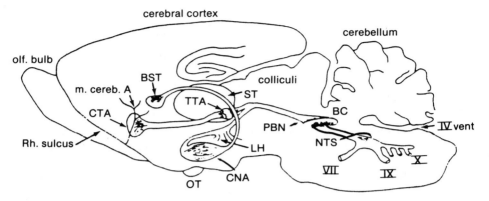

Figure 7.2 Synopsis of gustatory pathways. Basic pathways of the central gustatory system superimposed on a parasagittal section of the rat brain. Abbreviations: BC, brachium conjunctivum; BST, bed nucleus of the stria terminalis; CNA, central nucleus of the amygdala; CTA, cortical taste area; IV vent., fourth ventricle; IX, glossopharyngeal nerve; LH, lateral hypothalamus; m. cereb. A, middle cerebral artery; NTS, nucleus of the solitary tract; olf. bulb, olfactory bulb; OT, optic tract; PBN, parabrachial nuclei; Rh. sulcus, rhinal sulcus; ST, stria terminalis; TTA, thalamic taste area; VII, intermediate (facial) nerve; X, vagus nerve. (From Norgren, 1977.)

pharyngeal (IX), and vagal (X) cranial nerves. Gustatory fibers from these sources synapse in the anterior end of the nucleus of the solitary tract, in the lateral division. From this nucleus, fibers carrying gustatory information project ipsilaterally in the reticular formation to cells in the caudal parabrachial area, located between the principal and mesencephalic trigeminal nuclei. This pontine taste area receives gustatory information from both anterior and posterior tongue fields. From this dorsal pontine area, axons ascend in the central tegmental bundle to the thalamic "taste" areas on the medial edge of the posterior ventrobasal complex.

Thalamic cells that respond to thermal and tactile stimuli from the tongue are interposed between the "taste relay" medially and the remainder of the trigeminal projection target cells laterally. In addition to synapsing in the thalamus, gustatory axons from pontine nuclei also pass ventrally through the subthalamus, penetrating the internal capsule. Rostral to the internal capsule, fascicles from this projection branch into individual fibers, which orient laterally through the substantia innominata, and appear to end in the central nucleus of the amygdala. Some fibers, however, course through the stria terminalis to terminate in the bed nucleus of the stria. From the thalamic relay nucleus, fibers project rostrally and laterally to end in the gustatory neocortex.

Figure 7.3 shows the classic view of gustatory responsiveness in the tongue. Gustatory receptors, or taste buds, on the anterior tongue and palate are

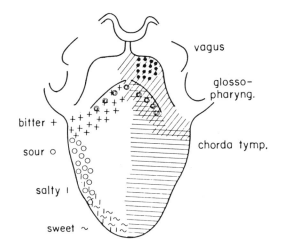

Figure 7.3 Classical view of gustatory responsiveness on the tongue. (From Denton, 1984.)

innervated by the chorda tympani and greater superficial petrosal nerves, respectively. These nerves pass into the medulla via the intermediate nerve, which is the visceral afferent fiber bundle part of the facial nerve complex. The lingual branch of the glossopharyngeal nerve innervates the posterior portions of the tongue. Afferents from epiglottal and other laryngeal taste buds course in the superior laryngeal branch of the vagus.

The sense of taste plays an important role in food selection and palatability, as well as in the reflexive control of swallowing. The differences between the facial and vagal systems that mediate the different roles of taste are especially clear in the catfish. In this animal, taste buds located most externally, innervated by the facial nerve, play a role in food selection and appreciation, while taste buds located closest to the alimentary canal, innervated by the vagus, are concerned with ingestive and protective reflexes. The neuroanatomic distinction may extend to mammals, in which gustatory nerves innervating the tongue project to the rostral solitary nucleus, whereas nerves innervating taste buds on the palate and pharynx, closer to the alimentary canal, project to the caudal solitary nucleus.

These taste systems interact with trigeminal (V) somatosensory innervation of the mouth and face. Trigeminal deafferentation severely disrupts food intake in several species. The perceived palatability of taste stimuli is altered after deafferentation. Positive taste responses to sapid stimuli are strongly diminished, while negative responses to aversive tastes are unaffected or only slightly diminished. We can therefore conclude that taste palatability is not independent of somatosensation, in that trigeminal input interacts with gustatory information to enhance primarily the positive aspects of palatability.

Pathways that subserve gustatory processing interact with other brain areas, especially in circumventricular organs that respond to angiotensin with an increase in firing rate of their intrinsic cells, to regulate sodium balance. Several reports, for example, have linked the area postrema, a circumventricular organ in the dorsal medulla, to the control of sodium regulation. Rats with lesions in the area postrema consume excess amounts of sodium chloride solutions. The behavior is specific for sodium; intake of potassium chloride or glucose remains unchanged. Because of the proximity of the area postrema to the solitary nucleus, there was some question that the lesion had encroached, but the increased ingestion of salt only occurred when the solitary nucleus was undamaged.

Lesions to other circumventricular organs affect sodium intake, but not necessarily in the same way. Ablation of the periventricular tissue around the anterior part of the third ventricle (OVLT) results in reduced consumption by rats of sodium solutions, along with adipsia, even while the animals are maintained on a reduced-sodium chow. There is, however, no corresponding reduction in diuresis. The animals with this lesion are not insensitive to sodium levels; they respond with increased sodium intake after being given injections of formalin, which is a standard means of lowering body sodium levels.

Several investigators have focused on the control of saline intake by neurons in the classic gustatory circuit. Gustatory information appears to reach the lateral hypothalamus of the rat only through a dorsal route, the ascending gustatory pathway, which courses from the pontine taste area (parabrachial nucleus) to the ventral thalamus via the midbrain reticular formation and subthalamus. This pathway also has terminals in the zona incerta and subthalamus. The zona incerta thus connects three principal gustatory areas: lateral hypothalamus, ventral thalamus, and midbrain reticular formation.

Electrical stimulation of the zona incerta increases the intake of both saline and water. Correspondingly, lesions of the zona incerta produce reliable impairments of need-related sodium appetite. Horizontal knife cuts dorsal to the zona incerta, separating it from the ventral thalamus, or ventral to the zona incerta, separating it from the hypothalamus, also result in severe impairments in sodium appetite. Lesions of the zona incerta, positioned as it is at a critical juncture for gustatory pathways, usually produce greater impairments in need-related sodium appetite than lesions of the ventral thalamic taste relay. It is not surprising that lesions of the lateral hypothalamus also produce impairment in the behavioral regulation of sodium intake.

The hierarchic distinction between behavioral regulation of sodium intake and internal mechanisms of sodium homeostasis can also be viewed from an anatomic perspective. Chronic decerebrate rats, similarly to intact controls, excrete comparable levels of excess sodium 24 hours after a sodium load. Decerebrate rats also reduce their urine sodium output, as do intact controls, when placed on a sodium-deficient diet. The behavioral aspects of sodium homeostasis, however, are completely absent in decerebrate rats. Treatments that deplete sodium in decerebrate rats alter neither the intake of sodium chloride nor the frequency of positive ingestive responses to applications of sodium, as they do in intact rats. The behavioral, as opposed to hormonal, compensatory responses that follow changes in the internal sodium state are therefore dependent upon forebrain mechanisms ascending from the pontine taste area.

It should be mentioned that the ventral thalamic nuclei that relay gustatory information do not act only for "primary" tastes such as salt, but may act at a more fundamental level to relay information about the regulation of other nutrients. For example, parathyroidectomized rats show a sharp increase in calcium ingestion unless the ventral thalamic nuclei have been destroyed. This finding could be construed to suggest that taste has an important role in self-selection for dietary calcium, even if such a taste is not classically defined as primary.

In more rostral areas, electrical stimulation of the medial or lateral septal area reduces the intake of saline in a two bottle preference test. This effect is specific for saline; it does not affect the intake of 5% glucose or 1% potassium chloride. Lesions of the septum produce an increased sodium appetite and an augmented drinking response to colloid treatment. Septal lesions also apparently sensitize a rat's brain to the stimulating effects of angiotensin II on sodium appetite.

The behavioral control of sodium appetite can be viewed even further in terms of an anatomic hierarchy. For example, rats with anterolateral neocortical damage—in the gustatory neocortex—initially display similar feeding and drinking deficits to rats with lateral hypothalamic damage. These rats, however, exhibit normal feeding responses to food deprivation and glucoprivation, and they also drink normally in response to hypertonic saline ingestion.

Because this gustatory cortical zone (Figure 7.4) exists within the ventral primary somatosensory facial areas, the original suggestion was that it influenced perception or appreciation of gustatory stimuli. This suggestion proved untenable, however, as it became clear that the gustatory neocortex is necessary for the normal associative learning processes involved in taste-guided responses.

In conditioned taste aversion learning, animals associate a taste (e.g., salt) as a conditioned stimulus with an illness produced, for example, by an injection of lithium chloride. Surgical ablation of this area of cortex produces major deficits in the acquisition and retention of a taste aversion established preoperatively. This area of cortex can be further divided functionally in that prepiriform and insular lesions produce acquisition deficits, whereas lesions in gustatory neocortex alone produce no such acquisition deficits. It is particularly important that such lesions only disrupt the conditioning process; they do not disrupt the ability of rats to detect or respond to the positive behavioral attributes of any of the taste modalities.

A

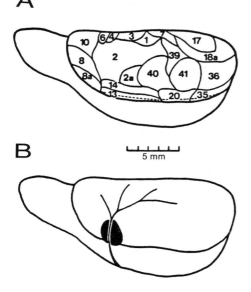

B

5 mm

Figure 7.4 Gustatory cortical zone. (From Lasiter et al., 1985.)

As a result of these cortical lesions, degenerating axonal by-products are evident in the ventral and ventromedial thalamic nuclei. This raises the question of whether lower-level thalamic systems are involved in the "higher level" learning processes. Lesions of the medial ventrobasal thalamic complex, which includes thalamic gustatory nuclei, attenuate taste reactivity to sucrose, citric acid, and quinine, but not to sodium chloride (in the absence of need). Moreover, there is a marked attenuation of conditioned taste aversion learning to salty tastes in these animals, but no such deficits in animals with lesions of the mediodorsal periventricular thalamic nuclei. Eventually, however, these animals can acquire a conditioned taste aversion, most likely through a modal switch to olfactory cues. These results indicate that the thalamus is important for directing the modality of the cues to the cortex, where taste conditioning takes place: In the absence of fiber connections for one food modality, the cortex can still subserve conditioning if another modality is intact.

The behavioral regulation of sodium intake is also controlled by the amygdala. Application of acetylcholine to the amygdala in sodium-deprived rats increases sodium chloride intake, while decreasing it in thirsty and satiated subjects. This result suggests possible interactions between dietary choline and the regulation of sodium. Bilateral transection of stria terminalis or the ventral amygdalofugal tract, both of which connect the amygdala with the hypothalamus, decreases saline intake in deprived rats. Rats with amygdala lesions also show less sodium appetite than controls in response to stimulating doses of deoxycorticosterone acetate. These results indicate that impulses from the amygdala to the hypothalamus are critical for behavioral regulation of sodium homeostasis.

The amygdala also has a role in other regulatory behavior. Lesions to various amygdalar nuclei impair acquisition of conditioned taste aversions to "salty" tastes. When lesions are created after rats have learned an aversion, a complete loss of the aversion results. Given the projections of the amygdala to olfactory tubercle, subthalamic nucleus, and parabrachial complex, food aversion deficits caused by amygdala lesions could be the result of impaired olfactory, gustatory, or gastrointestinal processing in various parts of the brain.

Localization and Binding of Sodium-Regulatory Hormones

The CNS sites for eliciting physiologic actions of angiotensin II include the area postrema, nucleus submedialis, organum vasculosum lamina terminalis (OVLT), the subfornical organ, and the medial preoptic area. The circumventricular organs are sites in which the blood brain barrier is not complete, and in which it is anticipated that circulating angiotensin has a resulting effect on the CNS. These areas are thus important in linking central and peripheral regulation of water and salt intake and blood pressure. Sites in which maximal specific binding for angiotensin is high include the area postrema, midbrain, thalamus, hypothalamus, and septum.

Angiotensin II is also found in the central amygdala, spinal trigeminal nuclei, and the sympathetic lateral column and substantia gelatinosa of the spinal cord. Substantial angiotensin II immunoreactivity occurs in the paraventricular and the perifornical nuclei of the hypothalamus. The arcuate median eminence region shows a dense plexus of angiotensin II fibers. Many of these angiotensin cells and fiber tracts are connected with the subfornical organ.

Neurons in the deep cerebellar nuclei and brainstem are studded with angiotensin II immunoprecipitate. Within fiber projections of the hippocampus, angiotensin II precipitate shows up in the nucleus of the diagonal band of Broca, the lateral olfactory tract, and hippocampal pyramidal cells. Angiotensin II reactivity in hippocampal efference is evident in alveus, cingulate gyrus, precommissural fornix, and fimbria. Angiotensin II has also been demonstrated in pericapillary pinealocytes, posterior pituicytes, and third-ventricle tanycytes.

Regional uptake of mineralocorticoids and glucocorticoids is similar, with the highest uptake in hippocampus, followed by septum and amygdala. Receptors bind both adrenal cortical hormones, but recent evidence supports the existence of at least two distinct subtypes, with glucocorticoid receptors having a wider distribution. Aldosterone autoradiograms of adrenalectomized animals show several labelled neurons, primarily in limbic structures. Within the hippocampus, labelling includes the pyramidal layer, subiculum, and dentate granule cells. Extensive labeling is also found in amygdala, entorhinal and piriform cortex, and in cingulate gyrus.

Functionally, however, aldosterone and corticosterone may have different targets. For example, hippocampus is not primarily an aldosterone target, whereas it is a target for corticosterone. Hippocampal lesions do not affect the salt appetite induced by adrenalectomy. Moreover, administration of corticosterone, which would take up the available hippocampal sites, fails to suppress saline intake and does not block aldosterone's action on saline intake.

*B*ehavior and Salt Appetite

Human neonates (< 4 months) do not differentially ingest water and sodium chloride. From 4 to 24 months, however, infants exhibit heightened acceptance of saline in preference to water. Behavioral development of a particular appetite such as this is consistent with the hypothesis of a postnatal maturation of peripheral or central systems underlying the response. This maturation is no doubt specific to species: 2-day old naive chicks rapidly restore their serum sodium concentrations to normal levels by water ingestion after dehydration and diuresis after overhydration. Though on a different developmental timetable, the chicken shows an osmoregulatory capability similar to the human's in its independence of learning or sensory experience.

An older study by Davis (1928) of diet selection in newly weaned infants is interesting in documenting a robust ability to regulate nutrient intake once the regulatory systems have matured sufficiently. Davis allowed newly weaned infants to choose their own foods in whatever quantities they desired from a wide range of commonly used natural food materials that were unmixed and unseasoned, and generally unaltered, except in some cases by simple cooking. She assembled data on the foods consumed and on the general condition of the infants, who had been admitted to the hospital with various diseases including rickets, colds, and chicken pox.

All of the infants chose their own foods in such quantity and variety as to maintain themselves, and to improve their conditions. The child with rickets, a vitamin D deficiency disease, healed without further treatment in a short period of time. The children were generally omnivorous, with a liking for fruits and cereals, as well as fish and meats. They ate salt occasionally, never spitting it out, and often going back for more. The patterns of their behavior indicated a tendency to eat certain foods in waves. There were, for example, "meat jags," "egg jags," or "cereal jags." There were also no symptoms of overeating, or of temporary disgust. Raw beef was preferred to cooked beef, but oatmeal and wheat were preferred cooked. Eggs, carrots, and peas were eaten either way. There was no evidence of discomfort or abdominal pain. In general, the infants showed adequate nutrient regulatory behavior when left to choose the foods they were offered. There was, by the way, no clue as to whether they were attracted by color or odor.

Studies of regulatory behavior later focused upon single nutrients, especially after Richter et al. (1938) showed elegant experimental methods for understanding a nutrient regulatory system. Although sodium, because of its primary taste qualities, has been most intensively studied, considerable work on potassium and its interactions with the sodium system also exists.

A greater proportion of young rats deprived of potassium and given a single brief preference test demonstrate a preference for potassium chloride, compared with controls who show no such preference. The preference occurs during the first 5 minutes or less of exposure, which lends support to the hypothesis that the specific hunger for potassium is innate. Appetite for potassium can be reversed by prior intragastric potassium repletion, but not with salts of sodium. Potassium appetite, however, does not appear to be completely specific for potassium itself in that depletion results in increased ingestion of solutions of NaCl, KCl, CaCl$_2$, and quinine sulfate in concentrations that are unacceptable to normal rats. In fact, potassium-deprived animals also drink large quantities of an aversive NaCl solution, indicating that potassium appetite may be subserved by a more general salt appetite, which by typical co-occurrence would usually serve to alleviate almost any "salt" deficiency.

Animals show a very clear sodium appetite in many ways. For example, within seconds after initial sampling, a rat subjected to a body sodium deficiency for the first time will avidly ingest salts of sodium, rejecting nonsodium salts. Rhesus monkeys placed on a low-sodium diet and given injections of furosemide to promote sodium loss show enhanced intake of sodium. Rats rapidly depleted of body sodium by subcutaneous injections of formalin, and without prior experience with salt, will increase their rate of bar pressing for saline in proportion to the dosage of formalin injected. This dose-response to formalin indicates that rats without prior experience are able to discriminate between varying intensities of sodium need.

Such innate recognition is also seen in higher order behavior. An experiment by Krieckhaus (1979) provides an excellent example. Thirsty rats, with no need for sodium, were taught for several weeks to run to one arm of a T-maze for distilled water. The other arm contained a much less acceptable hypertonic sodium solution. The animals were then tested when not thirsty for preference. At this time, all solutions were removed from the maze, and the animals were either sodium "replete" or "deplete." If their sodium status was low, they had a highly reliable tendency to run to the arm that had previously contained sodium. This was not true if their sodium status was relatively normal. Moreover, there was no such tendency for animals trained with a KCl solution to run to that arm when they were now sodium depleted. It thus appears that rats are capable of learning where and what sodium is, without wanting it at the time.

Because salt is a "primary" taste, it is important to examine the contribution of taste responses to the need-related appetite for sodium. The evidence shows that unlike hunger and thirst salt appetite cannot be satiated in the absence of taste stimulation. This was later shown to be a more complex phenomenon. Repletion of body sodium in the absence of taste (i.e., by gavage) is not initially as satiating as drinking. As the interval between gavage repletion and testing lengthens, however, the satiating effect begins to increase until it equals that of drinking. Apparently, multiple regulatory systems control salt appetite. Taste happens to be an initial monitor.

In rats, taste motor reflexes, like fixed action patterns, can be studied directly (Figure 7.5). These reflect the palatability of the taste and can be classified as ingestive or aversive. These stereotyped taste patterns are modified by the physiological state of the animal. For example, if the animal is sodium-replete, there is a mixture of ingestive and aversive taste patterns to oral infusions of 0.5 M NaCl. If the animals are depleted of sodium, this pattern shifts to an exclusive set of ingestive responses, indicating an increase in the palatability of high-salt solutions in depleted animals. This shift in behavior is specific for the physiological state; if the depleted animals are tested with 0.01 M HCl, there is no such shift toward ingestive responses.

These changes in taste also reflect changes in the motivational state of the animal. When rats are thirsty, they are not interested in running down a runway for salty solutions. When they are rendered salt hungry by mineralocorticoid treatment, however, they run vigorously for salty tasting solutions as high as 24%. Moreover, running speed is correlated with the degree of mineralocorticoid treatment and salt concentration, and will decrease substantially if the salt need of the animal is reduced by the prior opportunity to consume sodium.

Changes in taste also characterize alterations in the physiological state of humans. For example, patients with adrenal cortical insufficiency exhibit increased taste sensitivity, and can detect minimal concentrations of sodium salts at least eight times more dilute than those detected by the most sensitive normal subjects. Treatment with steroids returns the thresholds to values

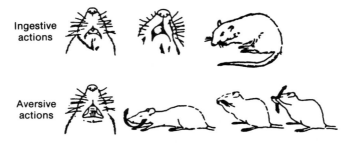

Figure 7.5 Taste reflexes in the rat. Ingestive actions include rhythmic tongue protrusion, lateral tongue protrusion (nonrhythmic), and paw licking. Aversive actions include gaping, headshaking, face washing, and forelimb flailing. (From Grill and Norgren, 1978.)

detected by normal subjects. Thus, changes in taste due to alterations in salt supply may reflect compensatory changes in the state of the pituitary adrenal system.

How are these changes in taste coded? After extended sodium deprivation in rats, whole and single nerve fiber chorda tympani responses to NaCl are smaller. The fibers naturally more responsive to sodium are most affected. Similarly, adrenalectomy, which results in excessive sodium loss, produces a large decrease in chorda tympani responsiveness to suprathreshold solutions of sodium. Thus the effect of sodium deprivation is a decrease in single strength over a labeled-line code for "saltiness." Deprived animals therefore sense strong sodium solutions as weak, and would not be so inclined to give aversive responses to the normally aversive solution.

A sensitive period exists for the influence of dietary sodium on functional taste receptor development. As Hill and Przekop (1988) have shown, sodium restriction of the material diet on or before embryonic day 8, but not 2 days later, in rats reduces the offspring's chorda tympani responses to sodium chloride by about 40%. Since this is before the initial formation of taste buds, it seems clear that the development of fault taste responses depends on other systemic interactions with maternal dietary sodium.

As we have seen, prior experience with taste is not necessary to elicit a need-dependent sodium appetite. Yet taste seems to be an important factor in monitoring sodium intake, and in calculating the changing sodium need. We have also seen that "higher-order" behaviors participate in the regulation of sodium status. Is taste critical for these behaviors, or do other systems subserve the behaviors?

Normal rats respond to natriuretic and mineralocorticoid treatments by increasing both saline and water intake. Rats with lesions centered in the thalamic taste relay do not increase saline intake in response to these treatments, but do increase their water intake. If, however, rats are permitted to drink saline prior to induction of the lesions, they show normal increases in both saline and water intake. Preoperative experience with sodium need alone does not protect rats against the taste relay lesion deficit. One simple hypothesis is that taste perception is required for the normal response to sodium need, except when the animals have the opportunity to learn something else.

What is this "something else?" If the location of the saline during postoperative testing is different from the location during preoperative training for some rats and not others, a difference in the protective effect of preoperative experience occurs. A protective effect is evident when the pre- and postoperative locations are the same, but not when they differ. The protective effect may therefore be due to place learning. Rats can remember tasting saline in a particular place and can then return there when they are in a state of sodium need. The "higher-order" learning ability can thus mediate normal taste-dependent responses to sodium need.

Beyond the need for sodium, there appear to be rather strong preferences for salt in humans and several other species. In the United States, people consume about 6-18 g salt every day, which is an order of magnitude more than the presumed requirement. These preferences can be readily modified. Beauchamp (1987) reports an experiment in which a group of young adults were placed on a self-maintained, lowered sodium diet for 5 months. Their taste responses to salt in various foods were monitored during a 2-month baseline period, as well as during the experimental period. A control group allowed to consume salt freely was similarly monitored. The actual amount of salt consumed was determined by unannounced urine collections. The results showed that the preferred salt level in food is alterable by contact with available salt. Preferred concentrations of salt fell in experimental subjects, but not in controls.

Pathology

Pica is defined as a perversion of the appetite. The word derives from the Latin for magpie, a bird that eats a variety of items to satisfy its hunger. Several kinds of pica have been distinguished: geophagia—eating dirt or clay; amylophagia—laundry starch; trichophagia—hair; and lithophagia—stone or gravel. The ingestion of soot or burned matches has also been observed. Otherwise normal children and adults of both sexes engage in one or more of these practices. Those who indulge form neither a distinct nor homogeneous population. The practices are not restricted to nation or climate.

Pica probably represents a particular mineral appetite. During medieval times, the simultaneous existence of pica and anemia was recognized, and a mode of iron therapy was prescribed. Currently, conditions associated with pica include iron deficiency anemia, intestinal obstruction, and parotid gland enlargement. Treatment with iron has been reported to reverse pica under some conditions.

Recent studies of geophagic clay from a village in Nigeria indicates that it is sold widely in the markets of West Africa. Mineralogic analysis of this clay reveals a kaolinitic composition quite similar to that of the clays in the pharmaceutical Kaopectate. In the pharmaceutical, these clays are designed to counteract gastric upset and irritated intestines. Kaolinite absorbs toxins and bacteria, and has been reported to form a protective coat on the mucous membranes of the digestive tract. At least one form of pica can thus be defined as a therapeutic practice.

Experimental studies of pica, however, suggest that nutrients may play a part. Weanling rats fed a low calcium diet ingest lead acetate solutions in much greater proportions than iron-deficient or control weanlings. This behavior occurs even with high concentrations of lead acetate that normal weanlings find aversive. There is apparently no regulatory system for lead per se, since injections of lead acetate into these animals do not alter their lead ingestion. Calcium deficiency may thus be one cause of lead pica. This is particularly important because lead pica has often been cited as a result of poor supervision or emotional support, and not as a result of nutritional factors.

Supplements of minerals have varying abilities to cure allotriophagia (pica). Iron supplements have a spotty history in curing pagophagia (ice eating) and other forms of pica. Grazing animals are often seen eating bones or other substances when their grazings lack minerals, especially phosphorus. The regulatory system may not be especially complete for these minerals as for salt, and such action may reflect a fortuitous repletion through chewing on nontypical items. There are observations that cattle do not select phosphorus preferentially when their grazings lack the mineral. They do not even take in enough phosphorus to prevent aphosphorosis. The concept that a lack of some minerals results in aberrant intake of other minerals needs further study, especially since this is in contrast to the specificity of salt.

Because regulatory systems for salt and water are complementary, and because blood pressure is a function of fluid volume, the influence of salt on hypertension is a natural line of study. Excess salt consumption has been implicated in the increasing prevalence of hypertension in West African countries. Historical evidence about salt supplies in this area suggests that availability was not uniform. For example, salt production in Senegal and Gambia has been extensive since ancient times, whereas the population of ancient Nigeria has had to depend upon a meager supply of vegetable salts or imports. Reports of lower blood pressure in Senegalese and Gambians than Nigerians may reflect the historical differences in salt supply, perhaps indicating a differential evolution of physiological means to conserve the precious mineral.

Renin and angiotensin levels are high in some forms of hypertension. Angiotensin, in addition to stimulating aldosterone secretion, exerts a potent vasopressor action by constricting peripheral arterioles. In several species, angiotensin exerts a greater effect on blood pressure when infused into vertebral arteries than when given intravenously, which suggests that central sites of action (e.g., area postrema) are important in the angiotensin action on blood pressure.

In animals given deoxycorticosterone, provision of sodium chloride or other sodium halides induces hypertension. How might sodium, other than through its action on regulatory hormones, influence blood pressure directly? Existing data indicate that sodium attenuates the affinity of α_2-adrenergic receptors for agonists, which have a profound hypotensive action. This could result in a disinhibition of neurons that normally inhibit the sympathetic nervous system. For example, microinjection of hypertonic saline into the solitary nucleus, a site of α_2 receptor action on blood pressure, produces a robust and lasting pressor response.

Can reduction of dietary sodium produce a lasting reduction in blood pressure? Sodium depletion in dogs produces little overall change in blood pressure, although individual components of the cardiovascular system are altered. Cardiac output and central venous pressure fall, but total peripheral resistance and heart rate increase. The compensatory action of the renin angiotensin system thus may tend to counteract any beneficial effect of a reduction in dietary sodium. These findings resemble those seen in humans after sodium depletion. Low sodium intake in rats, however, will prevent hypertension produced by administration of deoxycorticosterone.

Evidence suggests that focus on a single nutrient is inappropriate. The blood pressure of spontaneously hypertensive rats is lower with a high-calcium/high-sodium diet than with a high-calcium/low-sodium diet.

Sodium appetite in hypertensive individuals may be more of a symptom than a cause. Hypertensive individuals, compared to controls, tend to perceive suprathreshold salt stimuli as less intense. Using hedonic ratings, the same salt stimuli are also perceived as tasting more pleasant to hypertensives than to controls. The evidence therefore suggests that hypertensive humans, similarly to sodium deficient rats, are less sensitive to the taste of suprathreshold amounts of salt and tend to react to such stimuli more positively, which may account for why these two groups consume more salt. Atrial natriuretic factor attenuates the preference for hypertonic saline in hypertensive rats, while not having an effect in normotensive rats, and may therefore play a role in the increased salt appetite in those with hypertension.

*S*ummary

Salt is so necessary to our health and well-being that economic and semantic references to it are ingrained in several cultures. Several physiologic systems control body salt content, but we usually operate at a level well above any "set point" value. Aldosterone, which is secreted by the adrenal cortex, serves to stimulate salt retention. Aldosterone and angiotensin both appear to act on sodium appetite. Angiotensin further acts on the brain to produce a variety of interrelated effects, including elevation of blood pressure, stimulation of drinking, and increased secretion of vasopressin and corticotropin. Vasopressin inhibits renin secretion, thereby controlling the further production of angiotensin. Atrial natriuretic factor counteracts the forces of sodium retention through its natriuretic and diuretic actions.

The gustatory pathways in the brain are active in the behavioral relations of salt, in part because of their importance in food selection and palatability. Brain pathways that subserve taste interact with circumventricular organs that are responsive to the hormones that regulate salt. These brain pathways can be viewed in terms of a hierarchy in which forebrain mechanisms subserve "higher-order" salt regulation behaviors while brainstem mechanisms subserve "lower-order" behavior.

Animals have several behaviors that subserve sodium appetite. These behaviors include "simple" taste reflexes as well as mechanisms of learning. Humans have a preference for sodium that extends far beyond need.

Pica, which is a perversion of the appetite, may represent a particular mineral appetite, or at least an attempt to dose oneself with materials that act as pharmaceuticals for certain ailments. Because blood pressure is a function of fluid volume, and regulatory systems for salt and water are complementary, the influence of salt on hypertension is a natural line of study. Angiotensin levels are high in some forms of hypertension and may counteract any beneficial effect of a reduction in dietary sodium. Sodium appetite in hypertensive people may also be more of a symptom than a cause: Salt is perceived as tasting more pleasant in hypertensive people. Atrial natriuretic factor may play a role in treatment of hypertension.

References

Beauchamp, G.K. The human preference for excess salt. *American Scientist, 75,* 1987, 27–33.

Davis, C.M. Self selection of diet by newly weaned infants. *American Journal of Diseases of Children, 36,* 1928, 651–679.

Denton, D. *The hunger for salt.* New York: Springer-Verlag, 1984.

Epstein, A.N. Mineralocorticoids and cerebral angiotensin may act together to produce sodium appetite. *Peptides, 3,* 1982, 493–494.

Ganten, D. & Speck, G. The brain renin-angiotensin system: A model for the synthesis of peptides in the brain. *Biochemical Pharmacology, 27,* 1978, 2379–2389.

Grill, H.J. & Norgren, R. The taste reactivity test: I. Mimetic response to gustatory stimuli in neurologically normal rats. *Brain Research, 143,* 1978, 263–279.

Hill, D.L. & Przekop, P.R., Jr. Influences of dietary sodium on functional taste receptor development: A sensitive period. *Science, 241,* 1988, 1826–1828.

Hollenberg, N.K. Set point for sodium homeostasis: surfeit, deficit, and their implications. *Kidney International, 17,* 1980, 423–429.

Krieckhaus, E.E. "Innate recognition" aids rats in sodium regulation. *Journal of Comparative and Physiological Psychology, 73,* 1970, 117–112.

Lasiter, P.S., Deems, D.A., & Glanzman, D.L. Thalamocortical relations in taste aversion learning: I. Involvement of gustatory thalamocortical projections in taste aversion learning. *Behavioral Neuroscience, 99,* 1985, 454–476.

Norgren, R. A synopsis of gustatory neuroanatomy. In LeMagnen, J. & MacLeod, P. (Eds.), *Proceedings of the sixth international symposium on olfaction and taste,* Washington, DC: Information Retrieval, 1977, pp. 225–232.

Richter, C.P. Increased salt appetite in adrenalectomized rats. *American Journal of Physiology, 115,* 1936, 155–161.

Richter, C.P. Self regulatory functions during gestation and lactation. In C.A. Villee (Ed.), *Second conference on gestation.* New York: Josiah Macy Jr. Foundation, 1955.

Richter, C.P. & Barelare, B., Jr. Nutritional requirements of pregnant and lactating rats studied by the self-selection method. *Endocrinology, 23,* 1938, 15–24.

Richter, C.P., Holt, L.E., Jr., & Barelare, B., Jr. Nutritional requirements for normal growth and reproduction in rats studied by the self-selection method. *American Journal of Physiology, 122,* 1938, 734–744.

Suggested Readings

Adam, W.R. & Dawborn, J.K. Effect of potassium depletion on mineral appetite in the rat. *Journal of Comparative and Physiological Psychology, 78,* 1972, 51–58.

Ahern, G.L., Landin, M.L., & Wolf, G. Escape from deficits in sodium intake after thalamic lesions as a function of preoperative experience. *Journal of Comparative and Physiological Psychology, 92,* 1978, 544–554.

Antusses-Rodrigue, J., McCann, S.M., & Samson, W.K. Central administration of atrial natriuretic factor inhibits saline preference in the rat. *Endocrinology, 118,* 1986, 1726–1728.

Avrith, D.B. & Fitzsimons, J.T. Increased sodium appetite in the rat induced by intracranial administration of components of the renin-angiotensin system. *Journal of Physiology, 301,* 1980, 349–364.

Barelare, B. & Richter, C.P. Increased sodium chloride appetite in pregnant rats. *American Journal of Physiology, 121,* 1938, 185–188.

Bealer, S.L. & Johnson, A.K. Sodium consumption following lesions surrounding the anteroventral third ventricle. *Brain Research Bulletin, 4,* 1979, 287–290.

Beauchamp, G.K., Cowart, B.J., & Moran, M. Developmental changes in salt acceptability in human infants. *Developmental Psychobiology, 19,* 1986, 17–25.

Berridge, K.C. & Fentress, J.C. Trigeminal-taste interaction in palatability processing. *Science, 228,* 1985, 747–750.

Berridge, K.C., Flynn, F.W., Schulkin, J., & Grill, H.J. Sodium depletion enhances salt palatability in rats. *Behavioral Neuroscience, 98,* 1984, 652–660.

Blaine, E., Covelli, M.D., Denton, D.A., Nelson, J.F., & Shulkes, A.A. The role of ACTH and adrenal glucocorticoids in the salt appetite of wild rabbits [*Dryctolagus cuniculus* (L)]. *Endocrinology, 97,* 1975, 793–801.

Changaris, D.G., Severs, W.B., & Keil, L.C. Localization of angiotensin in rat brain. *The Journal of Histochemistry and Cytochemistry, 26,* 1978, 593–607.

Chiaraviglio, E. Amygdaloid modulation of sodium chloride and water intake in the rat. *Journal of Comparative and Physiological Psychology, 76,* 1971, 401–407.

Contreras, R.J. Salt taste and disease. *American Journal of Clinical Nutrition, 31,* 1978, 1090–1099.

Contreras, R.J. & Frank, M. Sodium deprivation alters neural responses to gustatory stimuli. *Journal of General Physiology, 73,* 1979, 569–594.

Contreras, R.J. & Stetson, P.W. Changes in salt intake after lesions of the area postrema and the nucleus of the solitary tract in rats. *Brain Research, 211,* 1981, 355–366.

Conway, J., Hatton, R., Keddie, J., & Dawes, P. The role of angiotensin in the control of blood pressure during sodium depletion. *Hypertension, 1,* 1979, 402–409.

Covelli, M.D., Denton, D.A., Nelson, J.F., & Shulkes, A.A. Hormonal factors influencing salt appetite in pregnancy. *Endocrinology, 93,* 1973, 423–429.

Dalhouse, A.D., Langford, H.G., Walsh, D., & Barnes, T. Angiotensin and salt appetite: Physiological amounts of angiotensin given peripherally increase salt appetite in the rat. *Behavioral Neuroscience, 100,* 1986, 597–602.

Emmers, R. & Nocenti, M.R. Role of the thalamic nucleus for taste in modifying calcium intake in rats maintained on a self-selection diet. *The Physiologist, 6*, 1963, 176.

Epstein, N., Fitzsimons, J.T., & Johnson, A.K. Peptide antagonists of the renin-angiotensin system and the elucidation of the receptors for angiotensin-induced drinking. *Journal of Physiology, 238*, 1974, 34P–35P.

Ermisch, A. & Ruhle, H.J. Autoradiographic demonstration of aldosterone-concentrating neuron populations in rat brain. *Brain Research, 147*, 1978, 154–158.

Felix, D. & Akert, K. The effect of angiotensin II on neurons of the cat subfornical organ. *Brain Research, 76*, 1974, 350–353.

Finger, T.E. & Morita, Y. Two gustatory systems: Facial and vagal gustatory nuclei have different brainstem connections. *Science, 227*, 1985, 776–778.

Fischer-Ferraro, C., Nahmod, V.E., Goldstein, D.J., & Finkielman, S. Angiotensin and renin in rat and dog brain. *Journal of Experimental Medicine, 133*, 1971, 353–361.

Fregly, M.J. & Waters, I.W. Effects of mineralocorticoids on spontaneous sodium chloride appetite of adrenalectomized rats. *Physiology & Behavior, 1*, 1966, 65–74.

Gavros, H. How does salt raise blood pressure? A hypothesis. *Hypertension, 8*, 1986, 83–88.

Gentil, C.G., Mogenson, G.J., & Stevenson, J.A.F. Electrical stimulation of septum, hypothalamus, and amygdala and saline preference. *American Journal of Physiology, 220*, 1971, 1172–1177.

Gordon, J.G., Tribe, D.E., & Graham, T.C. The feeding behavior of phosphorus-deficient cattle and sheep. *Animal Behaviour, 2*, 1954, 72–78.

Grijalva, C.V., Kiefer, S.W., Gunion, M.W., Cooper, P.H., & Novin, D. Ingestive responses to homeostatic challenges in rats with ablations of the anterolateral neocortex. *Behavioral Neuroscience, 99*, 1985, 162–174.

Grill, H.J., Schulkin, J., & Flynn, F.W. Sodium homeostasis in chronic decerebrate rats. *Behavioral Neuroscience, 100*, 1986, 536–543.

Henkin, R.I., Gill, J.R., Jr., & Bartter, F.C. Studies on taste thresholds in normal man and in patients with adrenal cortical insufficiency: The role of adrenal cortical steroids and of serum sodium concentration. *Journal of Clinical Investigation, 42*, 1963, 727–735.

Hirose, S., Yokosawa, H., & Inagami, T. Immunochemical identification of renin in rat brain and distinction from acid proteases. *Nature, 274*, 1978, 392–393.

Israel, A. & Barbella, Y. Diuretic and natriuretic action of rat atrial natriuretic peptide (6-33) administered intracerebroventricularly in rats. *Brain Research Bulletin, 17*, 1986, 141–144.

Itoh, H., Nakao, K., Katsuura, G., Morii, N., Shiono, S., Sakamoto, M., Sugawara, A., Yamada, T., Saito, Y., Matsushita, A., & Imura, H. Centrally infused atrial natriuretic polypeptide attenuates exaggerated salt appetite in spontaneously hypertensive rats. *Circulation Research, 59*, 1986, 342–347.

Iwasaki, K. & Sato, M. Taste nerve responses in mice. *Proceedings of the Japanese Symposium of Taste and Smell, XV*, 1981, 109–112.

Jalowiec, J.E. & Stricker, E.M. Sodium appetite in adrenalectomized rats following dietary sodium deprivation. *Journal of Comparative and Physiological Psychology, 82*, 1973, 66–77.

Keith, L., Brown, E.R., & Rosenberg, C. Pica: The unfinished story. Background: Correlations with anemia and pregnancy. *Perspectives in Biology and Medicine, 13*, 1970, 626–632.

Kiefer, S.W., Cabral, R.J., & Garcia, J. Neonatal ablations of the gustatory neocortex in the rat: Taste aversion learning and taste reactivity. *Behavioral Neuroscience, 98*, 1984, 804–812.

Kosten, T. & Contreras, R.J. Adrenalectomy reduces peripheral neural responses to gustatory stimuli in the rat. *Behavioral Neuroscience, 99*, 1985, 734–741.

Krieg, W.J.S. Connections of the cerebral cortex: I. The albino rat. A. Topography of cortical areas. *Journal of Comparative Neurology, 84*, 1946, 221–275.

Kurtz, T.W. & Morris, R.C., Jr. Sodium-chloride dependent hypertension. *Hypertension, 8*, 1986, 359–360.

Lasiter, P.S. Thalamocortical relations in taste aversion learning: II. Involvement of the medial ventrobasal thalamic complex in taste aversion learning. *Behavioral Neuroscience, 99*, 1985, 477–495.

Lasiter, P.S. & Glanzman, D.L. Cortical substrates of taste aversion learning: dorsal prepiriform (insular) lesions disrupt taste aversion learning. *Journal of Comparative and Physiological Psychology, 96*, 1982, 376–392.

Lasiter, P.S. & Glanzman, D.L. Cortical substrates of taste aversion learning: Involvement of dorsolateral amygdaloid nuclei and temporal neocortex in taste aversion learning. *Behavioral Neuroscience, 99*, 1985, 257–276.

Lasiter, P.S., Deems, D.A., Detting, R.L., & Garcia, J. Taste discriminations in rats lacking anterior insular gustatory neocortex. *Physiology & Behavior, 35*, 1985, 277–285.

McEwen, B.S., Lambdin, L.T., Rainbow, T.C., & DeNicola, A.F. Aldosterone effects on salt appetite in adrenalectomized rats. *Neuroendocrinology, 43*, 1986, 38–43.

Michell, A.R. Sodium 'need' and sodium appetite during the estrous cycle of sheep. *Physiology & Behavior, 21*, 1978, 519–523.

Milner, P. & Zucker, I. Specific hunger for potassium in the rat. *Psychonomic Science, 2*, 1965, 17–18.

Nachman, M. & Ashe, J.H. Effects of basolateral amygdala lesions on neophobia, learned taste aversions, and sodium appetite in rats. *Journal of Comparative and Physiological Psychology, 87*, 1974, 622–643.

Nishimura, H. Physiological evolution of the renin-angiotensin system. *Japanese Heart Journal, 19*, 1978, 806–822.

Norgren, R. & Pfaffman, C. The pontine taste area in the rat. *Brain Research, 91*, 1975, 99–117.

Paulus, R.A., Eng, R., & Schulkin, J. Preoperative latent place learning preserves salt appetite following damage to the central gustatory system. *Behavioral Neuroscience, 98*, 1984, 146–151.

Phillips, M.I. Angiotensin in the brain. *Neuroendocrinology, 25*, 1978, 354–377.

Quartermain, D., Miller, N.E., & Wolf, G. Role of experience in relationship between sodium deficiency and rate of bar pressing for salt. *Journal of Comparative and Physiological Psychology, 63*, 1967, 417–420.

Reid, I.A. Interactions between the renin-angiotensin system and the brain. In Johnson, J.A. & Anderson, R.R. (Eds.), *The renin angiotensin system*. New York: Plenum Press 1980, pp. 257–291.

Reul, J.M.H.M & DeKloet, E.R. Two receptor systems for corticosterone in rat brain: Macrodistribution and differential occupation. *Endocrinology, 117*, 1985, 2505–2511.

Richter, C.P. & Eckert, J.F. Increased calcium appetite of parathyroidectomized rats. *Endocrinology, 21*, 1937, 50–54.

Schulkin, J. Mineralocorticoids, dietary conditions, and sodium appetite. *Behavioral Biology, 23*, 1978, 197–205.

Schulkin, J. & Fluharty, S.J. Further studies on salt appetite following lateral hypothalamic lesions: Effects of preoperative alimentary experiences. *Behavioral Neuroscience, 99*, 1985, 929–935.

Schulkin, J., Arnell, P., & Stellar, E. Running to the taste of salt in mineralocorticoid-treated rats. *Hormones and Behavior, 19,* 1985, 413–425.

Schulkin, J., Leibman, D., Ehrman, R.N., Norton, N.W., & Ternes, J.W. Salt hunger in the rhesus monkey. *Behavioral Neuroscience, 98,* 1984, 753–756.

Simpson, F.O., Ledingham, J.M., Paulin, J.M., & Purves, R.D. Body sodium in rats: response to DOCA, adrenalectomy, changes in salt intake, and a salt load. *American Journal of Physiology, 250,* 1986, F551–F558.

Snowdon, C.T. & Sanderson, B.A. Lead pica produced in rats. *Science, 183,* 1974, 92–94.

Stricker, E.M. Thirst and sodium appetite after colloid treatment in rats with septal lesions. *Behavioral Neuroscience, 98,* 1984, 356–360.

Stricker, E.M. & Sterritt, G.M. Osmoregulation in the newly hatched domestic chick. *Physiology & Behavior, 2,* 1967, 117–119.

Stricker, E.M. & Verbalis, J.G. Hormones and behavior: The biology of thirst and sodium appetite. *American Scientist, 76,* 1988, 261–267.

Travers, J.B. & Norgren, R. Electromyographic analysis of the ingestion and rejection of sapid stimuli in the rat. *Behavioral Neuroscience, 100,* 1986, 544–555.

Vermeer, D.E. & Ferrell, R.E., Jr. Nigerian geophagical clay: A traditional anti-diarrheal pharmaceutical. *Science, 227,* 1985, 634–636.

Walsh, L.L. & Grossman, S.P. Electrolytic lesions and knife cuts in the region of the zona incerta impair sodium appetite. *Physiology & Behavior, 18,* 1977, 587–596.

Weisinger, R.S., Denton, D.A., McKinley, M.J., & Nelson, J.F. ACTH induced sodium appetite in the rat. *Pharmacology Biochemistry, & Behavior, 8,* 1978, 339–342.

Wilson, T.W. History of salt supplies in West Africa and blood pressures today. *The Lancet, 8484,* 1986, 784–785.

Wolf, G., McGovern, J.F., & Dicara, L.V. Sodium appetite: some conceptual and methodological aspects of a model drive system. *Behavioral Biology, 10,* 1974, 27–42.

Wolf, G., Schulkin, J., & Simson, P.E. Multiple factors in the satiation of salt appetite. *Behavioral Neuroscience, 98,* 1984, 661–673.

Chapter 8

Glucose:
The Blood Sugar
Signal

Models of foraging behavior teach us that a general principle underlying mechanisms of hunger and satiety is the need to regulate a balance between energy input and output. The emphasis on caloric homeostasis does not preclude an analysis of individual nutrients. From historical and metabolic perspectives, glucose has been the prime focus as a putative feedback signal to receptors involved in the initiation or limitation of feeding.

When the environment places a greater demand on an individual's energy, carbohydrates are the first substrate to be depleted. On the other side of energy regulation, protection against excessive blood glucose occurs by conversion of carbohydrates to fat, and by increased combustion of carbohydrates. Mayer (1955) postulated the existence of glucoreceptors on mechanisms that act to integrate behavioral and humoral control of blood glucose levels. This glucostatic theory was not, however, the first systematic theory of feeding.

Prior to Mayer's analysis, Cannon (1963) had proposed an account of the control of feeding based upon stomach contractions. This theory was supplanted in the 1940s and 1950s with a dual-center model, based upon stereotaxic manipulation of the ventral hypothalamus. This model held that the lateral hypothalamic area was a "hunger center," while the ventromedial area was a "satiety center." Additional support accrued for this model when it was shown that these areas of the hypothalamus could sense levels of blood glucose, and that gold thioglucose seemed to destroy ventromedial areas preferentially. Investigators later found little support that administration of glucose directly to the hypothalamus had direct effects on feeding. Moreover, electrical stimulation of "feeding" areas produced stimulus-bound gnawing and drinking. As Novin (1985) has reviewed, a third model developed when it became clear that (1) these hypothalamic areas may not be "centers" in the classic sense; and (2) peripheral organs that regulate glucose homeostasis may provide key signals for the behavioral counterpart of the regulation.

As Novin has indicated, it is now recognized that the optimal utilization and storage of nutrients involve an orchestrated action of the alimentary tract, viscera, and brain. Recent evidence has explicated the brain's control of feeding, and shown its interactions with viscera through the autonomic nervous system. Increased understanding of this coordination has led to improved theory and treatment for two pathologic conditions associated with blood sugar and mechanisms of hunger: diabetes mellitus and obesity.

*B*iochemistry and Physiology

Glycolysis

The pathways of glycolysis occur with only minor variation in most forms of life, indicating evolutionary conservation of this important energy-yielding pathway. As Figure 8.1 shows, glycolysis occurs in two major stages. In the first stage, two ATP molecules are expended to phosphorylate the 1 and 6 positions of the hexose, thus providing it with a favorable energy configuration for further breakdown. This stage has been termed one of collection, because a number of different hexoses are all transformed by these pathways to glyceraldehyde 3-phosphate. In the second stage of glycolysis—a common pathway for all sugars—four molecules of ATP are formed, leaving a net yield of two ATP molecules per hexose unit.

The first step in the breakdown of glucose is the formation of glucose

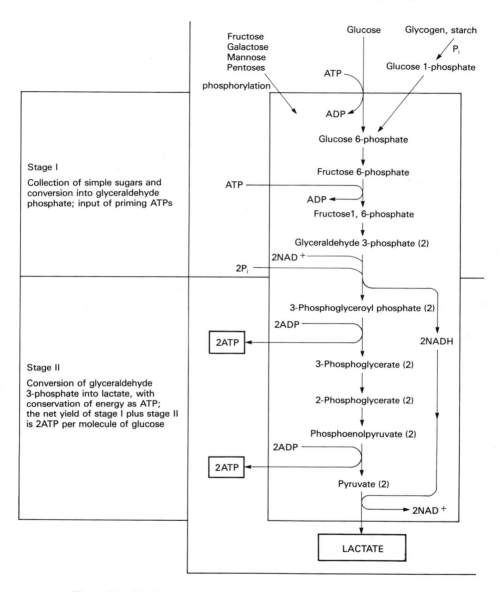

Figure 8.1 Biochemical steps in the sequence of glycolysis. (From Lehninger, 1976.)

6-phosphate. This step is catalyzed by either hexokinase or glucokinase, which enzymes differ in their distribution and sugar specificity. Hexokinase is the more widely distributed in tissues, and acts on many hexoses and hexose derivatives. Glucokinase, which is present in liver but not in muscle or adipose tissue, shows a much greater specificity for glucose. In liver, this enzyme has a lower K_m than does hexokinase, is not inhibited by its phosphorylated product, and has a maximal activity 15 times greater than hexokinase. Both hexokinase and glucokinase require manganese or magnesium, suggesting an interaction between the individual's energy metabolism and the nutrient status of these metals.

Prior to the second addition of an energy-rich phosphate, glucose 6-phosphate is converted to fructose 6-phosphate by the action of glucose phosphate isomerase, which is specific for substrate and product, and proceeds in either direction. The second phosphate addition produces fructose 1,6-diphosphate by the action of 6-phosphofructokinase. This enzyme is regulated in part by concentration of ATP, which, when high, slows the reaction.

The hexose diphosphate is then cleaved to form two triose phosphates: glyceraldehyde 3-phosphate and dihydroxyacetone phosphate. The former continues along the glycolytic pathway, but the latter can be converted to glyceraldehyde 3-phosphate by the action of an isomerase. The second stage of glycolysis is now ready to begin.

Glyceraldehyde 3-phosphate is then oxidized by its dehydrogenase. The other important component of this reaction is NAD^+. The product is 3-phosphoglyceroylphosphate, which is now the substrate for a reaction with ADP, catalyzed by phosphoglycerate kinase. From this reaction, 2 molecules of ATP are formed. The product, 3-phosphoglycerate, proceeds in the next reaction to transfer the position of the phosphate. This particular reaction also requires magnesium. The 2-phosphoglycerate is then dehydrated by enolase, which also requires magnesium or manganese. The product, phosphoenolpyruvate, is converted to pyruvate by pyruvate kinase. This reaction also requires manganese or magnesium. In this reaction, 2 molecules of ADP are converted to 2 ATPs.

In the last step of glycolysis, pyruvate is converted to lactate by a dehydrogenase, regenerating NAD^+ in the process. The overall balance sheet for glycolysis thereby leaves 2 molecules of lactate, 2 molecules of ATP, and 2 molecules of water, for every molecule of glucose. The final reaction would therefore be: Glucose $+ 2P_i + 2ADP \Rightarrow 2$lactate $+ 2$ATP $+ 2H_2O$, where P_i is an inorganic orthophosphate.

Gluconeogenesis

Most of the reactions along the pathway from pyruvate to glucose 6-phosphate are catalyzed during a reversal of the glycolytic sequence by the same enzymes. Glycolysis, however, has three irreversible steps that cannot be utilized during gluconeogenesis (see Figure 8.2). It should not be surprising that these steps each involve interconversion of ADP and ATP, given that each reaction sequence must have a favorable energy.

The first of these alternate steps is the phosphorylation of pyruvate to

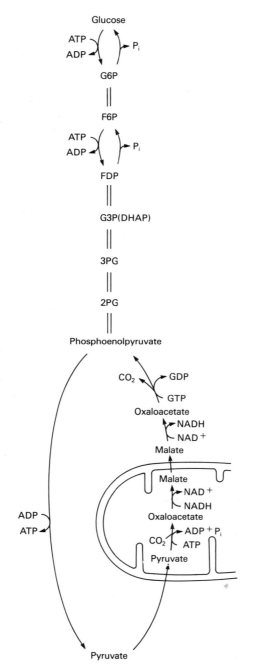

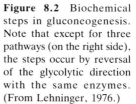

Figure 8.2 Biochemical steps in gluconeogenesis. Note that except for three pathways (on the right side), the steps occur by reversal of the glycolytic direction with the same enzymes. (From Lehninger, 1976.)

phosphoenolpyruvate. This reaction sequence takes place in both cytosol and mitochondrial compartments of liver cells because the intermediate, oxaloacetate, is unable to pass through the mitochondrial membrane in the liver. It must be transformed first into malate, which can be transported into the cytosol. The malate is subsequently reoxidized to oxaloacetate before being converted to phosphoenolpyruvate. During this sequence, phosphate is liberated by the conversion of ATP to ADP, which reverses the energy flow from glycolysis.

The next set of interconversions from phosphoenolpyruvate to fructose 1,6-diphosphate occur by a reversal of the glycolytic sequence using the same enzymes at each step. The second major change in the gluconeogenic sequence now occurs in the transformation of the diphosphate into the monophosphate by the enzyme fructose diphosphatase, which liberates an inorganic orthophosphate. The conversion to glucose 6-phosphate then proceeds by the reverse of the glycolytic reaction.

The final liberation of the phosphate to form glucose does not occur by reversal of the kinase reaction, but is brought about by glucose 6-phosphatase and occurs mainly in the liver. This enzyme is dependent upon the presence of magnesium.

This pathway from pyruvate to glucose can incorporate precursors from the tricarboxylic acid cycle, which enter by undergoing oxidation to oxaloacetate. This biochemical pathway for glucose formation becomes more important during fasting or other means of glucose loss. For example, when rats are fasted or given a drug that blocks glucose reabsorption by the kidney, they form glucose with relative efficiency after being fed succinate or other tricarboxylic acid cycle intermediates. Under some conditions, gluconeogenesis can be promoted by the transamination of amino acids into alpha-ketoglutarate and oxaloacetate, which then enter into the glucose formation sequence.

The important regulatory enzymes of the opposing biochemical sequences of glycolysis and gluconeogenesis are controlled largely by the energy state of the animal. When the energy charge is low and respiratory fuels are not readily available, the shift is to the acceleration of glycolysis and the inhibition of gluconeogenesis. When cells have ample levels of ATP or respiratory fuels, gluconeogenesis is promoted while glycolysis is inhibited. These shifts occur because the important regulatory enzymes in the opposing sequences do not catalyze reversible reactions at those particular steps in the sequence. The enzymes at those steps are different, thereby permitting independent regulation by various products and cofactors.

Systemic

Contact and interaction of the biological system with nutrients is considered to begin with chemoreception in the olfactory and oral cavities. Alimentation, digestion, absorption, and transport then follow. As a nutrient signal, glucose appears to have an effect on the organism's subsequent behavior at each of these steps along the interaction. In the discussion of behavior in this chapter, we will consider chemoreception and alimentation as factors in the control of blood glucose. Examination of the visceral factors in the control of blood glucose and of behavior presently follows.

Stomach and gut.   Prior to the focus on nutrients, Cannon's model of feeding held that large stomach contractions produced "hunger pangs" and that quiescence of the stomach produced "satiety." With the failure of stomach denervation, or even removal, to affect feeding behavior in any significant way, the hypothesis fell into disrepute. More recently, Deutsch (1982) revived the hypothesis, showing that the stomach is a major source of signals controlling feeding. He showed that rats compensated for ingestion of a nutritive substance even if the ingesta was siphoned off by gastric cannulae, or prevented from leaving the stomach by inflation of a pyloric cuff. He also showed that vagotomy below the diaphragm abolishes satiety produced by gastric distention even if rats remain responsive to the satiety signals produced by nutrients. His work implied that nutrients need never be absorbed from food for satiety to be observed. What remains clear, however, in spite of these findings, is that nutrients, particularly glucose, play a strong role in the control of ingestive behavior.

Glucose per se is rarely ingested. It is usually present as a moiety within a larger saccharide chain. Sucrose, for example, is a disaccharide containing residues of glucose and fructose (Figure 8.3). Moreover, sugars are typically present in foods with substantial quantities of other nutrients and non-nutritive substances. Although glucose is readily absorbed, its presence in larger complexes together with other nutrients delays its entry into the bloodstream to some extent, especially in comparison with direct gastric or duodenal infusion. When glucose (0.3 M) is infused into the duodenum of rabbits or rats at a relatively slow rate (1 ml/min) to mimic a more natural absorption, the animals show decreased subsequent food intake.

Food and nutrient stimuli in the small intestine release a gut peptide called cholecystokinin (CCK), which, when administered experimentally into the peritoneum, produces a strong signal for satiety. This satiety mechanism is dependent upon signals from the vagus; abdominal vagotomy eliminates the signal.

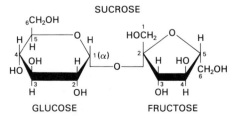

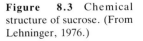

Figure **8.3** Chemical structure of sucrose. (From Lehninger, 1976.)

Once absorbed into the bloodstream, glucose has a variety of effects. After it is transported to various tissues, it is glycolized to produce ATP in energy-needy systems. As for being a signal to limit hunger, a number of glucose-receptive and -sensitive sites are candidates to transduce the nutrient signal into a behavioral one.

Liver. One prime candidate is the liver. The liver is the principal organ of storage in the post-absorptive period. It functions to maintain blood glucose and other nutrient levels during the interval between meals. Early in starvation the liver is the body's only endogenous source of glucose and ketone bodies.

Glucose is transported into the liver by a carrier-mediated mechanism. In contrast to adipose tissue and muscle, however, the transport system for glucose in the liver is not as sensitive to insulin. This transport system operates quite rapidly, thus acting to equalize the concentration of glucose inside and outside of cells. Glucose uptake by the liver is therefore determined primarily by the rate of further metabolism.

Other humoral factors regulate the liver's control of glucose. For example, fight or flight reactions require quick mobilization of glucose. Epinephrine, released by the adrenal medulla, is able to mobilize considerable amounts of glucose quickly through an amplification cascade in liver cells (Figure 8.4). Through a series of catalyzed phosphorylations, each epinephrine molecule can release approximately 3 million glucose molecules. Moreover, epinephrine also inhibits glycogen synthesis, thus directing action toward glucose availability.

In addition to epinephrine, glucagon is a glycogenolytic hormone. Glucagon, a polypeptide hormone of the pancreas, is secreted by the alpha cells of the islets of Langerhans whenever the blood glucose level drops below a normal baseline level. Similarly to epinephrine, glucagon acts through a phosphorylation cascade, but unlike epinephrine its effect is limited primarily to liver cells. Because the stimulus for glucagon release is a drop in blood glucose levels, it is considered to be the hormone that counterbalances insulin, which causes the opposite effect on blood glucose by facilitating its uptake into tissues.

Vagal afferents in the liver are quite capable of encoding information about the status of glucose, since the firing rate of single vagal fibers varies inversely with the concentration of blood glucose. Information about blood glucose, encoded by vagal fibers in the liver, reaches the brain's gustatory system via vagal connections with the nucleus tractus solitarius (NTS). Coordination with gustatory information about sugars is thus possible (see discussion of behavior).

Infusion of 2-deoxyglucose, a glucose analogue, produces glucoprivation because, while recognized and taken up as glucose by cells, it can not be fully metabolized as glucose. Infusions of 2-deoxyglucose into the hepatic portal system increase feeding far more effectively and with shorter latency than

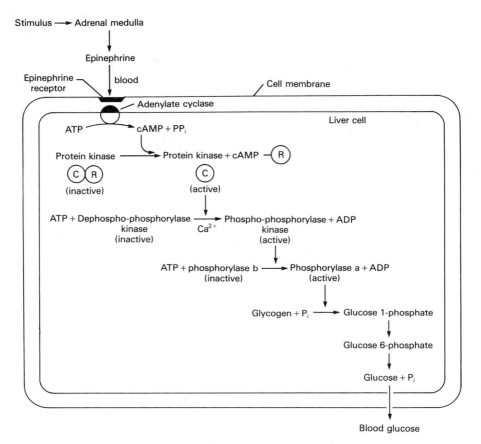

Figure 8.4   Epinephrine stimulation of glycogenolysis by amplification cascade in liver cells. (From Lehninger, 1976.)

similar infusions into the jugular vein. This result suggests that a decrease in glucose delivery to the liver may provide a "hunger" signal. Moreover, elimination of signals from the liver by vagotomy or by direct current blockade attenuates food intake produced by liver glucoprivation or food deprivation.

As an organ of satiety, the liver is less effective when it is isolated experimentally than when considered along with organs of taste, alimentation, and digestion. Glucose infusion directly into the liver has minimal suppressive effects on subsequent glucose intake. The elevation of blood glucose levels by oral intake, or by gastric or duodenal infusion, has much greater suppressive effects than glucose infusion into the bloodstream.

These findings, however, show some variation between species and experiments. In contrast to rats, food-deprived dogs show a reliable suppression of food intake when glucose is administered into the hepatic portal vein. Administration of epinephrine to the hepatic portal system, which also mobilizes a considerable amount of glucose, suppresses food intake. Moreover, mobilization of glucose by administration of pancreatic glucagon also suppresses food intake, but only when the glycogen content of the liver is relatively high, as occurs during less active times in the rat's daily cycle.

Of these two hormones that mobilize glucose, glucagon has more relevance to feeding. This relative importance can be seen upon hepatic vagotomy, which eliminates glucagon's suppressive result but has no effect on epinephrine's suppression. Moreover, glucagon may itself have a suppressive effect independent of glucose. Injection of antibodies to glucagon into the peritoneal cavity increases meal size and duration at the onset of the first meal after deprivation, without affecting the prandial increase in portal vein blood glucose, which suggests that glucagon is necessary for the normal termination of meals.

Russek (1976) has proposed a theoretical equation of intake control based upon liver glucoreceptors. The equation takes into account the robust inverse linear correlations between food intake and (1) the hepatic concentration of reducing sugars; (2) concentration of liver glycogen; (3) hepatocyte membrane potential; and (4) the calculated glucose output. The equation neatly predicts the food intake of an animal under various experimental manipulations that produce a real change in feeding. For example, when all the variables present in a satiated animal are calculated, the equation gives a small negative number for the food intake value. The equation will further respond with a small increase in feeding to dilution of body fluids and to insulin, and with a large increase in food intake as a response to cooling. These changes correspond with experimental findings.

Developmental evidence also exists for the liver's involvement in the glucose regulation of feeding. Rats first suppress feeding to glucose on day 14 of life. The liver and gut enzymes glucokinase and hexokinase appear at about this time (14-16 days). This finding provided the strongest developmental correlation showing a relationship between the appearance of nutrient suppression of feeding and the onset of liver and gut enzymes for utilization. The onset of glucoprivic feeding produced by 2-deoxyglucose did not occur until the rats reached 30 days, suggesting developmental delineation of two separate systems of "hunger" and "satiety."

Pancreatic islets and adrenal medulla.   From the point of view of hormones, fuel homeostasis is considered to be controlled by opposing actions of secretion products of the islets of Langerhans. Insulin, which engenders fuel availability, is secreted by beta cells lying deep within the islet. Insulin regulates and directs movement of exogenous fuels into cells for storage or subsequent liberation of energy. Alpha cells in the outer layer of the islets secrete glucagon when exogenous fuels are not present. These cells therefore regulate production of endogenous fuels (e.g., glucose), principally through glucagon's action on the liver.

The islets might be viewed as a complete organ, responsible for fuel distribution in the organism. Islet cells act as a coupled unit, releasing more insulin than glucagon during times of exogenous fuel excess (i.e., meals), and more glucagon than insulin when endogenous fuel production is needed. Sensing the individual's fuel status appears to be done by glucoreceptors on islet cells. This view of the islets' function, however, must be tempered by knowledge of their interaction with other systems. Pancreatic vagotomy, for example, decreases levels of plasma insulin in adrenalectomized rats, and electrical stimulation of the pancreatic vagus increases levels of insulin, which in turn lowers blood carbohydrates. A vagal mechanism therefore modulates the secretion of insulin.

Insulin, in addition to lowering blood glucose, provokes a compensatory response from the adrenal medulla. Epinephrine is released, stimulating hepatic glucose output (i.e., glycogenolysis). Fructose, a hexose that cannot cross the blood brain barrier or be oxidized in brain, cannot suppress the rise in epinephrine secretion, which suggests that the compensatory reaction to insulin may originate in the CNS. But the behavioral result of administration of insulin—an increase in feeding—is abolished by fructose, which suggests a normal peripheral effect of hexoses, most likely in the liver.

An interesting response in the adrenal medulla during fasting dissociates the sympathetic, energy-using component associated with epinephrine release from the compensatory action of epinephrine on the liver. The Landsberg group (Young et al., 1984) has shown that hypoglycemia leads to a suppression of the sympathetic nervous system (SNS) in virgin and pregnant rats, but there is clear evidence for adrenal medullary stimulation during fasting. The suppression of the SNS, with the consequent decrease in metabolic rate, contributes to a conservation of calories at a time of diminished energy intake. The small amounts of epinephrine released are unlikely to affect thermogenesis, but can greatly stimulate glycogenolysis through amplification in liver cells, thus supporting the mobilization of substrates without increasing the expenditure of energy.

Adrenal cortex.   Glucocorticoids from the adrenal cortex are under secretory control by adrenocorticotropic hormone (ACTH) from the anterior pituitary, which is controlled by humoral factors released from the medial basal hypothalamus. The principal glucocorticoid, corticosterone, is highly active in the induction of enzymes involved in gluconeogenesis in the liver, particularly the enzyme that converts oxaloacetate to phosphoenolpyruvate. Glucocorticoids are also important for the induction of enzymes required to convert the carbon skeletons of specific amino acids into glucose (e.g., tyrosine aminotransferase).

Circadian rhythms, entrained by light, are expressed through the hypothalamo-pituitary-adrenocortical axis to produce a rhythm in corticosterone output. The glucocorticoid rhythm coincides with the rhythm in blood glucose levels, both of which correspond to variation in feeding behavior. Indeed, behavior and hormonal physiology appear to combine to mobilize fuels during an animal's active period.

Honma's (1984) data illustrate the correspondence. The principal peak in corticosterone appears to be related to the time span in controlled feeding from the preceding meal. The hormone level spontaneously peaks about 20 hours after the first meal following a fast. When the time span to the next meal is less than 20 hours, the hormone rise is masked by the preceding meal and is not manifest. When that time span is greater than 30 hours, the hormone rise is far ahead of the following meal. When the feeding cycle is within the 24 hour (circadian) range, there is a self-sustaining oscillation in corticosterone. Thus, there is normally a prefeeding hormone peak, which would serve to mobilize fuels just prior to exogenous intake, producing a generalized rise in blood glucose to coincide with the onset of the active period.

Central Nervous System

A number of arguments suggest that visceral factors are more important than central factors to the regulation of feeding by glucose. The principal argument, according to Stricker and McCann (1985), is that the increased food intake of hypoglycemic rats is inhibited by intravenous infusion of fructose, a hexose that cannot nourish cells in the CNS. Several observations support this argument. First, gastric emptying increases during hypoglycemia induced by insulin, and this effect is eliminated by the administration of fructose. Furthermore, hepatic vagotomy abolishes this inhibitory effect of fructose. Second, gastric emptying decreases in rats with severe diabetes, as in intact rats, in proportion to an increasing dose of a glucose load. Calories empty in these rats, however, more rapidly than normal, regardless of the concentration of the load. Finally, rats with varying degrees of chemical damage of the pancreatic islets eat more food than intact rats after an overnight fast; individual intakes are proportional to the induced glucose intolerance (i.e., the inability of the animals to secrete insulin in response to a glucose load). These observations support the hypothesis that food intake is controlled by satiety signals related to delivery of utilizable calories to the liver.

Mayer's glucostatic theory holds that increased utilization of glucose is sensed by glucoreceptors that act to inhibit feeding. Conversely, decreased glucose utilization should activate feeding. Considerable evidence, however, indicates that direct infusions of glucose into the CNS, particularly in the ventromedial (VM) hypothalamus, do not inhibit feeding in the short term but reduce food intake over periods longer than 19 hours. Moreover, direct infusions of 2-deoxyglucose into the VM hypothalamus are ineffective in eliciting feeding. However, when 2-deoxyglucose is injected into the lateral ventricles, producing a more general neuroglucopenia, robust feeding results.

These observations support the concept of multiple kinds of "hunger," as well as multiple limitors that produce "satiety." This is not to mention that many of the early studies focused on a global concept of food intake, whereas it is now recognized that appetites for particular nutrients exist. These individual appetites may have impelled animals to eat a composite food when such a food was the only one available in these studies. Moreover, the logic extends to satiety: If there are different appetites for individual nutrients, there must also be a limitor for each of these nutrients.

The glucostatic dual center hypothesis (Figure 8.5) was based on observations regarding ventromedial (VM) and lateral hypothalamic (LH) areas. The original findings were that damage to VM nuclei can disinhibit feeding and produce obesity, while destruction of LH areas reduces feeding and a variety of other regulatory processes. The notion that these feeding "centers" operate on a regulatory signal provided by glucose was strengthened by experiments with gold thioglucose, a substance that is taken up by glucose-receptive sites and destroys them with its toxic effect. In these experiments, peripheral administration of gold thioglucose resulted in a relatively selective

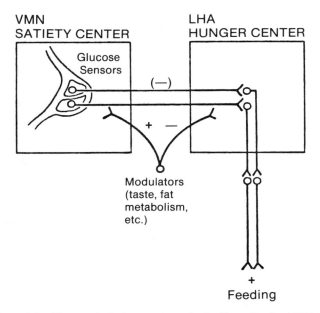

Figure 8.5   Glucostatic dual center hypothesis. (From Novin, 1985.)

destruction of VM hypothalamic neurons. Subsequent electrophysiological experiments identified glucose sensitive neurons in the LH, as well as in the VM hypothalamus. These neurons sensitive to glucose were further shown to be directly receptive to glucose upon iontophoresis, which altered their activity.

The model suffered, however, upon increasing recognition that the concept of "center" was misleading. The hidden assumption in the adoption of the concept, possibly based on the utilization of cell-staining methods, was that clusters of brain cells have discrete function. Two principal areas of intense research converged to invalidate this assumption, thereby defeating the concept. First, the concept of *interconnectedness* emphasized circuits and entire pathways from sensory reception to production of behavior. This research contributed to the notion that large scale destruction of "centers" disrupts fibers that pass through these areas en route to other functionally important areas of the brain. For example, destruction of substantia nigra, or of its dopamine fibers that pass through the LH en route to the striatum, results in aphagia and adipsia much like that produced by destruction of the LH.

The second area of research, in *neural plasticity*, emphasized the regenerative potential of the brain and thereby challenged the notion that these centers were the sole source of a function. For example, "recovered" VM damaged animals can still respond normally to homeostatic challenges.

If we conceive of the regulation of feeding and energy homeostasis as engaging multiple systems with redundant rerepresentations, it becomes easy to emphasize the importance of each of these systems without specifying the locus of control. Thus, we are not saying that feeding is controlled by the stomach, the liver, or the hypothalamus. We then no longer neglect the importance of any system when its destruction fails to abolish control of the behavior. Systems can be recognized for the input they contribute to the whole.

VMH and LH.   The connectedness of central and peripheral systems in the control of glucose regulation can be seen especially upon stimulation of various sites. Stimulation of VM areas results in an increase in activity of one of the key gluconeogenic enzymes—phosphoenolpyruvate carboxykinase—and a decrease in the liver glycolytic enzyme, pyruvate kinase. It is no surprise, then, that such stimulation also produces a rapid rise in blood glucose. The disappearance of a dose of labeled glucose remains unaltered by such stimulation, indicating that the hyperglycemia is a result of hepatic glucose output. In terms of the coordination of systems, it is particularly interesting that despite hyperglycemia, plasma insulin remains at basal levels. This inhibition of a normal insulin response is eliminated by adrenalectomy.

Stimulation of the LH, on the other hand, decreases the activity of the carboxykinase, and is ineffective in producing a change in glucose output.

However, when current is passed through LH electrodes that have previously been shown to elicit feeding, a distinctive biphasic hyperglycemia can be blocked by methods that suppress the action of epinephrine, indicating that this hyperglycemia results from glycogenolysis. Continual stimulation of these LH-feeding sites produces excessive food intake and obesity, with the accompanying rise in blood glucose, but no change in plasma insulin during stimulation. If food is withheld during stimulation, there is still a large increase in blood glucose, but now a decrease in insulin level. Thus, the control of blood glucose by the LH appears to be independent of the control of insulin release.

It is also instructive to look at the single-unit activity of neurons in the hypothalamus in relation to nutrients, particularly glucose, that normally affect feeding. An increase in ambient glucose alters the activity of a sizable proportion of VM neurons, primarily in the direction of facilitation. This finding supports the theory that views VM hypothalamus as participating in satiety. Norepinephrine (NE), which usually stimulates feeding, inhibits VM "satiety" neurons. The interaction between signals provided by NE and by glucose is seen in the related finding that NE affects more neurons responsive than unresponsive to glucose.

The link between VM hypothalamus and adrenocortical mechanisms was especially emphasized by Dallman (1984). Glucocorticoids generally stimulate appetite and promote glucose production. The primary "job" of the VM hypothalamus is to inhibit food intake, insulin secretion, and adrenocortical function. Lesions to these neurons result in nonrhythmic food intake, hyperinsulinemia, nonrhythmic adrenocortical function, and obesity. Adrenalectomy prevents or reverses these effects of VM lesions; replacement with corticosterone restores them.

The LH and VM hypothalamus may be responsive to substances other than glucose or the classic hormones that have an effect on feeding. In particular, Oomura (1986) performed analyses of the blood of fasted rats, and revealed two endogenous sugar acids that might be related to the control of food intake. These substances, 2-deoxytetronic acid (2-DTA) and 3-deoxypentanoic acid (3-DPA), appear to have opposite functions. Injection of 2-DTA into the third ventricle reduces food intake for 24 hours in rats deprived of food for 72 hours. It also depresses single-unit activity in the lateral hypothalamus, which is in keeping with theories of LH function. In contrast, the same amounts of 3-DPA elicit feeding at levels dependent upon dose, and increase unit activity in the LH. Moreover, electrophoretic application of these sugar acids produces suppression (2-DTA) and excitation (3-DPA) only in LH neurons sensitive to glucose, indicating a system coordinated with the monitoring of glucose. In the VM hypothalamus, the effects of these sugar acids were simply reversed. These findings by Oomura give credence to the notion that 2-DTA may be an endogenous satiety substance, while 3-DPA may be a hunger substance. As yet, unfortunately, the source(s) of production of these sugar acids is unknown.

Amygdala. The amygdala, as a site of reception for gustatory pathways, is also involved in feeding behavior and the monitoring of blood glucose. Glucose-sensitive neurons in the centromedial amygdala of the monkey decrease firing during a bar-pressing response on which the availability of food is contingent. Normally, glucose-sensitive neurons in the amygdala are identified by their decrease in activity in response to glucose. Feeding behavior and body weight of rats are altered after neurochemical damage to the amygdala. Manipulations that produce a high DA/NE ratio result in increases in body weight and feeding, while low ratios are associated with the opposite effects.

Brainstem. Evidence shows that while forebrain mechanisms are important in the control of feeding, they are not essential. In decerebrate rats, in which the experimental cut has eliminated the contribution from all neural mechanisms forward to the brainstem, insulin treatment still produces hypoglycemia and enhances ingestion of sucrose, but does not augment water consumption. Taste reflexes also are the same in decerebrate and intact rats, which suggests that the caudal brainstem is the neural substrate of ingestion and rejection responses. Infusion of 5-thioglucose (5-TG), a recognizable glucose like 2-DG that can not be fully metabolized, into either the lateral or fourth cerebral ventricles results in increased feeding and hyperglycemia. If the cerebral aqueduct is obstructed so that the lateral ventricles cannot communicate with the fourth ventricle in the hindbrain, infusion of 5-TG into the lateral ventricles has no effect. Under these conditions, however, 5-TG in the fourth ventricle still increases feeding and blood glucose levels. These results further suggest that glucoreceptors mediating feeding and hyperglycemia in response to glucoprivation are located in the caudal hindbrain. Moreover, glucose infused into the cisterna magna increases insulin in plasma, a response that is abolished by vagotomy. That these effects occur without significant changes in blood glucose suggests the importance of central glucoreceptors.

NE and the paraventricular hypothalamus. The regulation of nutrient intake and blood glucose has been linked to the activity of central NE systems, thus implicating phenylalanine and tyrosine in these mechanisms (see Chapter 4). From the vantage point of the periphery, infusion of nutrients directly to the duodenum alters the neurochemistry of the hypothalamus. Nutrient infusion enhances the synaptic release of NE in lateral sites, but suppresses it in medial hypothalamus, and this increased efflux is suppressed by the addition of glucose. Moreover, glucoprivation by administration of 2-DG enhances release of NE in these medial sites.

These observations are consistent with the results of NE infusion into the hypothalamus, as exemplified by the considerable body of data from the Leibowitz laboratory at The Rockefeller University. For the most part, infusion of NE into the LH attenuates eating in the deprived animal, whereas infusion into the medial hypothalamus elicits eating in the sated animal. Leibowitz has further delimited these findings.

In extensive mapping studies, she has shown that the paraventricular nucleus (PVN) in the hypothalamus (Figure 8.6) is the most sensitive site for the elicitation of feeding by NE. Upon injection, both the rate of and the time spent feeding increase. The lateral perifornical hypothalamus is the most sensitive site for injections of NE to suppress feeding in hungry animals. Furthermore, this lab has shown that postsynaptic α_2-adrenergic receptors mediate feeding induced by PVN injections of NE or by the agonist clonidine. In particular, the feeding response is blocked by α_2 antagonists, but is unaffected by other specific receptor antagonists.

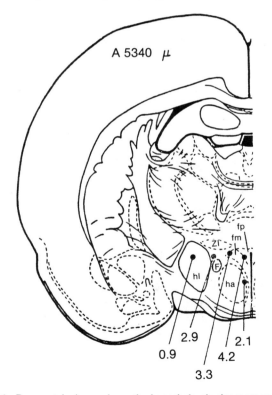

Figure 8.6 Paraventricular nucleus, the hypothalamic site most sensitive to NE's stimulatory effects on feeding. (From Leibowitz, 1978.)

This feeding response, elicited by NE activity in the PVN, is especially important in the control of carbohydrate regulation. Animals injected with NE in the PVN, and presented with 3 pure nutrients—carbohydrate, fat, and protein—show enhanced consumption of the carbohydrate, with little or no feeding on fat or protein. In fact, animals increase consumption of carbohydrate whether or not the substance is sweet, and prefer sucrose to saccharin. Indeed, the "feeding" response to injections of NE in the PVN may really be a carbohydrate response.

It is particularly interesting that the principal gluconeogenic hormone, corticosterone, is necessary for the full expression of the NE feeding response. Food consumption elicited by injection of NE into the PVN is severely attenuated by adrenalectomy or hypophysectomy. Replacement with corticosterone, but not with mineralocorticoids or sex steroids, restores the NE feeding response. In fact, the feeding response to PVN injections of NE is also dependent upon the endogenous rhythm of corticosterone production, occurring with greater strength at the onset of the dark phase, at which time corticosterone is reaching its natural peak, and when the animal is most vigorously seeking food. Moreover, this is also a time when α_2 NE receptor activity is at its highest in the PVN. Peripheral and central systems thus coordinate the intake and production of glucose at the phase of the cycle when the animals are most active.

A relationship between hypothalamic NE activity and blood glucose independent of the effects of corticosterone also exists. Activation of hypothalamic NE activity following stress is associated with concurrent increase in plasma glucose, even when the animals are adrenalectomized or hypophysectomized (with the epinephrine mechanism left intact). Glucose, however, may be acting to inhibit hypothalamic NE responses to stress; there is an inverse relationship between glucose and NE under other conditions. In fact, glucoprivation by 2-DG increases NE activity in the medial hypothalamus. Thus, there appears to be a monitored relationship between hypothalamic NE and blood glucose. Moreover, increased NE activity caused by 2-DG results in a hyperglycemia that is dependent upon sympathetic innervation of the viscera, but is not dependent upon corticosterone production.

Recent work in the Leibowitz laboratory (Chafetz et al. 1986) focused on the relationships between circulating glucose and the activity of the α_2 receptor. Specifically, we were interested in whether alterations in serum glucose levels might affect the receptors, thereby altering a system responsible for the intake of carbohydrates. We first showed that food deprivation produces a specific relationship between blood sugar levels and hypothalamic α_2 receptor activity: the lower the blood sugar levels, the lower the receptor activity. Then, by utilizing tolbutamide, a potent hypoglycemic agent that acts by releasing insulin, we were able to show that specific manipulation of blood glucose resulted in a direct effect on receptor activity: Decreases in blood glucose produced by this method lowered the rate of α_2 binding. Furthermore, by administering glucose along with tolbutamide, we were able to block the reduction of receptor activity, which indicated that the effect was specific to glucose.

Considerable work suggests that fluctuation of endogenous glucose provides a clear signal for feeding. For example, a 3-hour deprivation period induces a fall in blood glucose that differs not only between night and day but between the beginning and the end of daytime. There is a high correlation between subsequent intake and the time-dependent fall in blood glucose. From these observations, it can be concluded that rats eat at a rate just required to prevent hypoglycemia under conditions of plentiful food. After food deprivation, they increase this rate of feeding to correct the fall in blood glucose, perhaps to reestablish the supply of glucose to tissues.

By using continuous measurement of glucose in free-feeding rats, Campfield et al. (1985) have been able to provide a finer analysis of glucose. They have shown that blood glucose declines only a few minutes prior to a meal, and that a meal is initiated just as the glucose concentration is beginning to return to baseline. That the premeal decline in glucose is causally related to the initation of a meal is suggested by the "glucose clamp" experiments, in which glucose is infused during the continuous measurement of behavior and blood glucose. Such an infusion partially blocks the premeal decline in blood glucose and delays the subsequent meal. The time element in these studies is entirely consistent with the short time it took in our experiments for tolbutamide both to lower levels of blood glucose and to alter receptor activity.

Figure 8.7 summarizes our model of NE regulation of feeding and blood glucose. A fall in blood glucose, the critical signal prior to a meal, stimulates carbohydrate feeding by increasing the activity of NE systems, affecting in turn endocrine and autonomic systems that regulate blood glucose. As a consequence of this increased turnover and release of NE, the α_2 receptors in the hypothalamus are down-regulated. This is why a decrease in receptor activity is measured when glucose falls; it is a consequence of the monitoring of glucose by NE.

With regard to drugs that affect NE systems, work from the laboratory of Paul and Skolnick (Angel et al., 1985; Hauger et al., 1986) suggests a

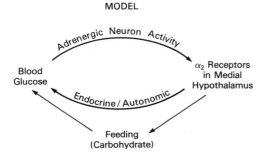

MODEL

Adrenergic Neuron Activity

Blood Glucose

α_2 Receptors in Medial Hypothalamus

Endocrine / Autonomic

Feeding (Carbohydrate)

Figure 8.7   Model of findings showing interactions between blood glucose, hypothalamic NE activity, and α_2-receptor binding. (From Chafetz et al., 1986.)

regulation of feeding and blood glucose. Amphetamine, which is a strong inhibitor of food intake, binds to specific receptors in hypothalamic slices. The addition of d-glucose, but not l-glucose or 2-DG, to the binding medium, or when administered parenterally to the rat, results in a dose- and time-dependent stimulation of amphetamine binding. Poisoning of the energy-dependent regulatory enzyme for cellular Na and K (Na/K ATPase) regulation with ouabain inhibits the glucose stimulation of amphetamine binding. Moreover, incubation of hypothalamic slices with glucose increases Na/K ATPase activity, a result also obtained by administering doses of amphetamine that produce anorexia. The data suggest that amphetamine binding to specific sites in the hypothalamus, linked to mechanisms controlling food intake, is regulated by glucose. The mechanism appears to entail an energy-dependent enzyme that hydrolyzes the net energy product of glycolysis.

Serotonin

Activation of serotonin (5-HT) receptors, by administration of 5-HT or its precursors, or of 5-HT agonists, reduces eating in food-deprived animals. In Chapter 3, we noted that this reduced food intake may be specific for carbohydrates. Studies by the Wurtman (1979) laboratory suggested that insulin secretion, stimulated by food intake and rising blood glucose, facilitates the entry of amino acids into peripheral tissues, except for tryptophan, which is bound to albumin. The relative rise in plasma tryptophan increases the brain's uptake of tryptophan and its consequent production of 5-HT, which then depresses carbohydrate intake, the initial stimulus for the mechanism. Recent studies in the Leibowitz lab have shown that 5-HT is active in the PVN to depress food intake, suggesting a balance in control of food intake by NE and 5-HT innervation of the hypothalamus.

Dopamine and the Striatum

The behavioral syndrome immediately following damage to the LH includes global motivational inertia and decreased vigilance. Interaction with all biologically relevant stimuli—including food, water, temperature, and other animals—diminishes. Destruction of the LH, however, does not destroy only a small group of neurons located at the electrode tip. Dopamine (DA) fibers originating in the substantia nigra pass through the LH en route to the striatum. Destruction of substantia nigra cells, or of the DA fibers passing through the LH, results in a behavioral syndrome essentially similar to that produced by LH destruction.

As an animal feeds, efflux of DA in the striatum increases. This increased DA output may in part be influenced by insulin, which produces an immediate rise in DA efflux upon administration. The hypothesis that central DA mechanisms mediate positive reinforcement with various stimuli, particularly the natural rewards of food and sweet solutions in food-deprived animals, is especially relevant. Selective receptor antagonists of the D_2 subclass of dopamine receptors decrease the sham intake of a sweet solution of 10% sucrose. These observations are consistent with the idea that dopaminergic activation of a central D_2 receptor is necessary for the positive reinforcing effect of sucrose.

DA fibers also innervate the perifornical hypothalamus (PFH), where injections of DA suppress feeding in animals deprived of food. The ingestion of food may stimulate the release of DA, not only initiating the reinforcing properties of food but also setting into motion mechanisms acting to control subsequent intake.

Acetylcholine

Cholinergic activation of muscarinic receptors in the CNS plays a role in the regulation of hepatic glucose output. Agonists of the muscarinic acetylcholine (ACh) receptor, when injected into the third ventricle, cause a dose-dependent increase in hepatic venous glucose concentration, which is suppressed in a dose-dependent way by atropine. Injection of cholinesterase inhibitors, which increase endogenous levels of ACh, result in increased levels of glucagon, epinephrine, and NE in hepatic venous plasma. The elevation of glucose does not occur in adrenalectomized rats, suggesting that ACh may act through autonomic mechanisms controlling epinephrine secretion, which then acts directly on the liver to increase glucose output.

Behavior

Wyrwicka (1969) has asked: Why does an animal eat over and above caloric needs and become obese when palatable food is available (for example, on pig farms)? Or: Why does an animal refuse to eat less palatable food in spite of a need for nutrients? The answers, she suggests, may lie in the hedonistic aspect of eating related to the oro-pharyngeal contact with food.

As reviewed in Chapter 7, information about taste qualities of food arrives at the rostral end of the NTS, which then projects to the parabrachial nucleus, and from there to other gustatory receptive areas, including the PVN of the hypothalamus. The NTS also receives visceral information (e.g., from the liver) via vagal connections to its more caudal regions. It is therefore a key player in linking oro-pharyngeal information about the tastes of food with visceral information about physiological conditions. As Novin et al. (1985) have shown, infusion of glucose into the liver alone has minor effects on subsequent glucose intake. Likewise, oral intake of glucose has minor effects on glucose intake. When these two signals—oral and liver glucose—are combined in the same experimental treatment, a reliable suppression of subsequent glucose intake occurs. These observations suggest that information provided by oro-pharyngeal contact with foods must be coordinated with visceral information to have effects on behavior.

This coordination may be seen in another way. The satiety effect of CCK released from the gut during ingestion may also act through oral factors. CCK does not inhibit intake of water until tastents are added. The inhibition of intake is related to the tastent concentration. For example, the magnitude of the suppression in ingestive behavior by CCK covaries with the concentration of sucrose. Because vagotomy blocks this effect, it is believed that coordination of gustatory and visceral factors in the NTS may play a role.

In addition to the coordination of oral and visceral factors, blood glucose may have a direct effect on NTS neurons to inhibit further gustation. A rise in blood glucose will depress NTS responses to sweet, salty, sour, and bitter tastes, with the largest depression of responses occurring to sweet (glucose) and salty tastes, and the least suppression to bitter tastes. Glucose may thus have a "short loop" mechanism for inhibiting further food intake by decreasing oral sensations.

Mechanisms in the oral cavity have a clear influence on insulin release. Measurement of blood glucose and insulin in undisturbed and free-moving rats support this. In the first minute after the start of food intake, insulin levels rise. Glucose levels begin to rise only in the third minute, suggesting that the prior rise in insulin is due to factors occurring prior to digestion (i.e., oral sensation). This suggestion is further supported by observations that the same early insulin release can be observed if carbohydrate-free food is used. Moreover, if the same quantity of food ingested orally is injected into the stomach in the same time it takes for the animals to eat the food, the insulin release is delayed consistent with the rise in blood glucose. The oral cavity thus plays a major role in an initial phase of insulin release.

In human subjects, lingual application of glucose produces a dose-dependent release of insulin. The magnitude of the insulin release produced by the α anomer is different from that produced by the β anomer in subjects who could not differentiate the sweetness of the two anomers. The recognition of sweetness per se is therefore unrelated to the release of insulin, which occurs in response to gustatory stimulation of vagal mechanisms.

Taste factors alone, especially for sugars, are important in the regulation of ingestion. Investigators have shown that the chorda tympani, the primary carrier of taste information, responds differently to different sugars. In the hamster, the order of effectiveness for sugars to elicit chorda tympani responses is: sucrose > fructose > glucose > maltose > galactose. With sham drinking, the relative preferences for solutions of these sugars closely parallels their effectiveness in eliciting these responses from the chorda tympani.

Beyond taste, oral somatosensory factors play a role in dietary selection.

When rats are subjected to partial trigeminal deafferentation, depriving them of somatosensation from the lower anterior portion of the oral cavity but leaving gustation and olfaction intact, intake of carbohydrates and proteins is reduced. Although protein intake recovers somewhat, the ratio of protein to total intake remains reduced. These animals are also impaired in their responses to nutritional stresses such as food deprivation; they do not increase their intakes as do controls.

Other oral factors are important in regulating ingestion. Rats that have drunk a concentrated glucose solution to satiety, and who will drink no more even if access is prolonged, will return to vigorous ingestion if offered carbohydrate powder or laboratory chow. This particular "glucose satiety" does not reflect orosensory factors per se, as it is maintained even when the initial glucose load is delivered directly to the stomach, bypassing oral stimuli. It is also not a response to palatability, as both chow and glucose power are less palatable than a glucose solution. The argument put forth by Mook and colleagues (1986) is that postingestive inhibition robs the solution of its reinforcing properties, so that the oral lapping behavior undergoes temporary extinction. Because a different food requires a different oral consummatory response (e.g., chewing), this response has not undergone extinction. A different food requiring a different oral response can thus reinstate ingestion, even in the face of "satiety" for the nutrient.

Stricker (1981) has argued that conditioning mechanisms may play a part in the initiation of feeding. You will recall considerable evidence that a drop in blood glucose immediately prior to a meal may be a strong signal for the initiation of that meal. From the evidence presented above, however, it is clear that oral factors prior to ingestion can produce a release of insulin. Taking this one step further, Stricker argues that thoughts about food ("intentions to eat") can be conditioned to these taste factors that normally invoke insulin release. Insulin release can thus be evoked by conditioning to these "intentions." In this case, intentions to eat actually precede the observed changes in glucose levels, and therefore could not be a consequence of such changes. In general, according to Stricker, hunger may be a result not only of relative strengths of satiety factors, but also of excitatory stimuli associated with food. These stimuli include the thought of food and its taste and smell, and would stimulate animals to seek and consume food unless strong signals of satiety are present to inhibit them.

*P*athologic Conditions

Obesity

A constancy of body weight in adults appears to be reestablished after occasional weight gain or loss. But as LeMagnen (1983) has suggested, and the data in this chapter have indicated, body weight is not regulated per se.

If that were true, astronauts would gain several hundred pounds after a few months under conditions of weightlessness. Obesity, a condition of high, relatively stable body weight, appears to be the product of intake, activity, and metabolism. Each of these factors may be influenced, according to McMinn (1984), by a variety of psychosocial and physiological factors.

Metabolically, caloric expenditure increases and food fuel efficiency decreases with overfeeding, so that less weight is gained than would be expected from a strict computation of energy balance. In an adult rat under steady conditions, the cumulative amount of food eaten in a given time matches its energy output plus the caloric cost of a small weight gain.

Studies of obesity have shown not only that genetically obese rodents have metabolic defects contributing to their obesity, but that humans have genetic tendencies for obesity. In genetically obese rodents, as opposed to their lean littermates, there is considerable elevation of pituitary ACTH, the hormone that controls corticosterone secretion from the adrenal cortex. Both ACTH and β-endorphin share a common precursor molecule, and there also are elevated levels of the endorphin in these animals. Corticosterone acts to increase glucose levels (and is permissive for other mechanisms of food intake), and endorphin acts to cause an increase in food intake. Moreover, β-endorphin also acts on the pancreas to stimulate the release of insulin, which contributes to the obesity. Courtney and Woods (1984) have found that vagotomy is able to prevent much of the weight gain of genetically obese rats, which suggests that the visceral signaling that provides behavioral and nutrient information to the animal is altered in obese individuals. Centrally, the levels of NE are altered in the hypothalami of obese rats, indicating that hypothalamic processes that influence food intake and body weight gain may be altered.

Stunkard and colleagues (1986a, 1986b) have provided strong evidence of the heritability of human obesity. They show that concordance rates for different degrees of being overweight are twice as high for monozygotic as for dizygotic twins. The genetic influence extends to height, weight, and a body-mass index. They also show a strong relationship between the weight class of adoptees and the body-mass index of biologic, but not adoptive, parents. This relationship extends across the whole range of body fatness. It is clear from these studies that family environment alone has no effect on obesity.

Fat and lean individuals also differ in their selection of diets. Many obese individuals consume more than half of their total daily calories as carbohydrates, predominately in the form of sweet snacks, especially during times of stress. There is recent evidence that sugar consumption leads to increased β-endorphin production, particularly in obese subjects. In rodents, there is evidence that obesity produced by a palatable diet is blocked by opiate antagonists (that block β-endorphin), suggesting that the stress-induced release of endorphins may enhance the intake of sweets, which in turn enhances the production of endorphins. Obesity thus results and continues from an inability to break what is apparently a pathologic cycle. A similar, self-reinforcing cycle has been noted by Novin (1984), who argued that overeating can lead to hyperinsulinemia. The greatly raised insulin level worsens the obesity by directing nutrients into fat storage, while retarding access to the stored fats. The tendency to eat is also increased because of the reduction of readily available nutrients.

Obese rats consistently select a diet higher in fat and lower in protein than the diets selected by lean rats, and the former generally eat more calories per day. Prior feeding of diets variable in protein content does not alter the selections of obese rats. In fact, when given access to sucrose, these animals increase their total caloric intake, independent of the protein content of the diet. Genetic obesity thus is more powerful in controlling food and caloric intake than is dietary history. This form of obesity, with concomitantly higher intake of dietary fat, appears to depend upon corticosterone production. Surgical removal of the adrenals lowers fat consumption in these obese rats, while corticosterone replacement restores it.

Humans appear to have an innate preference for sweet tastes, as well as an adult preference for high fat foods (somewhat resembling a rat's preference for a greasy diet). When 1-day-old infants are tested for their responses to sweet tastes, they consume more fluid when it is sweetened. When solutions are made sweeter by increasing the saccharide concentration, the infants respond by taking proportionately more of the solution. Moreover, "sweeter" sugars such as sucrose and fructose are more effective in eliciting consumption than are the "less sweet" sugars, glucose and lactose. When adults are tested, a similar response to sweet tastes occurs, indicating that a varied dietary experience does not alter the basic responsiveness to sweet tastes. Considerable individual variation occurs, however, not in the preferences for sweet tastes, but in the levels at which sweetness is preferred (preference-aversion function). Studies of twins indicate no evidence that these preference-aversion functions are under genetic control. Whatever mechanism establishes an individual's responses to sweets is apparently operating before birth, and it continues to set the individual's responses to sweets throughout development.

Alas, our preferences for fatty foods contribute no less to a behavioral tendency to overconsume. Indeed, the already high acceptance of high-fat dairy products is greatly enhanced by the addition of a small amount of sucrose. If a small amount of sucrose is added to a dairy product that has so much fat added as to be rated less "pleasant" than the same product with less fat (e.g., heavy cream with added oil), the ratings will change positively: the new taste will be rated as more pleasant. Apparently, the addition of sweet tastes to foods that are on the "aversive" side of an individual's hedonic ratings function can shift the function, thereby eliciting additional consumption.

With all the tendencies, predispositions, and self-reinforcing phenomena, whether there can be some measure of control imposed on the development of obesity remains as a question. It is beyond the scope of this work to discuss the enormous body of clinical literature on the topic. I will therefore include a few examples of metabolic and behavioral findings closely related to the discussion in this chapter.

Hirsch and his colleagues (Faust et al., 1977) at The Rockefeller University have shown that the metabolism of fat cells (adipocytes) is important in the development of obesity. There are apparently strong controls for the regulation of adipocyte size. In humans and rats who have undergone lipectomy, and in whom adipocyte size remains constant, there is less food consumption and body fat accumulation than in controls offered the same highly palatable diet. This work suggests that adipocyte resistance to enlargement is responsible at least in part for restraining excessive feeding and weight gain, and that an abnormality in this resistance contributes to obesity. In forms of obesity in which there is an increase in fat cell number, lipectomy may afford some relief.

The rate and quality of intake may influence subsequent behavior. The work of Geiselman and Novin (1982) showed that slow infusion of glucose into the duodenum of rabbits produces a satiety signal. Fast infusion (3 ml/min), however, results in the opposite effect: The rabbits nearly double their intake during the first half hour after infusion. Glucose thus produces hunger when it arrives at the duodenum quickly and is absorbed at a rapid rate. The suggestions from this work extend beyond simple recommendations to avoid consumption of sugars on an empty stomach. For example, ingestion of a diet high in fiber might be a means of avoiding glucose-induced hunger, because fiber increases gastric viscosity, delaying gastric emptying into the duodenum.

Finally, there is work currently examining the effects of acarbose, a complex oligosaccharide that inhibits the action of carbohydrate digestive enzymes, α-amylase, maltase, and sucrase, thereby slowing the rate of glucose absorption. When it is mixed in a diet containing high amounts of sucrose, it inhibits the elevations of body weight, insulin level, and lipid deposition that normally occur as a result of such a diet, even in the face of increased food intake.

Diabetes

The term *diabetes mellitus* was originally used to label a disorder characterized by the passage of sweet urine, excessive urination and thirst, and excessive hunger and weight loss, which results in death when left untreated over the course of several months. It has been recognized for over 100 years that the disease appears in primarily two forms: one affecting mainly obese adults and the other found more frequently among younger people.

Diabetic individuals are currently classified as having one of three major subclasses of the disease: insulin-dependent, non-insulin-dependent, and other types. Insulin-dependent diabetics are deficient in available insulin for a variety of reasons: a reduced amount of islet tissue, defective insulin formation, defective releasing mechanisms for insulin (perhaps lacking a normal response to glucose), or abnormally high rates of insulin destruction. Non-insulin-dependent diabetics are resistant or insensitive to the insulin they possess, perhaps due to overproduction of opposing hormones such as glucagon, or to a problem with insulin receptors. Insulin may still be used as treatment in these individuals to prevent ketosis.

The primary diagnosis is based on unequivocal elevation of plasma glucose concentrations together with typical symptoms; elevated fasting glucose levels on more than one occasion; and elevated plasma glucose concentration after an oral glucose challenge. That diabetes is essentially a disease of hyperglycemia can be shown by the changes in glucose metabolism and excretion: increased glycogenolysis, decreased glycogenesis, and increased gluconeogenesis. Impaired glucose transport across the membranes of skeletal muscles and other tissues also occurs. Another major aberration of glucose metabolism is the almost complete suppression of the conversion of glucose into fatty acids via acetyl-CoA (formed in the mitochondria by the oxidative decarboxylation of pyruvate). Moreover, there is the attendant glycosuria, polyuria, polydipsia, and polyphagia. Figure 8.8 summarizes these metabolic problems in diabetics.

There are several animal models of diabetes. As Mordes and Rossini (1981) have reviewed, spontaneous diabetes in animals is a common occurrence, but it has been well characterized in only a few species, principally rodents. For example, the Bio-Breeding laboratories in Canada discovered a spontaneous mutation of the Wistar rat that has an acute syndrome of hyperglycemia, hypoinsulinemia, and ketoacidosis (elevation of ketone bodies with a decrease in blood pH). In these insulin-dependent animals, there are increases in the plasma levels of glucagon, somatostatin, glucose, free fatty acids, and branched chain amino acids. These animals have a marked reduction of β cells.

The use of chemical agents to produce diabetes, primarily by preferentially destroying β cells, permits controlled study of physiological events that occur in the diabetic state. For example, rats given streptozotocin, an antibiotic, show varying degrees of glucose intolerance ranging from mild to pronounced symptoms of diabetes. These animals also exhibit one of the primary characteristics of diabetics: an enhanced food intake that appears to depend upon their degree of glucose intolerance. The findings suggest that feeding by these animals depends inversely on their glucose utilization: the less glucose that can be utilized, the "hungrier" the animals are. The behavior occurs despite elevations in blood glucose levels and is not simply a compensatory response to the increased loss of glucose in urine (e.g., glucose transport in the brain

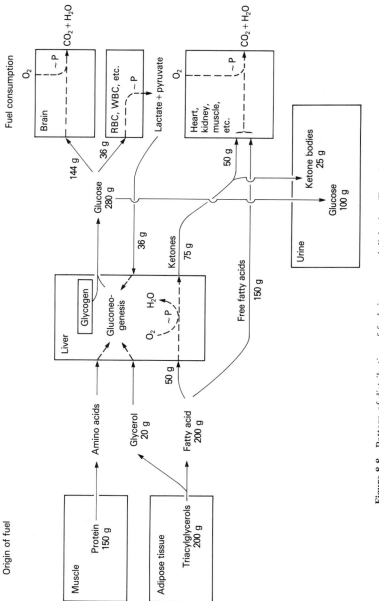

Figure 8.8 Pattern of distribution of fuels in untreated diabetics. (From Lehninger, 1976.)

is depressed). Lindberg et al. (1984) have suggested that in the diabetic, as in the normal individual, feeding may occur owing to periodic decreases in the signal for satiety associated with insulin's biological actions in the periphery.

Related to the dependence of amphetamine's anorexia-inducing actions on a mechanism involving glucose and Na/K ATPase is a recent finding that glucose competes with an amphetamine mechanism for the induction of stereotypy (i.e., glucose shifts the amphetamine dose-response curve for stereotypy to the right). Diabetic rats, however, are relatively unresponsive to most of the actions of amphetamine, including anorexia, enhanced locomotion, and stereotypy. It is therefore possible that the mechanism acting to reduce eating via an action on amphetamine receptors fails in diabetics, perhaps due to lack of insulin, thereby increasing food intake in these individuals. Considerable work is underway to test these and other related hypotheses about the changes related to glucose in diabetics.

Summary

Glucose is an important signal for the regulation of our desire to eat. The breakdown of glucose—glycolysis—occurs with only minor variation in most forms of life. Glycolysis liberates energy in the form of ATP, and the balance between glycolysis and new glucose formation—gluconeogenesis—is regulated by energy and nutrient flow.

As a nutrient signal, glucose has an effect on behavior at each stage of the organism's processing of food. The presence of glucose in the stomach or duodenum inhibits food intake. The firing rate of vagal afferents to the liver varies inversely with the concentration of blood glucose, but the liver is less effective as an organ of satiety when isolated experimentally than when considered along with organs of taste, alimentation, and digestion. Hormones from the pancreatic islets regulate and direct the movement of glucose. Epinephrine from the adrenal medulla stimulates hepatic glucose output. Corticosterone from the adrenal cortex stimulates gluconeogenesis in the liver.

Visceral factors with regard to glucose are probably more important than central factors in the regulation of feeding. Fructose, which cannot nourish cells in the CNS, inhibits food intake in hypoglycemic rats. However, central factors are quite important. Medial and lateral areas of the hypothalamus control levels of blood glucose and respond to changes in glucose that normally affect feeding. α_2 receptors in the paraventricular nuclei regulate carbohydrate intake and vary with the blood glucose level. Since changes in glucose usually occur under normal feeding conditions, it is likely that central and visceral factors act together to regulate feeding and the control of blood glucose.

That changes in blood glucose levels and carbohydrate intake occur when classic neurotransmitters are manipulated suggests an influence of transmitter precursors on these variables. Much work remains to establish these links.

Sugars are important in the regulation of oral factors, which can influence subsequent ingestive behavior. Oral factors may also play a part in a conditioning that invokes insulin release. Thoughts about food, and its taste and smell, may all play a part in this conditioning.

Evidence has accrued to show that obesity is inherited. Obesity involves increased preferences for sweets and fats and altered hormone production. Self-reinforcing cycles are also evident in which increased consumption leads to hormone responses that stimulate further consumption.

The use of chemical agents to produce diabetes permits the controlled study of the diabetic state. Experimental diabetic animals show enhanced food intake that depends on their degree of glucose intolerance.

References

Angel, I., Hauger, R.L., Do Luu, M., Giblin, B., Skolnick, P., & Paul, S.M. Glucostatic regulation of $(+)$-[^{3}H] amphetamine binding in the hypothalamus: Correlation with Na K -ATPase activity. *Proceedings of the National Academy of Sciences, USA, 82,* 1985, 6320–6324.

Campfield, L.A., Brandon, P., & Smith, F.J. On-line continuous measurement of blood glucose and meal pattern in free-feeding rats: The role of glucose in meal initiation. *Brain Research Bulletin, 14,* 1985, 605–616.

Cannon, W.B., *Bodily changes in pain, hunger, fear, and rage.* New York: Harper, 1963.

Chafetz, M.D., Parko, K., Diaz, S., & Leibowitz, S.F. Relationships between medial hypothalamic α_2-receptor binding, norepinephrine, and circulating glucose. *Brain Research, 384,* 1986, 404–408.

Courtney, N.D. & Woods, S.C. Vagotomy reduces body weight of genetically obese (Zucker) female rats and their lean littermates. *Nutrition and Behavior, 2,* 1984, 1–7.

Dallman, M.F. Viewing the ventromedial hypothalamus from the adrenal gland. *American Journal of Physiology, 246,* 1984, R1–R12.

Deutsch, A.J. Controversies in food intake regulation. In Hoebel, B.G. & Novin, D. (Eds.), *The neural basis of feeding and reward.* Brunswik, ME: Haer Institute, 1982, pp. 137–148.

Faust, I.M., Johnson, P.R., & Hirsch, J. Surgical removal of adipose tissue alters feeding behavior and the development of obesity in rats. *Science, 197,* 1977, 393–396.

Geiselman, P.J. & Novin, D. Sugar infusion can enhance feeding. *Science, 218,* 1982, 490–491.

Hauger, R.L., Hulihan-Giblin, B., Skolnick, P., & Paul, S.M. Glucostatic regulation of hypothalamic and brainstem [^{3}H]$(+)$-amphetamine binding during food deprivation and refeeding. *European Journal of Pharmacology, 124,* 1986, 267–275.

Honma, K-I., Honma, S., & Hiroshige, T. Feeding associated corticosterone peak in rats under various feeding cycles. *American Journal of Physiology, 246,* 1984, R721–R726.

Lehninger, A.L. *Biochemistry*, New York: Worth Publishers, 1976.

Leibowitz, S.F. Paraventricular nucleus: A primary site mediating adrenergic stimulation of feeding and drinking. *Pharmacology, Biochemistry & Behavior, 8,* 1978, 163–175.

Leibowitz, S.F. & Rossakis, C. Mapping study of brain dopamine- and epinephrine-sensitive sites which cause feeding suppression in the rat. *Brain Research, 172,* 1979, 101–113.

Leibowitz, S.F. & Stanley, B.G. Neurochemical controls of appetite. In Ritter, R., Ritter, S., & Barnes, C.D. (Eds.), *Feeding behavior: Neural and humoral controls*. New York: Academic Press, 1986, pp. 191–234.

Leibowitz, S.F., Brown, O., Tretter, J.R., & Kirschgesser, A. Norepinephrine, clonidine, and tricyclic antidepressants selectively stimulate carbohydrate ingestion through noradrenergic system of the paraventricular nucleus. *Pharmacology, Biochemistry, & Behavior, 23,* 1985, 541–550.

Leibowitz, S.F., Weiss, G.F., Yee, F., & Tretter, J.B. Noradrenergic innervation of the paraventricular nucleus: Specific role in control of carbohydrate ingestion. *Brain Research Bulletin, 14,* 1985, 561–567.

LeMagnen, J. Body energy balance and food intake: A neuroendocrine regulatory mechanism. *Physiology Reviews, 63,* 1983, 314–386.

Lindberg, N.O., Coburn, P.C., & Stricker, E.M. Increased feeding by rats after subdiabetogenic streptozotocin treatment: A role for insulin in satiety. *Behavioral Neuroscience, 98,* 1984, 138–145.

Mayer, J. Regulation of energy intake and body weight: The glucostatic theory and the lipostatic hypothesis. *Annals of the New York Academy of Sciences, 63,* 1955, 15–43.

McMinn, M.R. Mechanisms of energy balance in obesity. *Behavioral Neuroscience, 98,* 1984, 375–393.

Mook, D.G., Dreifuss, S., & Keats, P.H. Satiety for glucose solution in rat: The specificity is postingestive. *Physiology & Behavior, 36,* 1986, 897–901.

Mordes, J.P. & Rossini, A.A. Animal models of diabetes. *The American Journal of Medicine, 70,* 1981, 353–360.

Novin, D. Obesity: A self-reinforcing phenomenon. *Nutrition and Behavior, 2,* 1984, 89–93.

Novin, D. The nature and integration of signals controlling food intake. In H. Weiner (Moderator), Psychobiological and neurobiological mechanisms in gastric function and ulceration. *Western Journal of Medicine, 143,* 1985, 207–222.

Novin, D., Robinson, K., Culbreth, L.A., & Tordoff, M.G. Is there a role for the liver in the control of food intake? *American Journal of Clinical Nutrition, 42,* 1985, 1050–1062.

Oomura, Y. Feeding regulation by endogenous sugar acids through hypothalamic chemosensitive neurons. *Brain Research Bulletin, 17,* 1986, 551–562.

Russek, M. A conceptual equation of intake control. In Novin, D., Wyrwicka, W., & Bray, G.A. (Eds.), *Hunger: Basic mechanisms and clinical implications*, New York: Raven Press, 1976, pp. 327–348.

Stricker, E.M. Factors in the control of food intake. *Behavioral and Brain Sciences, 4,* 1981, 591–592.

Stricker, E.M. & McCann, M.J. Visceral factors in the control of food intake. *Brain Research Bulletin, 14,* 1985, 687–692.

Stunkard, A.J., Foch, T.T., & Hrubec, Z. A twin study of human obesity. *Journal of the American Medical Association, 256,* 1986a, 51–54.

Stunkard, A.J., Sorenson, T.I.A., Hanis, C., Teasdale, T.W., Chakraborty, R., Schull,

W.J., & Schulsinger, F. An adoption study of human obesity. *New England Journal of Medicine, 314*, 1986b, 193–198.

Wurtman, J.J. & Wurtman, R.J. Drugs that enhance central serotoninergic transmission diminish elective carbohydrate consumption by rats. *Life Sciences, 24*, 1979, 895–904.

Wyrwicka, W. Sensory regulation of food intake. *Physiology & Behavior, 4*, 1969, 853–858.

Young, J.B., Rosa, R.M., & Landsberg, L. Dissociation of sympathetic nervous system and adrenal medullary responses. *American Journal of Physiology, 247*, 1984, E35–E40.

Suggested Readings

Alvarez-Buylla, R., Rojas, M., de Alvarez-Buylla, E.R., & Faria, N. Effects of intracisternal glucose or insulin injections on glucose homeostasis in cat. *Diabetes, 35*, 1986, 826–831.

Bartness, T.J. & Waldbillig, R.J. Cholecystokinin-induced suppression of feeding: An evaluation of the generality of gustatory-cholecystokinin interactions. *Physiology & Behavior, 32*, 1984, 409–415.

Bennett, P.H. Classification of diabetes. In Ellenberg, M. & Rifkin, H. (Eds.) *Diabetes Mellitus*, New York: Medical Examination Publishing Co., 1983, 409–414.

Berthoud, H.R. & Mogenson, G.J. Ingestive behavior after intracerebral and intracerebroventricular infusions of glucose and 2-deoxy-D-glucose. *American Journal of Physiology, 233*, 1977, R127–R133.

Bhakthavatsalam, P. & Leibowitz, S.F. α_2-noradrenergic feeding rhythm in paraventricular nucleus: relation to corticosterone. *American Journal of Physiology, 250*, 1986, R83–R88.

Booth, D.A., Coons, E.E., & Miller, N.E. Blood glucose responses to electrical stimulation of the hypothalamic feeding area. *Physiology & Behavior, 4*, 1969, 991–1001.

Castonguay, T.W., Dallman, M., & Stern, J.S. Corticosterone prevents body weight loss and diminished fat appetite following adrenalectomy. *Nutrition and Behavior, 2*, 1984, 115–125.

Castonguay, T.W., Rowland, N.E., & Stern, J.S. Nutritional influences on dietary selection patterns of obese and lean Zucker rats. *Brain Research Bulletin, 14*, 1985, 625–631.

Crane, P.D., Braun, L.D., Cornford, E.M., Nyerges, A.M., & Oldendorf, W.H. Cerebral cortical glucose utilization in the conscious rat: Evidence for a circadian rhythm. *Journal of Neurochemistry, 34*, 1980, 1700–1706.

Cruce, J.A.F., Thoa, N.B., & Jacobowitz, D.M. Catecholamines in the brains of genetically obese rats. *Brain Research, 101*, 1976, 165–170.

Desor, J.A., Maller, O., & Greene, L.S. Preference for sweet in humans: infants, children, and adults. In Weiffenbach, J.M. (Ed.) *Taste and development: The genesis of sweet preference*. Maryland: National Institute of Health, 1976, pp. 161–172.

Drewnowski, A. & Greenwood, M.R.C. Cream and sugar: Human preferences for high-fat foods. *Physiology & Behavior, 30*, 1983, 629–633.

Flynn, F.W. & Grill, H.J. Insulin elicits ingestion in decerebrate rats. *Science, 221*, 1983, 188–190.

Fox, P.T., Raichle, M.E., Mintun, M.A., & Dence, C. Non-oxidative glucose consumption during focal physiologic neural activity. *Science, 241*, 1988, 462–464.

Frohman, L.A. & Bernardis, L.L. Effect of hypothalamic stimulation on plasma glucose, insulin, and glucagon levels. *American Journal of Physiology, 221,* 1971, 1596–1603.

Fullerton, D.T., Getto, C.J., Swift, W.J., & Carlson, I.H. Sugar, opioids, and binge eating. *Brain Research Bulletin, 14,* 1985, 673–680.

Giza, B.K. & Scott, T. R. Blood glucose selectively affects taste-evoked activity in rat nucleus tractus solitarius. *Physiology & Behavior, 31,* 1983, 643–650.

Glick, Z. & Bray, G.A. The α-glucosidase inhibitor acarbose stimulates food intake in rats eating a high carbohydrate diet. *Nutrition and Behavior, 1,* 1982, 15–20.

Goldman, C.K., Marino, L., & Leibowitz, S.F. Postsynaptic α$_2$ noradrenergic receptors mediate feeding induced by paraventricular nucleus injection of norepinephrine and clonidine. *European Journal of Pharmacology, 115,* 1985, 11–19.

Gonzalez, M.F. & Deutsch, J.A. Vagotomy abolishes cues of satiety produced by gastric distension. *Science, 212,* 1981, 1283–1284.

Grill, H.J. & Norgren, R. Chronically decerebrate rats demonstrate satiation but not bait shyness. *Science, 201,* 1978, 267–269.

Grossman, S.P., Dacey, D., Halaris, A.E., Collier, T., & Routtenberg, A. Aphagia and adipsia after preferential destruction of nerve cell bodies in hypothalamus. *Science, 202,* 1978, 537–539.

Iguchi, A., Gotoh, M., Matsunaga, H., Yatomi, A., Honmura, A., Yanase, M. & Sakamoto, N. Mechanism of central hyperglycemic effect of cholinergic agonists in fasted rats. *American Journal of Physiology, 251,* 1986, E431–E437.

Jefferson, L.S. & Neely, J.R. Intermediary metabolism. In Brodoff, B.N. & Bleicher, S.J. (Eds.), *Diabetes mellitus and obesity.* Baltimore: Williams & Wilkins, 1982, pp. 3–26.

Jhanwar-Uniyal, M., Roland, C.R., & Leibowitz, S.F. Diurnal rhythm of α$_2$-noradrenergic receptors in the paraventricular nucleus and other brain areas: Relation to circulating corticosterone and feeding behavior. *Life Sciences, 38,* 1986, 473–482.

Kow, L-M. & Pfaff, D.W. Actions of feeding-relevant agents on hypothalamic glucose-responsive neurons *in vitro. Brain Research Bulletin, 15,* 1985, 504–513.

Langhans, W., Zieger, U., Scharrer, E., & Geary, N. Stimulation of feeding in rats by intraperitoneal injection of antibodies of glucagon. *Science, 218,* 1982, 894–896.

Larue-Achagiotis, C. & LeMagnen, J. Feeding rate and responses to food deprivation as a function of fasting-induced hypoglycemia. *Behavioral Neuroscience, 99,* 1985, 1176–1180.

LeMagnen, J. The metabolic basis of dual periodicity of feeding in rats. *Behavioral Brain Sciences, 4,* 1981, 561–607.

Lenard, L. & Hahn, Z. Amygdalar noradrenergic and dopaminergic mechanisms in the regulation of hunger and thirst-motivated behavior. *Brain Research, 233,* 1982, 115–132.

MacIsaac, L. & Geary, N. Partial liver denervations dissociate the inhibitory effects of pancreatic glucagon and epinephrine on feeding. *Physiology & Behavior, 35,* 1985, 233–237.

Maggio, C.A., Yang, M-U., & Vasselli, J.R. Developmental aspects of macronutrient selection in genetically obese and lean rats. *Nutrition and Behavior, 2,* 1984, 95–110.

Margules, D.L., Moisset, B., Lewis, M.J., Shibuya, H., & Pert, C.B. β-endorphin is associated with overeating in genetically obese mice (ob/ob) and rats (fa/fa). *Science, 202,* 1978, 988–991.

McCaleb, M.L. & Myers, R.D. 2-Deoxy-D-glucose and insulin modify release of norepinephrine from rat hypothalamus. *American Journal of Physiology, 242,* 1982, R596–R601.

McCaleb, M.L. & Myers, R.D. Striatal dopamine release is altered by glucose and insulin during push-pull perfusion of the rat's caudate nucleus. *Brain Research Bulletin, 4,* 1979, 651–656.

McCaleb, M.L., Myers, R.D., Singer, G., & Willis, G. Hypothalamic norepinephrine in the rat during feeding and push-pull perfusion with glucose, 2-DG, or insulin. *American Journal of Physiology, 236,* 1979, R312–R321.

McCall, A.L., Fixman, L.B. Fleming, N., Tornheim, K., Chick, W., & Ruderman, N.B. Chronic hypoglycemia increases brain glucose transport. *American Journal of Physiology, 251,* 1986, E442–E447.

Miller, M.G. Oral somatosensory factors in dietary self-selection in rats. *Behavioral Neuroscience, 98,* 1984, 416–423.

Miller, M.G. & Teates, J.F. Oral somatosensory factors in dietary self-selection alter food deprivation and supplementation. *Behavioral Neuroscience, 98,* 1984, 424–434.

Myers, R.D. & McCaleb, M.L. Feeding: Satiety signal from intestine triggers brain's noradrenergic mechanism. *Science, 209,* 1980, 1035–1037.

Nakano, Y. Oomura, Y., Lenard, L., Nishino, H., Aou, S., Yamamoto, T., & Aoyagi, K. Feeding-related activity of glucose- and morphine-sensitive neurons in the monkey amygdala. *Brain Research, 399,* 1986, 167–172.

Novin, D. The integration of visceral information in the control of feeding. *Journal of the Autonomic Nervous System, 9,* 1983, 233–246.

Novin, D. & VanderWeele, D.A. Visceral involvement in feeding: There is more to regulation than the hypothalamus. *Progress in Psychobiology & Physiological Psychology, 7,* 1977, 193–241.

Panksepp, J. Central metabolic and humoral factors involved in the neural regulation of feeding. *Pharmacology, Biochemistry, & Behavior, 3,* 1975, 107–119.

Pauly, J.E. & Scheving, L.E. Circadian rhythms in blood glucose and the effect of different lighting schedules, hypophysectomy, adrenal medullectomy, and starvation. *American Journal of Anatomy, 120,* 1967, 627–636.

Pfaffman, C., Frank, M., & Norgren, R. Neural mechanisms and behavioral aspects of taste. *Annual Review of Psychology, 30,* 1979, 283–325.

Raskin, P. Glucagon. In Brodoff, B.N. & Bleicher, S.J. (Eds.), *Diabetes mellitus and obesity,* Baltimore: Williams & Wilkins, 1982, pp. 63–70.

Ritter, R.C., Slusser, P.G., & Stone, S. Glucoreceptors controlling feeding and blood glucose: Location in the hindbrain. *Science, 213,* 1981, 451–453.

Roland, C.R., Bhakthavatsalam, P., & Leibowitz, S.F. Interaction between corticosterone and α_2-noradrenergic system of the paraventricular nucleus in relation to feeding behavior. *Neuroendocrinology, 42,* 1986, 296–305.

Romsos, D.R. & Ferguson, D. Self-selected intake of carbohydrate, fat, and protein by obese (ob/ob) and lean mice. *Physiology & Behavior, 28,* 1982, 301–305.

Rowland, N. & Stricker, E.M. Differential effects of glucose and fructose infusions on insulin-induced feeding in rats. *Physiology & Behavior, 22,* 1979, 387–389.

Sakaguchi, T. & Yamaguchi, K. Effects of vagal stimulation, vagotomy, and adrenalectomy on release of insulin in the rat. *Journal of Endocrinology, 85,* 1980, 131–136.

Schneider, L.H., Gibbs, J., & Smith, G.P. D_2 selective receptor antagonists suppress sucrose sham feeding in the rat. *Brain Research Bulletin, 17,* 1986, 605–611.

Shimazu, T. & Ogasawara, S. Effects of hypothalamic stimulation on gluconeogenesis and glycolysis in rat liver. *American Journal of Physiology, 228*, 1975, 1787–1793.

Shor-Posner, G., Grinker, J.A., Marinescu, C., & Leibowitz, S.F. Role of hypothalamic norepinephrine in control of meal patterns. *Physiology and Behavior, 35*, 1985, 209–214.

Smith, G.P., Jerome, C., Cushin, B.J., Eterno, R., & Simansky, K.J. Abdominal vagotomy blocks the satiety effect of cholecystokinin in the rat. *Science, 213*, 1981, 1036–1037.

Smythe, G.A., Grunstein, H.S., Bradshaw, J.E., Nicholson, M.V., & Compton, P.J. Relationships between brain noradrenergic activity and blood glucose, *Nature, 308*, 1984, 65–67.

Steffans, A.B. Influence of reversible obesity on eating behavior, blood glucose, and insulin in the rat. *American Journal of Physiology, 228*, 1975, 1738–1744.

Steffans, A.B. Influence of the oral cavity on insulin release in the rat. *American Journal of Physiology, 230*, 1976, 1411–1415.

Storlien, L.H., Grunstein, H.S., & Smythe, G.A. Guanethidine blocks the 2-deoxy-D-glucose induced hypothalamic noradrenergic drive to hyperglycemia. *Brain Research, 335*, 1985, 144–147.

Vanderweele, D.A., Macrum, B.L., & Oetting, R.L. Glucagon, satiety from feeding and liver/pancreatic interactions. *Brain Research Bulletin, 17*, 1986, 539–543.

Vasseli, J.R., Haraczkiewicz, E., & Pi-Sunyer, F.X. Effects of acarbose (Bay g5421) on body weight, insulin, and oral glucose and sucrose tolerance in sucrose consuming rats. *Nutrition and Behavior, 1*, 1982, 21–32.

Weingarten, H.P. Conditioned cues elicit feeding in sated rats: A role for learning in meal initiation. *Science, 220*, 1983, 431–433.

White, N.M. & Blackburn, J. Effect of glucose on amphetamine-induced motor behavior. *Life Sciences, 38*, 1986, 2255–2262.

Yamazaki, M. & Sakaguchi, T. Effects of D-glucose anomers on sweetness taste and insulin release in man. *Brain Research Bulletin, 17*, 1986, 271–274.

Part IV
Micronutrients

Chapter 9
Zinc: A Trace of Nutrient Action

The diversity of research on zinc, its relation to dietary and other behaviors, and the growing realization that zinc deficiencies pose a major health problem in several areas of the world lead us to focus on zinc as representative of the trace element basis for behavior. We should keep in mind, however, that zinc's presence in enzymes and its regional distribution in the brain differ to a great extent from that of iron, copper, or other trace metals. The generality of these findings to other metals should therefore be regarded as a qualified example, meant only to illustrate this nutrient basis for behavior.

Trace elements usually act as catalytic or structural components of larger molecules. The physiological coordination with these larger molecules typically defines the function of the trace element. A trace element is considered essential when its deficiency consistently results in the impairment of these functions. Trace elements can be differentiated from macrominerals such as sodium, potassium, and calcium in that they are necessary only in minute amounts and are not distributed ubiquitously throughout bodily tissues.

Trace elements include those naturally occurring elements in the periodic table that are not bulk elements (hydrogen, carbon, nitrogen, oxygen, and sulfur) or macrominerals. The biologic functions of the trace element zinc, as a component of more than 50 enzymes, have been intensively and diversely investigated. Because of its high concentrations in specific regions of the brain, the role of zinc in neurobiologic function is coming under intense scrutiny.

Zinc's high concentration in the hippocampal formation has made the study of its functions a useful probe for insights into memory formation. Recent behavioral evidence is beginning to show behavioral adaptation as a means of altering zinc homeostasis. This evidence suggests the existence of neural mechanisms that recognize the body's zinc status and act to maintain adequate levels. Deficiency or excess of zinc have both been implicated in cognitive and behavioral disorders.

*B*iochemistry and Physiology

Haloenzymes are catalytically active complexes of enzymes and cofactors. When metal ions are used as cofactors, they can function as facilitators at the primary catalytic site, as bridging groups to bind the substrate and the enzyme through the formation of a coordinating complex, or as stabilizing agents for the catalytically active conformation of the enzyme protein. Examples of haloenzymes include cytochrome oxidase (copper), ferredoxin (iron), adenosine triphosphatase (magnesium), and alcohol dehydrogenase or glutamate dehydrogenase (zinc).

Glutamate dehydrogenase catalyzes the reversible reaction: α-ketoglutarate $+ NAD(P)H + NH_4 = $ l-glutamate $+ NAD(P) + H_2O$. Because α-ketoglutarate is an intermediate in the tricarboxylic acid cycle, this dehydrogenase enzyme is important in linking amino acid and carbohydrate metabolism. Deficiency in this enzyme's activity could therefore result in aberrations in intermediary metabolism and in amino acid function in tissues (e.g., brain) expressing high concentrations of the enzyme.

Zinc, as a nutrient, is required for fetal brain development. Deficiency can result in brain and behavioral anomalies that persist into adult life. Altered enzyme activity during development is one way through which a gestational or lactational deficiency produces these anomalies. Although gestational-lactational zinc deficiency does not result in a drop in the concentrations of glutamate dehydrogenase, it does diminish the activity of this enzyme. This form of zinc deficiency also produces a drop in the concentrations and activity of 2, 3-cyclic nucleotide 3-phosphohydrolase, which suggests a delay in myelination. Similarly, gestational-lactational copper deficiency results in reduced brain growth, as well as lowered content and activity of copper metalloenzymes. The development of normal brain biochemical functions of these enzymes is thus dependent upon the coordinated presence of their metal cofactors.

Zinc is important for the physiological activity of several enzymes in other tissues as well. Weanling rats maintained on a zinc-deficient diet for several weeks show diminished activity of alcohol dehydrogenase in liver, kidney, testis, and bone. There is also diminished activity of alkaline phosphatase in the kidney, testis, pancreas, bone, and thymus, and reduced activity of carboxypeptidase in the pancreas. This diminished biochemical function is specific for the restriction in zinc; no such changes are observed in manganese- or iron-dependent enzymes.

Zinc is also necessary for the synthesis of DNA, RNA, and protein, and is thus required for the genesis of certain cells. Sandstead and associates (1972) have shown that zinc deficiency during lactation in rats diminishes the incorporation of tritiated thymidine into DNA and of sulfur into protein. In keeping with zinc's role in myelination, these researchers have also shown a reduction in lipid concentration resulting from zinc deprivation.

If some of the proteins that bind and release zinc are actively involved in receptor function, the results of alterations of dietary zinc might be explained by a change in the binding of these proteins to their natural ligands. For example, in a series of studies examining the anorexia that results from zinc deficiency, it was shown that the deficient animals are resistant to opiate-induced feeding by dynorphin. Studies of naloxone binding in these zinc-deficient animals show that their brain proteins have a higher affinity for this opiate receptor blocker, which suggests that zinc plays an important role in the physiology of endogenous opiate receptor proteins.

It is also becoming clear that zinc has important interactions with other neurotransmitter systems. In the late 1950s and early 1960s, it was known that catechols and ethanolamines form relatively stable chelate bonds with metals. Recognizing the biologic significance of this coordination, Colburn and Maas (1965) later showed that divalent cations such as zinc, copper, iron, and magnesium form complexes with catecholamines and ATP, and that they do so primarily in synaptosome fractions of the brain. Figure 9.1 diagrams such a complex.

Further evidence that the complexes formed by metal ions and catecholamines are physiologically significant comes from work showing that chelating agents (used to bind metal ions, thereby removing them from the catecholamine complex) inhibit the storage of norepinephrine in synaptic vesicles. The potential for understanding the dietary coordination of this relationship between trace elements and energy distribution in the brain has remained

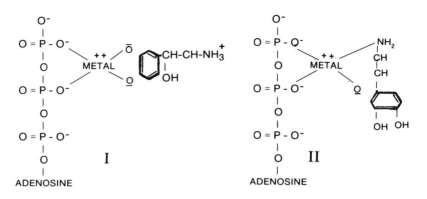

Figure 9.1 Diagram example of a ternary complex of catecholamine, ATP, and divalent cation. (From Colburn and Maas, 1965.)

relatively unexplored, although Wallwork and colleagues (1984) have shown that zinc deficiency results in elevation of catecholamines in specific regions of the brain. Pharmacologic evidence also shows that zinc deficiency reduces the animal's sensitivity to feeding induced by norepinephrine, which suggests an interaction between zinc and catecholamine receptors, perhaps of the α_2 subtype. This is particularly interesting in view of the staining for zinc in areas such as the paraventricular nuclei, which Leibowitz has shown to be sensitive to feeding induced by norepinephrine (see Chapters 4 & 8).

Zinc's interaction with glutamic acid decarboxylase and its modulation of GABA receptor proteins suggests its function in GABA physiology. At low levels, zinc stimulates the activity of the GABA synthesizing enzyme, and at high levels it inhibits the activity of the enzyme. Physiologic alterations of zinc thus have the potential for increasing and decreasing the synthesis of GABA. Zinc's physiological role for the normal binding of GABA to its receptors is suggested in the findings that zinc applied to fresh frozen membranes leads to an increase in sodium-dependent GABA binding sites at low doses and a reduction in GABA binding sites when applied at progressively higher doses. Pharmacologic evidence also shows that zinc deficient animals require higher doses of the GABA agonist muscimol to induce feeding, thus implicating the receptor function in a physiologic role. Further evidence for zinc's interaction with GABA systems comes from electrophysiological work showing that chelation of zinc alters inhibition of granule cell activity in the hippocampus by basket cells, which contain GABA. These data imply that steps should be taken only to maintain a normal balance of zinc; deviation above or below a normal range can alter neurotransmission.

Zinc probably has a normal function at central excitatory synapses. Peters and associates (1987) have shown that zinc selectively blocks the action of N-methyl-d-aspartate on cortical neurons. It also blocks aspartate receptor-mediated toxicity, but not toxicity produced by other analogs.

Zinc can also modulate neurotransmission through its actions on other metal ions. Wallwork and his associates (1983) have shown that deficiency of zinc leads to elevated copper concentrations in several brain areas, as well as alterations in the levels of calcium, magnesium, sodium, and potassium. In addition to altering general neuronal activity through a shift in the ionic balance, these effects could more specifically alter transmitter levels and receptor activity through activation or deactivation of receptor proteins and catabolic enzymes.

There is growing evidence that zinc may participate more directly in neurotransmission. Electron micrographs of labeled zinc autoradiography have shown that zinc is associated with synaptic vesicles (in zinc-rich areas of the brain) and not with other cellular components such as mitrochondria. Zinc is also enriched in synaptic fractions of the brain. According to Frederickson's group (1983), a finding of 66 ppm zinc in the dried hilar zone of the hippocampus implies a concentration of 220 uM zinc in wet tissue. The actual concentration could be higher, because the zinc-rich tissue does not completely fill the zone analyzed. Since in this region the concentration of glutamate is about 8 uM, norepinephrine about 20 uM, and the opiate metenkephalin about 2 uM, there is a considerable excess of zinc ions, suggesting that they are available for other functions.

Howell and Frederickson (1984) have shown zinc to have characteristics of other neurotransmitters. They find, for example, that zinc uptake into the hippocampus saturates with time and concentration, requires metabolic energy, and is sensitive to environmental temperature, indicating that the transport of zinc into nerve tissue is an active physiological process. Moreover, electrical stimulation of the nerve cells that normally contain high levels of zinc facilitates both the uptake and release of zinc. These findings suggest that in addition to its roles in modulating enzyme and receptor proteins, zinc may have a signaling function as a neurotransmitter. At the very least, zinc could act in conjunction with glutamate released from mossy fiber nerve endings—in which both substances are found—to modulate glutamate's interactions with its receptors.

In the context of nutrient homeostasis, it is particularly important to understand Kasarskis's work (1984) on the uptake of radioactive zinc (^{65}Zn) in various brain regions of animals deficient in zinc. He finds an increased concentration of labeled zinc in every brain region examined in deficient animals, compared to pair-fed (undernourished) controls. The most striking site of uptake is in choroid plexus, indicating a role for this tissue in the transport of zinc between plasma and cerebrospinal fluid.

Zinc has other peripheral biochemical functions that are important for the study of dietary interactions. Zinc deficiency diminishes prostaglandin synthesis and secretion, implicating zinc as an important factor in lipid metabolism. Some of the clinical manifestations of zinc deficiency even resemble those of essential fatty acid deficiency. Zinc also interacts with insulin in the pancreatic islets, controlling its solubility and storage, and thereby modulates the insulin response to changes in blood sugar. Zinc is also necessary for testicular integrity and output, and is therefore involved in controlling the amount of testicular steroids that interact in central and peripheral target tissues.

Anatomy

It has been known for over 100 years that sulfides precipitate colored salts of trace metals. If zinc had not been the exception, producing instead a white sulfide that is invisible in tissue, it might have been shown to be present in the central nervous system before the 1950s. By that time, the use of dithizone (diphenylthiocarbazone) enabled investigators to see a red zinc dithizonate in the nervous system. Model experiments showing that zinc dithizonate has an absorption peak at 535 nm indicated that the stained material in tissue was indeed from zinc and not other metals.

The use of dithizone to trace the anatomic distribution of zinc, however, has its problems. First, the complex is labile and does not permit continuous investigation over time. Second, the sensitivity is low because the complex does not amplify zinc well in tissue.

In the late 1950s, Timm (1958) developed a method for staining metals that is at least 100 times more sensitive than the dithizone method. It is based on the observation that metal sulfide molecules are able to catalyze the reduction of silver ions to metallic silver. To aid in the donation of a reducing electron, Timm used hydroquinone in the developer. The last stage of his method is therefore similar to a photographic process that uses "physical development." Because several silver atoms are required at a catalytic site, the method extensively amplifies the metals present in the tissue.

Neither the dithizone nor the Timm procedure is inherently specific for zinc. Considerable work with the use of dithizone, however, has shown that the stain in tissues is due to zinc. It is now widely believed that the Timm method also demonstrates zinc, at least in tissues where dithizone will stain, because intravital treatment with dithizone prior to application of Timm's method successfully prevents most of the silver staining.

Haug (1973) has used Timm's method widely to map the staining throughout the CNS. His work shows considerable staining of neuropil in the telencephalon (much more than in brainstem, spinal cord, and cerebellum) in a pattern with regional and laminar distribution. Cortical areas are widely stained in a banded pattern that converges at the level of the rhinal fissure. In a modification of the stain, the bands of silver deposition in cortex occur in layers II and IV-V, with streaks of silver grains connecting the layers through a lighter band of unstained pyramidal cells in between. With the traditional stain, nerve cells are also stained throughout the cortex, but the overall pattern is essentially the same.

Whichever method is used, the most intense stain for zinc is found in the hippocampal formation, particularly in the mossy fiber projection field. Mossy fibers make up the synaptic output from dentate granule cells, distributing to the CA_3 and CA_4 pyramidal cell fields of the hippocampus proper. Mossy fibers also extend collaterals to the neuropil within the hilus immediately subjacent to the granule cells. The nerve endings of mossy fibers are probably the largest in the nervous system, and several studies have indicated an enrichment or deposition of zinc in these endings, particularly associated with synaptic vesicles.

There are other areas of less intense, but generally dark, staining throughout the hippocampus, including the inner and outer third of the dentate molecular layer, which receive commissural and perforant path fibers, respectively. Stratum radiatum and stratum oriens of CA_1 and CA_3 receive both commissural and ipsilateral fiber projections, and are moderately stained by Timm's method. Both lateral and medial zones of the subiculum, and the presubiculum, are stained more intensely than the commissural and associational zones of the hippocampus, but not as intensely as the mossy fiber projections. Figure 9.2 shows the results of Timm's stain in the hippocampal formation.

Table 9.1 shows the strength of the Timm stain in various regions of the nervous system. As the table indicates, the stain is most dense in cortical

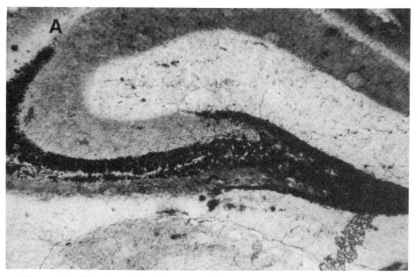

Figure 9.2 Timm's stain in hippocampal formation showing heavily stained mossy fiber zone and lighter stained commissural and associational zones. (From Chafetz, 1986.)

TABLE 9.1   Strength of Timm Stain In Selected Regions of the Brain
(Haug, 1973)

Brain Region	Stain Strength
Olfactory Bulbs	intense
anterior olfactory nucleus	Stain in fibrillary layer
	extends into glomeruli.
Olfactory tubercle	Stains throughout.
Septal Area	
medial areas	pale
lateral areas	darker
Bed Nucleus Stria Terminalis	darkly
Lateral Preoptic Region	poorly
Amygdala	
cortical, basal, parts of lateral and central nuclei	strong
parts of central and medial nuclei	weak
Hippocampus	
mossy fibers	most intense
dentate molecular layer (inner and outer thirds)	generally dark
stratum radiatum (CA$_1$ & CA$_3$)	moderate
stratum oriens (CA$_1$ & CA$_3$)	moderate
subiculum—lateral, medial, and presubiculum	more than radiatum, but less than mossy fibers
Neocortex	dense banded pattern converges at level of rhinal fissure—silver deposition layers II & IV-V
Striatum	
neuropil	dense—grains avoid fiber bundles
nerve cells	weakly
Diencephalon	
pineal	medium
medial habenula	strong
lateral habenula	pale
lateral thalamic nuclei	fine staining
anterior thalamic nuclei	less than lateral
dorsal thalamic nuclei	weak
midline and intralaminar thalamus	weak to moderate
geniculate bodies	weak
hypothalamus, except	uniform, finely grained
paraventricular and supraoptic nuclei	darkly
mamillary bodies cells	strong
neuropil	diffuse
Mesencephalon	
tectum, cells and neuropil	weak to moderate
several tegmental areas including dorsal and ventral nuclei	considerable
locus ceruleus	lightly

continued

TABLE 9.1 (Continued)

Brain Region	Stain Strength
Pons and Medulla	
reticular formation	lightly
motor cranial nerve nuclei—cells	fine grained
neuropil	enhanced
nucleus of solitary tract	same as motor cranial
Cerebellum	
cortex	moderate and uniform
molecular	lightly
granular layer and cerebellar nuclei	intermediate
Spinal Cord	
cells and neuropil	weak to moderate, more prominent in dorsal

areas. Except for the medial habenula and paraventricular and supraoptic nuclei, diencephalic areas stain weakly. Olfactory bulbs have an intense stain, as do parts of the amygdala. The neuropil of the striatum is densely stained. Most other areas of the nervous system show staining that is characterized as weak to moderate.

Having presented Haug's application of Timm's original staining method, we should also mention a more recent modification of Timm's method, along with Danscher's (1984a) selenium method. In my own laboratory (Chafetz, 1986), Timm's method was modified to react fresh frozen tissue with sulfides without perfusion. This procedure allows for observation of norepinephrine fluoresence in adjacent sections of tissue, as well as more controlled studies of post-mortem human tissue. Danscher's selenium method takes advantage of the chemical and physical resemblance between sulfur and selenium with the amplification process including a reduction of the selenite ion.

The two more recent methods are mentioned together because they result in a similar staining pattern that contrasts with Timm's original method. These methods produce results in cortical areas quite similar to the Timm method's results. But the modification and the selenium staining more closely resemble the part of the Timm staining that can be blocked by prior dithizone treatment, and these stain results are blocked by prior chelation. The differences, for example, are primarily seen in a lack of diencephalic staining. Whereas Haug has reported staining of cells in the paratenial and parafascicular thalamic nuclei, and in the mammillary bodies medial to the fornix, such a pattern is not seen with the newer methods. Figure 9.3 shows a sagittal section of a rat brain stained with the selenium method, with the cortical and basal ganglia staining intact, but with a distinct absence of diencephalic stain. Figure 9.4 shows a modified Timm stain of the human hilus.

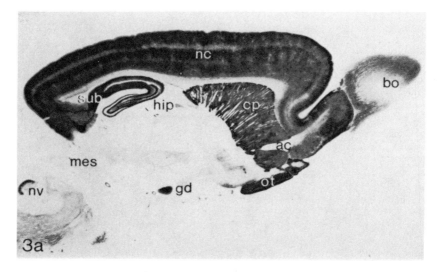

Figure 9.3 Sagittal section of rat brain stained with selenium method, showing intact cortical and basal ganglia stain, but a distinct absence of diencephalic stain. (From Danscher, 1984.)

Behavior

Zinc

The regional distribution of zinc in cortical areas, particularly in the mossy fiber region of the hippocampal formation, has stimulated research on zinc's role in learning and memory, and in other cognitive functions. This research is exemplified in the work of Ed Halas (1983, 1984), who has used Olton's distinctions regarding radial maze performance to study the effects of zinc deficiency.

You will recall from Chapter 5 that two types of memories are formed by animals performing on a radial maze. One is a *reference memory*, formed from the use of visual cues present in the same position every time the animal experiences the maze. The other is a *working memory*, which is more of a short-term storage of the sequence of arm entries the animal makes during each experience it has with the maze.

One of the best ways to differentiate these two types of memories is to use a 17-arm radial maze. In all trials with this maze, nine of the arms remain unbaited. Because this condition (lacking a food reward) is always present on these particular arms, the animals can learn to avoid them, thus forming

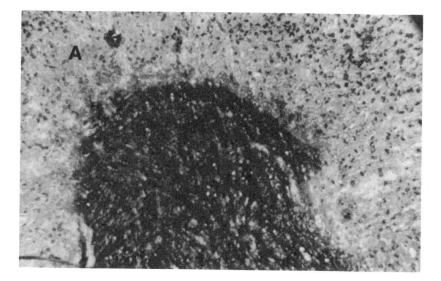

Figure 9.4   Modified Timm stain of human hilus showing mossy fiber region. (From Chafetz, 1986.)

a reference memory. The eight remaining arms are baited. Because the animal uses different sequences to enter these baited arms to search for food, it must hold the list of arms it has already entered in a short-term (working) memory, lest it repeat a trip to a recently depleted arm.

As Olton and colleagues (1978) have shown, damage to the hippocampal formation or to any of its extrinsic fiber connections—either efferent or afferent—results in a loss of the animal's ability to remember the list of baited arms. This indicates that working memory is dependent upon these neural systems. Because the animals are able to remember where the unbaited arms are so as to avoid them, the facility for reference memory formation must still be intact.

Halas (1983) hypothesized that a lactational zinc deficiency would deprive growing rat pups of the zinc necessary for optimal neuronal development and functioning of the hippocampal formation. If the hippocampal formation were malfunctioning as these animals matured, there should be impairments on the working memory component of the radial maze experiment.

That was indeed the finding. The animals deprived of zinc during development were impaired as adults in their working, but not reference, memories. This was in contrast to animals who were generally undernourished, but who performed adequately on both memory tasks. Moreover, it was later shown that the extent of impairment on working memory correlated with the severity in the deficit of granule cells, which normally concentrate high levels of zinc in their mossy fiber nerve endings.

Passive avoidance deficits in mice are also documented results of lesions to the hippocampal system. Gestational-lactational zinc deficiency, even if marginal, produces impairments on passive avoidance tasks. This also indicates that impaired development of the hippocampal system might be a functionally significant result of gestational-lactational zinc deficiency.

The Sandstead group (1977) has found that gestational-lactational zinc deficiency impairs the behavior of rats on an active avoidance task. This is in contrast to the findings in mice showing that strains with congenitally greater numbers of mossy fiber synapses on the basal dendrites of hippocampal pyramidal cells exhibit poor two-way avoidance, whereas mice with fewer synapses in this area exhibit superior performance. This latter finding, however, is in keeping with the notion that an imbalance of zinc in either direction results in a dysfunctional system.

These findings, showing that gestational and lactational deficiencies of zinc modify the developing brain, and thereby affect adult behavior, should be contrasted with the findings by Hesse and associates (1979) on zinc deficiency in adult animals. By the time the hippocampal formation has matured, there is little ability for zinc deficiency to alter the number of developing cells or their synaptic connections. This does not mean that hippocampal function cannot be impaired chemically or physiologically by acute zinc deficiency, only that the anatomical connections are likely to be intact.

Hesse measured a number of behaviors that are usually altered by damage to the hippocampal formation: open field activity, defensive immobility, T-maze alternation, appetitive approach latency, passive and active avoidance, and food consumption. These investigators showed that in every instance adult zinc deficiency altered behavior, but usually opposite to the effects of hippocampal damage. Comparison of the behavioral effects of zinc deficiency with those of adrenal steroid excess, however, showed close similarities. Hesse suggested that these similarities may be more than coincidental, given that zinc deficiency produces adrenal hypertrophy. Further work is obviously needed to show whether deficiency in adulthood produces behavioral changes by acting on corticosterone targets (e.g., hippocampus) or directly on systems that utilize zinc. It may well be that corticosterone targets such as the hippocampus, which take up and utilize high amounts of zinc, are especially sensitive to the effects of deficiency.

As Halas and Eberhardt (1987) have reviewed, deficiencies of iron or copper do not impair animals' abilities to the same extent. Rats fed an iron-deficient diet after weaning may suffer a long-lasting learning deficit that is not confounded with the general debilitation of the animals. In my laboratory

(Chafetz & Bernard, 1984) it was found that error scores of animals performing on a radial maze were correlated with hippocampal copper content: Animals with larger numbers of errors tend to have a lower concentration of copper.

Diet

Zinc's physiological association with proteins leads us to suspect that foods with a high protein content may contain relatively high concentrations of zinc. In fact, the foods containing the highest zinc levels are red meats and seafood, with oysters at 1,500 ppm topping the list. They contain some 30 times the quantity of zinc of their nearest competitors, the red meats, at 50 ppm. In contrast, vegetables and high-extraction wheat flour contain very little zinc.

Until recently, most studies on dietary zinc have focused either on zinc's role in cortical areas in memory function or on the pathologic signs, including anorexia, that result from zinc deficiency. These studies, as we will discuss, present the laboratory analogue of the cognitive and physical abnormalities seen in zinc-deficient individuals in many parts of the world. There has been little attention, however, to behavior in normal individuals that might serve to regulate dietary intake of zinc, or on the mechanisms of such regulation.

My approach to the study of zinc and behavior sought to remedy this deficit by focusing on the behavior in acutely deprived adult animals that would indicate an ability to regulate zinc intake (Chafetz et al., 1984). The idea was that acutely deprived rats should behave so as to be able to locate zinc on the arms of a radial maze, but only if zinc were present in the bait at the ends of the maze arms. This contrasted with the developmental deprivation studies of Halas in which neonatally deprived animals did not perform well on a radial maze, even when the bait contained zinc. In those developmental studies, the hippocampus was deprived of its normal connectional maturation; deficient animals should have shown the mnemonic deficit no matter what the bait contained. In our regulatory studies, we predicted that acutely deprived animals should be able to perform well only if they could find zinc-containing foods; otherwise, without the opportunity to regulate, there would be a behavioral deficit.

That was indeed the finding. Figure 9.5 shows that deficient animals performed as well as controls (phases I & IV) when the bait in the maze arms contained zinc. When deficient animals could not find zinc (phase II), they performed poorly compared to controls. That this effect was due to the micronutrient in the bait was suggested in phase III, during which the bait in half the arms contained zinc and when the controls performed as poorly as the deficient animals.

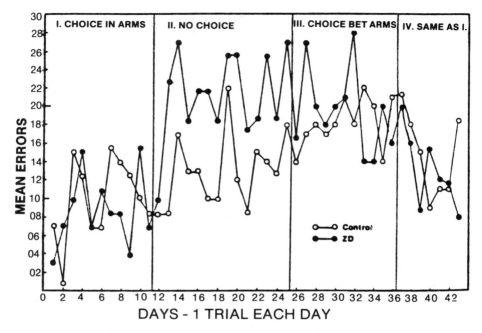

Figure 9.5 Results showing performance of adult zinc deprived and control animals in 8-arm radial maze. Deficient animals perform no differently from controls when bait in maze arms contains zinc, but poorly relative to controls when bait does not contain zinc. (From Chafetz et al., 1984.)

Although this work strongly suggested that animals could regulate their zinc intake by altering the quality of their maze performance, we could still argue that such performance was not conclusive. After all, we could never be certain about the deficiency status of deprived animals permitted to find foods that contain zinc, even when we could eliminate most of the available zinc from their environments. We therefore sought to remove zinc pharmacologically, so that no matter how much zinc the animals acquired from their experiences on the maze, we could be assured of their deficiency status.

The chelator that we used, however, did such an admirable job of removing zinc (Figure 9.6) that we probably disrupted hippocampal function severely, thereby impairing the animals' working memory abilities on the maze. Indicative of the severe disruption was the hyperreactivity we also witnessed in these animals. These were interesting findings in view of limbic system functions, but not subtle enough to show dietary regulation. We needed more subtle behavioral tasks to show regulation without significant impairment of other abilities.

In one study (Chafetz & Duhon, 1987), we trained animals to associate the taste of an unpleasant fluid (vinegar) with the amelioration of a zinc deficiency. Under these conditions, animals will seek out and consume the

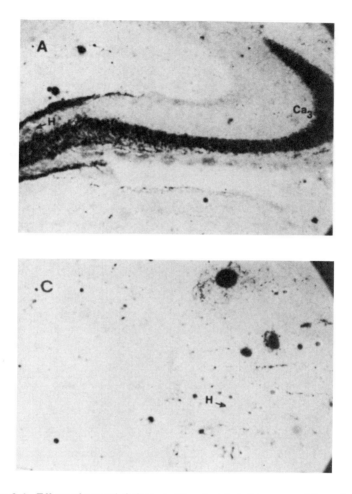

Figure 9.6   Effects of a metal chelator on Timm's stain in hippocampal formation. Lower photo is same view with chelator. (From Chafetz and Barbay, 1985.)

unpleasant vinegar solution, at least for a few days after it no longer contains zinc. When the vinegar is used as a reward for zinc-deficient animals on the radial maze (unpublished), there is no loss of performance. This indicates some regulatory ability without confounding the result by letting the animals find zinc in the maze arms.

The association of the taste of an unpleasant solution with the amelioration of a nutrient deficiency is called a *conditioned preference* and was used by Christensen and his associates (1974) to show regulatory ability for zinc. Zinc-deficient animals were provided with 0.2% acetic acid containing enough zinc to ameliorate their deficiencies. Within a short period of time, the animals consume the acetic acid, even though it is normally quite aversive. Acetic acid can then be given without zinc, and the animals will consume it for a period of days, indicating an association of the taste with the amelioration of their deficiencies. We were able to replicate these findings under slightly different conditions in which the acetic acid was not presented to the animals in a novel way: they were quite experienced with the aversive taste of the acetic acid, yet they consumed it when it contained zinc, and kept on consuming it (after conditioning) when it no longer contained zinc.

We were also able to show that animals can regulate zinc intake through behavior, without the benefit of taste-associative circumstances. In this experiment, the animals lived in operant chambers in which they always had a supply of food and distilled water. To get a pellet of food, they needed only to press a bar on one wall of the chamber.

By manipulating the mixture of deficient pellets in the food hoppers, we could alter the amount of zinc the animals were receiving from their environment, without making them clinically deficient. As you can see from Figure 9.7, the regulating animals differed from controls only when their supply of zinc was cut short. During these times, they consumed considerably more food than controls, in an apparent effort to reestablish their zinc supply. When all the zinc-normal food was cut from the hopper, and only deficient food was present, the animals did not consume more than controls. This

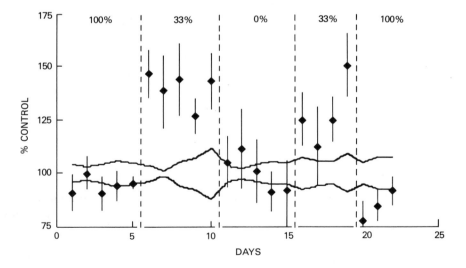

Figure 9.7 Apparent regulatory behavior for zinc. Regulating animals consume more pellets than controls when the content of zinc in their food supply is reduced. (From Chafetz and Duhon, 1987.)

behavior once again seems to present an example of a regulatory ability when the animals have the opportunity to regulate, and no attempt to regulate when there is no opportunity. It should be kept in mind that this apparent regulatory behavior occurred not when the animals were clinically deficient, but during the period of temporary dietary shortage. We therefore consider this finding to represent a behavioral analogue to the homeostatic changes in zinc uptake, absorption, and utilization that occur upon changes to the zinc supply in rats.

In this experiment, it was not likely that taste was a factor in the regulatory ability. A separate taste discrimination experiment showed that animals lacked the ability to discriminate deficient and normal pellets under the same conditions (partial zinc availability) in which apparent regulatory behavior was seen. The only time they could discriminate was during full zinc deprivation. The mechanism by which animals could regulate their zinc intake during partial zinc availability, though unknown, might therefore have been governed by postingestive consequences of altered zinc intake.

Zinc's physiological interactions with various proteins leads to speculation that proteins in the diet may have an influence on the regulation of zinc. Indeed, dietary protein intake affects the bioavailability of zinc. Studies of zinc balance have shown that increasing the protein content of the diet increases the absorption of zinc. This relationship, however, confounds the study of zinc deficiency because decreased elective consumption of deficient diets would alter the absorption of zinc. To get around the problem, Flanagan (1984) fed rats through intragastric tubes. Rats force fed a deficient diet in this manner grew as fast as rats fed a diet replete in zinc until the seventh day, after which the deficient rats rapidly lost weight and died. Flanagan suggested that it was likely that deficient rats allowed to eat freely tolerated the deficiency better because the lack of growth and protein build–up reduced the requirements for zinc.

In fact, the periodic drops in food consumption exhibited by deficient animals can be reduced or eliminated when animals are deprived of protein. Although this result was later qualified when it was shown that increased protein does not exacerbate the anorexia, the issue of a "floor" effect, or limit, on the diminished feeding was not addressed. Although the protein content of the food seems to be an important variable for the animal's adaptation to a zinc deficiency, it continued to be assumed that the diminished food intake in zinc-deficient animals represented a decreased consumption of protein. We therefore decided to determine whether deficient animals selectively reduce their intake of protein.

We offered zinc-deprived animals and controls a choice of low- or high-protein diets. The high-protein diet for half the animals was matched in carbohydrates to the low-protein diet; the high-protein diet for the other half was matched in calories. The results, however, were not consistent with the hypothesis that deficient animals choose less high protein. In fact, the deficient animals always chose less of the diet that had high carbohydrate content (especially the low-protein diet). Because the high-carbohydrate diets were more palatable, this result indicated that the diminished elective consumption of deficient animals has more to do with taste than with protein content. Several studies showing reduced taste acuity and an alteration in taste bud morphology in deficient animals support this conclusion.

Pathology

Growing clinical evidence indicates that dietary deficiencies of zinc exist in several parts of the world. There is extensive evidence of diet-related zinc deficiencies among adolescent village boys in Iran and in Egypt. Sandstead (1984) has also revealed evidence of zinc deficiency among infants from the lowest socioeconomic stratum in Egypt who have protein–calorie malnutrition. These observations gave impetus to much of the research on the developing behavioral status of rats and monkeys deprived of zinc during the neonatal period, in which deficiency impairs learning and memory abilities.

Zinc's role in cortical function, particularly in cognitive abilities, has also led to its implication in some cognitive disorders. Pick's disease, for example, is a degenerative senile or presenile dementia associated with severe cognitive and motor disorders. The pathologic neuronal changes that occur in this disease are found initially in the hippocampus before they spread to other cortical areas. Postmortem examination of tissue from patients with Pick's disease has shown increased zinc levels and more intense Timm staining in the hippocampus. It has therefore been suggested that alterations of glutamate and zinc in the hippocampus are responsible for the behavioral manifestations of this disorder.

Other investigators concerned with the role of zinc in hippocampal function have studied the relationships between zinc and convulsive disorders, especially ones similar to those seen in patients with Pick's disease. Elevation of zinc levels by intraventricular administration of zinc salts causes epileptic seizures in rats, characterized by running fits and tonic-clonic convulsions, indicating that the elevated zinc in Pick's disease may be at least partially responsible for the attending convulsive disorders. In keeping with this idea, there is the finding that electrically induced hippocampal granule cell seizure activity is associated with the loss of mossy fiber Timm staining. Because there is no granule cell damage with this experimental method, the simplest explanation for the loss of staining is that convulsive granule cell discharge results in a loss of synaptic metal via physiological release. This finding therefore indicates that convulsive discharges may result from an excess of zinc in the synaptic junction.

Iatrogenic zinc loss is also associated with cognitive and motor symptoms. Patients with progressive systemic sclerosis who were treated with the amino acid histidine showed a large decrease in serum zinc concentration. As a result of treatment the patients developed the anorexia and loss of taste acuity normally associated with zinc deficiency. They also developed cerebellar signs such as intention tremor and ataxia, suggesting that zinc's presence in cerebellum has a role in normal cerebellar function. Thought and speech interruptions were also observed. When zinc was administered to these patients, even with continued histidine administration, the signs and symptoms of deficiency all returned to or toward normal within 8 to 24 hours.

The anorexia observed as a result of zinc deficiency in several species has been likened to the condition observed primarily in young women (anorexia nervosa). Bakan (1979), noting the similarity, suggested that zinc therapy be used in anorectic patients. Indeed, the hidden assumption in the work showing that the anorexia in zinc-deficient rats is resistant to normal stimulants of feeding is that deficiency causes the condition.

This notion has only partial merit. Deficiencies of virtually every essential nutrient cause some form of anorexia. To name the loss of feeding "anorexia" tends to avoid the real issue of an understanding of the behavioral mechanism. In fact, animals form conditioned aversions to (deficient) foods that produce a general malaise. How these conditioned aversions relate to "anorexia" is largely unknown. Also, as a true anorectic becomes more and more deprived, nutrient deficiencies that may by themselves produce a form of "anorexia" become confounded with the cause of the original disorder.

However, the study of "anorexia" that results from trace metal deficiency may, as I have discussed elsewhere (Chafetz, 1984), be advantageous as an heuristic device. The heuristic model may involve, for example, some abnormality in a zinc metalloenzyme, so that a net "zinc deficiency" could occur despite adequate consumption of foods that contain zinc. In this form of the proposition, the anorectic does not have to be deprived of the essential nutrient to exhibit effects that normally occur as a result of deprivation. In other words, the cause could be an enzyme deficiency that "looks" like a zinc deficiency, because the enzyme happens to utilize zinc for its normal physiological function. With this proposition in mind, further studies of deficiency-related anorexias can be pursued without the hidden confounding factor.

Moreover, other attractive models of anorexia—notably the auto-addiction opioid model (Marrazzi & Luby, 1986)—can easily be linked. In this model, it is proposed that brain opioids mediate the physiologic and metabolic changes that occur in response to extreme food deprivation. The anorectic becomes addicted to these changes, and opiate blockade has been shown to be a useful therapeutic approach. We recall that zinc-deficient animals are resistant to the feeding induced by the opiate dynorphin. Potential endogenous changes in proteins (e.g., opiate receptors) that interact with zinc can thus be seen to result in the similar physiologic and behavioral consequences of zinc deficiency.

Summary

Zinc is one of 14 trace elements currently recognized as necessary to maintain normal metabolism, physiology, or growth in humans and animals. Zinc acts as a cofactor with enzymes and receptor proteins. In its function with proteins, it can act as a facilitator, bridging group, or stabilizing agent. Zinc is also necessary for the synthesis of DNA, RNA, and protein.

As a nutrient, zinc is required for fetal brain development. Deficiencies during development can result in brain and behavioral anomalies that persist into adult life. Zinc is also required for normal adult function. Acute deficiencies have effects on receptor binding and behavior. Zinc has been implicated in the normal function of opiate, GABA, aspartate, and NE transmitter systems, and zinc may act as a transmitter in its own right.

Zinc is found primarily in cortical tissues, especially in the hippocampal formation where it is highly concentrated in the mossy fiber terminal zone. The relatively high concentrations of zinc in cortical tissues that are important for learning and memory has implicated zinc in memory formation. Animals deprived of zinc during development show as adults impairment in working memory. This same impairment is found in animals who have disruption of the hippocampus or its fiber connections.

Animals can regulate their intake of zinc under conditions in which dietary zinc levels fluctuate. Animals consume more zinc when zinc levels in the diet are lowered. They also form conditioned preferences for tastes that are associated with the amelioration of a zinc deficiency.

Zinc-excess and -deficiency are both associated with pathologic conditions. Zinc-excess is associated with Pick's disease, while zinc-deficiency is associated with other cognitive disruptions, and with anorexia. The anorexia found in zinc-deficient animals does not correspond closely to anorexia nervosa, although aspects of zinc-deficiency can teach us more about the human disease state.

References

Bakan, R. The role of zinc in anorexia nervosa: Etiology and treatment. *Medical Hypotheses, 5,* 1979, 731–736.

Chafetz, M.D. Anorexia: A micronutrient model. *The Southern Psychologist, 2,* 1984, 39–47.

Chafetz, M.D. Timm's method modified for human tissue and compatible with adjacent section histofluorescence in the rat. *Brain Research Bulletin, 16*, 1986, 19–24.

Chafetz, M.D. & Bernard, D.L. Handling: Effects on eight-arm-maze behavior and hippocampal trace metals. *Physiological Psychology, 11*, 1984, 261–268.

Chafetz, M.D., Abshire, F.M., & Bernard, D.L. Zinc deficiency in adult rats alters foraging in a radial maze. In Frederickson, C.J. et al. (Eds.), *The neurobiology of zinc*, Part B. New York: Alan R. Liss, 1984, pp. 109–120.

Chafetz, M.D. & Barbay, S. Zinc deprivation and metal chelation effects on reactivity and eight-arm maze behavior. *Nutrition and Behavior, 2*, 1985, 213–224.

Chafetz, M.D. & Duhon, J. Evidence for behavioral regulation of dietary zinc intake. *Nutrition & Behavior, 3*, 1987, 279–290.

Christensen, C.M., Caldwell, D.F., & Oberleas, D. Establishment of a learned preference for a zinc-containing solution by zinc-deficient rats. *Journal of Comparative and Physiological Psychology, 87*, 1974, 415–421.

Colburn, R.W. & Maas, J.W. Adenosine triphosphate-metal-norepinephrine ternary complexes and catecholamine binding. *Nature, 208*, 1965, 37–41.

Danscher, G. Do the Timm sulphide silver method and the selenium method demonstrate zinc in the brain? In Frederickson, C.J. et al. (Eds.), *The Neurobiology of zinc*, Part A. New York: Alan R. Liss, 1984, pp. 273–287.

Danscher, G. Similarities and differences in the localization of metals in rat brains after treatment with sodium sulphide and sodium selenide. In Frederickson, C.J. et al. (Eds.), *The Neurobiology of zinc*, Part A. New York: Alan R. Liss, 1984, pp. 229–242.

Flanagan, P.R. A model to produce pure zinc deficiency in rats and its use to demonstrate that dietary phytate increases the excretion of endogenous zinc. *Journal of Nutrition, 114*, 1984, 493–502.

Frederickson, C.J., Klitenick, M.A., Manton, W.I., and Kirkpatrick, J.B. Cytoarchitectonic distribution of zinc in the hippocampus of man and the rat. *Brain Research, 273*, 1983, 335–339.

Halas, E.S. & Eberhardt, M.J. A behavioral review of trace element deficiencies in animals and humans. *Nutrition and Behavior, 3*, 1987, 257–271.

Halas, E.S. & Kawamoto, J.C. Correlated behavioral and hippocampal effects due to perinatal zinc deprivation. In Frederickson, C.J. et al. (Eds.), *The neurobiology of zinc*, Part B. New York: Alan R. Liss, 1984, pp. 91–108.

Halas, E.S., Eberhardt, M.J., Diers, M.A., & Sandstead, H.H. Learning and memory impairment in adult rats due to severe zinc deficiency during lactation. *Physiology & Behavior, 30*, 1983, 371–381.

Haug, F-M. S. Heavy metals in the brain: A light microscope study of the rat with Timm's sulphide silver method. Methodological considerations and cytological and regional staining patterns. *Advances in Anatomy, Embryology, and Cell Biology, 47*(4), 1973, 1–71.

Hesse, G.W., Hesse, K.A.F., & Catalanotto, F.A. Behavioral characteristics of rats experiencing chronic zinc deficiency. *Physiology & Behavior, 22*, 1979, 211–215.

Howell, G.A. & Frederickson, C.J. Electrical stimulation facilitates zinc turnover in hippocampal slices. In Frederickson, C.G. et al. (Eds.), *The neurobiology of zinc*, Part A. New York: Alan R. Liss, 1984, 141–155.

Kasarskis, E.J. Regulation of zinc homeostasis in rat brain. In Frederickson, C.J. et al. (Eds.), *The neurobiology of zinc*, Part A. New York: Alan R. Liss, 1984, pp. 27–38.

Marrazzi, M.A. & Luby, E.D. An auto-addiction opioid model of chronic anorexia nervosa. *International Journal of Eating Disorders, 5*(2), 1986, 191–208.

Olton, D.S., Walker, J.A., & Gage, F.H. Hippocampal connections and spatial discrimination. *Brain Research, 139*, 1978, 295–308.

Peters, S., Koh, J., & Choi, D.W. Zinc selectively blocks the action of N-methyl-d-aspartate on cortical neurons. *Science, 236*, 1987, 589–593.

Sandstead, H.H. Neurobiology of zinc. In Frederickson, C.J. et al. (Eds.), *The neurobiology of zinc*, Part B. New York: Alan R. Liss, 1984, pp. 1–16.

Sandstead, H.H., Fosmire, G.J., Halas, E.S., Jacob, R.A., Strobel, D.A., & Marks, E.O. Zinc deficiency: Effects on brain and behavior of rats and rhesus monkeys. *Teratology, 16*, 1977, 229–234.

Sandstead, H.H., Gillespie, D.D. & Brady, R.N. Zinc deficiency: Effect on brain of the suckling rat. *Pediatric Research, 6*, 1972, 119–125.

Timm, F. Zur Histochemie de Schwermetalle, das Sulfid-Silber-Ferfahren. *Dt. Z. ges gericht Med, 46*, 1958, 706–711.

Wallwork, J.C., Milne, D.B., & Sandstead, H.H. Distribution of minerals and catecholamines in rat brain: Effects of zinc deficiency. In Frederickson, C.J. et al. (Eds.), *The neurobiology of zinc*, Part B. New York: Alan R. Liss, 1984, pp. 49–64.

Wallwork, J.C., Milne, D.B., Sims, R.L., & Sandstead, H.H. Severe zinc deficiency: Effects on the distribution of nine elements (potassium, phosphorus, sodium, magnesium, calcium, iron, zinc, copper, and manganese) in regions of the rat brain. *Journal of Nutrition, 113*, 1983, 1895–1905.

Suggested Readings

Baraldi, M., Caselgrandi, E., & Santi, M. Effect of zinc on specific binding of GABA to rat brain membranes. In Frederickson et al. (Eds.), *The neurobiology of zinc*, Part A. New York: Alan R. Liss, 1984, pp. 59–71.

Chafetz, M.D. & Marx, E.S. Zinc deprivation effects on dietary self-selection in rats. unpublished paper.

Chesters, J.K. & Quarterman, J. Effects of zinc deficiency on food intake and feeding patterns of rats. *British Journal of Nutrition, 24*, 1970, 1061–1069.

Chesters, J.K. & Will, M. Some factors controlling food intake by zinc-deficient rats. *British Journal of Nutrition, 30*, 1973, 555–566.

Constantinidis, J. & Tissot, R. Role of glutamate and zinc in the hippocampal lesions of Pick's disease. In DiChiara, G. & Gessa, G.L. (Eds.), *Glutamate as a neurotransmitter*, New York: Raven Press, 1981, pp. 413–422.

Crawford, I.L. & Connor, J.D. Localization and release of glutamic acid in relation to the hippocampal mossy fibre pathway. *Nature, 244*, 1973, 442–443.

Dreosti, I.E., Manuel, S.J., Buckley, R.A., Fraser, F.J., & Record, I.R. The effect of late prenatal and/or early postnatal zinc deficiency on the development and some biochemical aspects of the cerebellum and hippocampus in rats. *Life Sciences, 28*, 1981, 2133–2141.

Ebadi, M., White, R.J., & Swanson, S. The presence and function of zinc-binding proteins in developing and mature brains. In Frederickson, C.J. et al. (Eds.), *The Neurobiology of zinc*, Part A. New York: Alan R. Liss, 1984, pp. 39–57.

Essatara, M'B., Levine, A.S., Morley, J.E., & McClain, C.J. Zinc deficiency and anorexia in rats: Normal feeding patterns and stress induced feeding. *Physiology & Behavior, 32*, 1984, 469–474.

Essatara, M'B., McClain, C.J., Levine, A.S., & Morley, J.E. Zinc deficiency and anorexia in rats: The effect of central administration of norepinephrine, muscimol and bromoerogocryptine. *Physiology & Behavior, 32*, 1984, 479–482.

Essatara, M'B., Morley, J.E., Levine, A.S., Elson, M.K., Shafer, R.B., & McClain, C.J. The role of the endogenous opiates in zinc deficiency anorexia. *Physiology & Behavior, 32*, 1984, 475–478.

Frederickson, C.J., Howell, G.A., & Kasarskis, E.J. (Eds.) *The neurobiology of zinc*, Part A: Physiochemistry, anatomy and techniques, Part B: deficiency, toxicity, and pathology. New York: Alan R. Liss, 1984.

Gentle, M.J., Dewar, W.A., & Wight, P.A.L. The effects of zinc deficiency on oral behavior and taste bud morphology in chicks. *British Poultry Science, 22*, 1981, 265–273.

Golub, M.S., Gershwin, M.E., & Vijayan, V.K. Passive avoidance performance of mice fed marginally or severely zinc deficient diets during post-embryonic brain development. *Physiology & Behavior, 30*, 1983, 409–413.

Golub, MS., Keen, C.L., Vijayan, V.K., Gerschwin, M.E., & Hurley, L.S. Early development of brain and behavior in mice fed a marginally zinc deficient diet. In Frederickson, C.J. et al. (Eds.), *The neurobiology of zinc*, Part B. New York: Alan R. Liss, 1984, pp. 65–76.

Gore, M.G. L-glutamic acid dehydrogenase. *International Journal of Biochemistry, 13*, 1981, 879–886.

Hambridge, K.M., Hambridge, C., Jacobs, M., & Baum, J.D. Low levels of zinc in hair, anorexia, poor growth, and hypogeusia in children. *Pediatric Research, 6*, 1972, 868–874.

Henkin, R.I., Patten, B.M., Re, P.K., & Bronzert, D.A. A syndrome of acute zinc loss. *Archives of Neurology, 32*, 1975, 745–751.

Lehninger, A.L. *Biochemistry*. New York: Worth Publishers, 1976.

Mahajan, S.K., Abraham, J., Hessburg, T., Prasad, A.S., Migdal, S.D., Abu-Hamdan, D.K., Briggs, W.A., & McDonald, F.D. Zinc metabolism and taste acuity in renal transplant recipients. *Kidney International, 24*, 1983, S-310–S-314.

Maske, H. Interaction between insulin and zinc in the Islets of Langerhans. *Diabetes, 6*, 1957, 335–341.

Mason, K.E., Burns, W.A., & Smith, J.C. Testicular damage associated with zinc deficiency in pre- and postpubertal rats: Response to zinc repletion. *The Journal of Nutrition, 112*, 1982, 1019–1028.

Mertz, W. The essential trace elements. *Science, 213*, 1981, 1332–1338.

Meydani, S.N. & Dupont, J. Effect of zinc deficiency on prostaglandin synthesis in different organs of the rat. *The Journal of Nutrition, 112*, 1982, 1098–1104.

Montano, C.Y., Kasarskis, E.J., & Savage, D.D. Quantitative histofluorescence of hippocampus mossy fiber zinc. *Society for Neuroscience Abstracts, 190.3*, 1987, p. 679.

Otsuka, N., Okano, H., & Yokoyama, K. A study on the mossy fiber endings in the hippocampal formation by electron microscopic autoradiography. *Acta Histochemistry Cytochemistry, 8*, 1975, 175–176.

Prasad, A.S. & Oberleas, D. Changes in activities of zinc-dependent enzymes in zinc-deficient tissues of rats. *Journal of Applied Physiology, 31*, 1971, 842–846.

Prohaska, J.R., Luecke, R.W., & Jasinski, R. Effect of zinc deficiency from day 18 of gestation and/or during lactation on the development of some rat brain enzymes. *The Journal of Nutrition, 104*, 1974, 1525–1531.

Rajan, K.S., Wiehle, R.D., Riesen, W.H., Colburn, R.W., & Davis, J.M. Effect of metal chelating agents on the storage of norepinephrine *in vitro* by cerebral synaptic vesicles. *Biochemical Pharmacology, 26*, 1977, 1703–1708.

Schwegler, H., Lipp, H.P., Van Der Loos, H., & Buselmaier, W. Individual hippocampal mossy fiber distribution in mice correlates with two-way avoidance performance. *Science, 214,* 1981, 817–819.

Shike, M. Trace elements in parenteral and enteral nutrition. *Current Concepts and Perspectives in Nutrition, 3,* 1984, 1–11.

Sloviter, R.S. A selective loss of Timm staining in the hippocampal mossy fiber pathway accompanies electrically induced hippocampal granule cell seizure activity in rats. In Frederickson, C.J. et al. (Eds.), *The neurobiology of zinc,* Part A. New York: Alan R. Liss, 1984, pp. 127–139.

Van Campen, D. & House, W.A. Effect of a low protein diet on retention of an oral dose of ^{65}Zn and on tissue concentrations of zinc, iron, and copper in rats. *Journal of Nutrition, 104,* 1974, 84–90.

Weigand, E. & Kirchgessner, M. Total true efficiency of zinc utilization: Determination and homeostatic dependence upon the zinc supply status in young rats. *The Journal of Nutrition, 110,* 1980, 469–480.

Yehuda, S., Youdim, M.E.H., & Mostofsky, D.I. Brain iron deficiency causes reduced learning capacity in rats. *Pharmacology, Biochemistry, & Behavior, 25,* 1986, 141–144.

Chapter 10
Vitamins: Ascorbic Acid (C) and Thiamine (B₁)

Many vitamins cannot be synthesized by animals, who must acquire them from the dietary environment. Without these vitamins, animals can develop deficiency diseases. That diets contain substances necessary to prevent deficiency diseases has been recognized since antiquity. However, it was not until the early 1900s that scientists proved experimentally that animals need more than protein, fat, and carbohydrate in the diet for normal growth. The name *vitamine* was coined at this time to denote an amine essential for life. Thiamine (B_1) was this first "vitamine," concentrated from rice husks, which alleviated symptoms of beriberi among Japanese sailors limited to a diet of milled or polished rice. Ascorbic acid (C) was not isolated until the early 1930s, though it had been recognized since Great Britain was a world sea power that consumption of limes prevented scurvy in British sailors ("limeys").

Vitamins are classified as being fat- or water-soluble. This chapter will focus on two of the water-soluble vitamins (Figure 10.1). This is not for historic reasons alone. Several lines of research provide us with relatively extensive knowledge of the behavioral mechanisms of thiamine regulation. This work is exemplary in showing how these mechanisms might operate for the intake of any nutrient for which there is not a primary appetite. More recent evidence indicates direct interaction of thiamine with central neurotransmitters, providing a possible line of inquiry for control of these behaviors. With regard to ascorbic acid, much of the relevant work has focused on this latter aspect: there is now considerable evidence of ascorbate's interactions with neurotransmitters that play an important part in behavioral control. For these insights—behavioral and neuroscientific—our discussion centers on vitamins B_1 and C.

*B*iochemistry and Physiology

Some enzymes depend only on their protein's characteristics for biochemical function. Other enzymes, however, require nonprotein components— cofactors—for activity. A cofactor may be a metal ion (see Chapter 9) or it

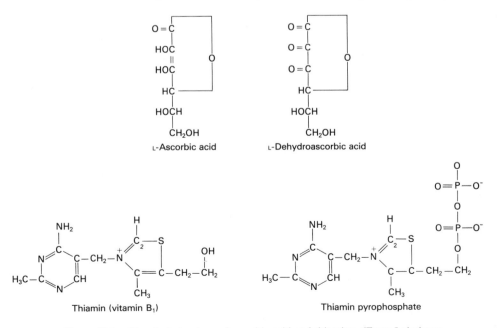

Figure 10.1 Chemical structure of ascorbic acid and thiamine. (From Lehninger, 1975.)

may be another organic molecule, called a coenzyme. Some enzymes require both. Coenzymes usually function as carriers of atoms, electrons, or molecules within the enzyme reaction. They contain at least a molecule of one of the vitamins as part of their structure.

The actions and functions of a vitamin can be studied at two general levels of inquiry: the affected functions that occur as a result of deficiency and restoration; and the specific biochemical reactions in which the vitamin is thought to play a part. It is often difficult to reconcile these two approaches, since the net results of the deficiency disease may have an indirect relationship to the specific biochemical functions of the vitamin. Nevertheless, both avenues of inquiry provide insight in the form of converging evidence and are therefore discussed in context.

Ascorbic Acid

Vitamin C has a biochemical role in mono-oxygenase (hydroxylase) reactions, which require copper, molecular oxygen, and a reductant such as ascorbate. In these reactions, ascorbate probably acts at the level of the metal to activate the oxygen, and not directly on the substrate. In this regard, ascorbate may be required for maintaining iron in the ferrous state. One mono-oxygenase reaction particularly important for our concerns is the hydroxylation of dopamine (DA) to norepinephrine (NE) (Figure 10.2). The enzyme, dopamine beta-hydroxylase (DBH) (see Chapter 4) contains 2-12 atoms of copper. The overall conversion in this reaction occurs with the transfer of two electrons to a suitable acceptor:

DA + ascorbate + $O_2 \rightarrow$ NE + dehydroascorbate + H_2O

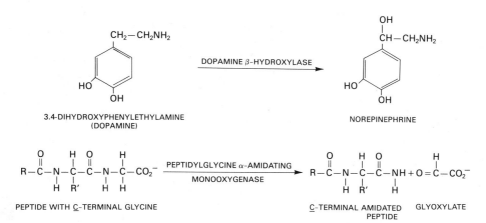

Figure 10.2 Monooxygenase reactions involving the use of ascorbate. (From England and Seifter, 1986.)

Ascorbate may therefore be an important factor in evaluating dietary effects of aspartame and tyrosine (see Chapter 4) on the brain and behavior. Interactions between *dietary* ascorbate and *dietary* precursors of catecholamine synthesis have not, to my knowledge, been investigated.

Many of the peptides active in the CNS and periphery have their carboxyl-terminal residue amidated as a common post-translational modification. The process is catalyzed by an enzyme (requiring copper) that cleaves the carboxyl-terminal residue with the use of molecular oxygen (Figure 10.2). This is not a simple hydrolytic cleavage, because the amino group at the terminal residue is retained in the final product as a terminal amide, while the remainder of the oxidized terminal group leaves as an aldehyde. Ascorbate is useful to this reaction analogously to the monooxygenase reaction: as a reductant for transfer of electrons. This utility broadens the significance of ascorbate in the CNS and periphery. For example, included among the peptides amidated are bombesin, calcitonin, corticotropin releasing factor, gastrin, growth hormone releasing factor, thryotropin releasing hormone, alpha-melanocyte stimulating hormone, neuropeptide Y, oxytocin, pancreatic polypeptide, substance P, vasoactive intestinal peptide, and vasopressin. Deficiency of vitamin C potentially affects all these neuroactive substances.

Ascorbic acid is found in several peripheral tissues, but its highest concentration is in the adrenal gland and pituitary. Ascorbate appears to be active in both adrenal cortex and medulla. In adrenal cortex, ascorbate appears to be a specific factor in the 11β-hydroxylase reaction (for the formation of corticosterone). For example, ascorbate protects against the loss of activity of 11β-hydroxylase induced by cortisol, which acts as a pseudosubstrate. Specificity is indicated; other biological antioxidants have no such protective effect. Another major function of ascorbate in adrenal cortex is as a protective compound for oxidative damage to cytochrome P450s.

Pituitary hormones not only regulate adrenal steroids but also play a role in ascorbic acid control. It has been known for several years that acute stress or injection of adrenocorticotropic hormone (ACTH) induces a 20-40% release of ascorbate from adrenals into the blood. After hypophysectomy, ascorbate levels decrease in adrenals, liver, blood, and urine. In the hypophysectomized animal, ACTH still has its normal action, inducing an equivalent percentage release of ascorbate. Replacement with corticosteroids does not restore adrenal ascorbate, which indicates that lack of such steroids is not the cause of decreased ascorbate. Administration of ascorbic acid by itself will not restore adrenal ascorbate; therefore, some other factor(s) must regulate its uptake. Both growth hormone and prolactin may serve this role, since they both elevate ascorbate in adrenals but not in blood. Thus, pituitary hormones play antagonistic roles in the uptake and release of adrenal ascorbate.

Ascorbic acid has an uneven regional distribution in the brain: the hypo-

thalamus accumulates more than other bra
sized in brain, and must first be transporte
urable transport system. The overall concent
brain is 1-2 mM, which is a relatively high l
regional content, the concentration of ascorl
at approximately 250 uM. Homeostatic m
"compartmentalizing" ascorbate concentrati
play several roles, any of which are potentia

Ascorbate's association with hydroxylase
examination of ascorbate's interactions with c
from drug injection studies in which ascorb   ......oxidant
suggested (on the basis of control injections of ascorbate vehicle) that ascorbate was active itself in producing or antagonizing behavioral effects of the drugs being tested. The evidence thus began to accrue that ascorbate's roles in the CNS go well beyond participation in enzyme activity. Because the original drug tests were related to DA activity in the striatum, much of the focus of ascorbate CNS research has been on striatal interactions, although ascorbate may act independently of DA receptors.

For example, an increase in the concentration of ascorbate in the extracellular fluid of rat striatum occurs with systemic administration of amphetamine. Electrolytic lesions in the crus cerebri of the striatonigral pathway abolish this effect. Moreover, these lesions abolish the effect of systematic amphetamine ipsilateral to a lesion, but not contralateral. The releases of striatal ascorbate by amphetamine administration may thus be controlled by a feedback pathway from the striatum.

Although amphetamine is an active stimulant of DA activity in the striatum, and may thus costimulate DA and ascorbate release, there is little evidence for ascorbate's interactions with presynaptic DA receptors. For example, electrical stimulation of the nigrostriatal pathway releases DA, which can be measured by voltammetry in anesthetized rats. Metoclopramide increases DA release, whereas apomorphine decreases DA release. Pretreatment of rats with ascorbate triples striatal ascorbate levels in extracellular fluid, but affects neither electrically stimulated DA release nor the effects of drugs on DA release. The administration of ascorbate to an incubation medium, however, does inhibit the binding of DA agonists to brain plasma membranes, indicating some interaction with postsynaptic receptors.

Evidence is accruing for ascorbate's interaction with glutamate (GLU) systems. In one study, iontophoresis of ascorbate (physiological concentrations) increased the firing rate of one-third of the neurons tested in the neostriatum of anesthetized rats. When administered to neostriatal neurons activated by the simultaneous injection of GLU, ascorbate excited more than two-thirds of the cells. This link to GLU has been further strengthened in

oltammetry to measure the release of ascorbate in various
he relative amplitude of the ascorbate signal corresponded to
density of excitatory amino acid transmission determined by other
s. Moreover, GLU and aspartate cause the release of ascorbate from
ptosomes.

Because of its antioxidant properties, ascorbate may play a role as scavenger for free radicals. The neurotoxic actions of methamphetamine and 1-methyl-4-phenyl pyridinium (MPP^+) have been attributed, at least in part, to the generation of free radicals. These drugs enhance auto-oxidation of DA to 6-hydroxydopamine, which destroys DA nerve terminals, thereby depleting DA at the site of injection. If ascorbate is administered just prior to injection, the depletion of DA caused by these drugs is significantly attenuated in a dose-response manner, indicating that ascorbate acted to prevent the oxidation of DA.

Developmental studies by Kratzing and associates (1984, 1985) suggest that ascorbate's anti-free radical role may be important to an organism during a time of maximal cell proliferation. Ascorbate levels in fetal rat brain increase almost 100% from the 15th to 20th day of gestation. There is an 18% drop from this plateau after birth. Even though DA and NE systems are developing at this time, it is unlikely that ascorbate is increasing solely as a requirement for developing catecholamine enzymes. Ascorbate increases only twofold, whereas the catecholamines increase 15-fold during the same period. Furthermore, the levels of ascorbic acid in the brains of growing rats are not influenced by efforts to accelerate neural activity, including administration of caffeine or placement of the animal in a complex environment. Such manipulations presumably increase catecholamine activity, indicating again that ascorbate may have independent functions.

Thiamine

Thiamine pyrophosphate (TPP), a coenzyme containing the vitamin thiamine, participates in several important biochemical reactions. It is part of the pyruvate dehydrogenase complex, which catalyzes the oxidation of pyruvate to acetyl-CoA. This reaction is obligatory for entry of all carbohydrates into the tricarboxylic acid cycle. Moreover, acetyl-CoA is one of two precursors for the formation of acetylcholine (see Chapter 5). The oxidation of alpha-ketoglutarate to succinyl-CoA is a similar reaction and also occurs through the use of TPP by a dehydrogenase (for alpha-ketoglutarate). TPP also acts as an intermediate carrier of a glycolaldehyde group in reactions catalyzed by transketolase. That thiamine is important in carbohydrate metabolism is underscored by the fact that one prominent reaction catalyzed by transketolase is the reversible conversion between two intermediates of the phosphogluconate pathway and two intermediates of the glycolytic pathway (Figure 10.3). Furthermore, TPP participates in the activities of hexokinase, phospho-fructokinase, and glutamate dehydrogenase.

Brain slices and homogenates from animals deficient in thiamine show the physiologic significance of thiamine's participation in enzyme activity. Although brain slices from deficient animals show relatively normal glucose metabolism, producing CO_2 and acetylcholine from glucose at rates similar to controls, there is a severe decline in the K^+-induced increase in the formation of these compounds. In brain homogenates from deficient animals, activities of TPP-dependent enzymes—transketolase and alpha-ketoglutarate dehydrogenase—decrease precipitously, though there is no change in pyruvate dehydrogenase. When pyruvate dehydrogenase activity is studied in midbrain and pons (lateral vestibular nucleus), however, there is a selective reduction in its activity by 15-30%. Treatment with thiamine for 7 days restores glucose oxidation, acetylcholine synthesis, and dehydrogenase activity

```
        CH2OH
         |
         C = O
         |
       HOCH           D-Xylulose
         |            5-phosphate
       HCOH
         |
       CH2OPO3²⁻

         +

        CHO
         |
       HCOH            D-Erythrose
         |             4-phosphate
       HCOH
         |
       CH2OPO3²⁻

         ↕ transketolase

        CH2OH
         |
         C = O
         |
       HOCH
         |             D-Fructose
       HCOH            6-phosphate
         |
       HCOH
         |
       CH2OPO3²⁻

         +

        CHO
         |              D-Glyceraldehyde
       CHOH             3-phosphate
         |
       CH2OPO3²⁻
```

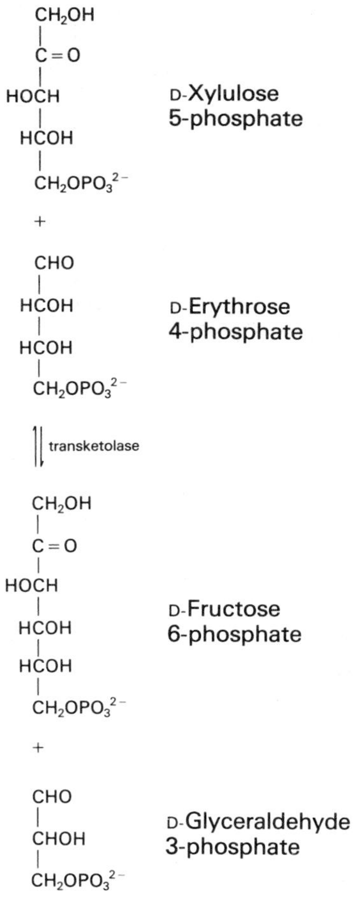

Figure 10.3 Transketolase reaction involving the use of thiamine. (From Lehninger, 1975.)

to normal, though transketolase activity remains lower than control levels. Activities of hexokinase, phosphofructokinase, and glutamate dehydrogenase are approximately normal in deficient animals.

A major metabolic consequence of thiamine deficiency is a widespread reduction in cerebral glucose utilization. In several CNS structures, glucose utilization declines with diminishing concentrations of cerebral thiamine.

There are relatively high concentrations of thiamine in brain tissue, and thiamine in brain appears to be differentially distributed. The highest thiamine content in normal animals has been measured in cerebellar vermis and in the caudate nucleus. Other brain areas having measurable thiamine levels include cortex, thalamus, hypothalamus, pons, and medulla. Dietary deficiency reduces, and administration of thiamine (or the pyrophosphate) reverses, thiamine content in each of these areas.

Thiamine is transported into the CNS by two separate mechanisms. One is a saturable, high-affinity process, that at physiologic levels of plasma thiamine accounts for 91% (cerebral cortex) to 95% (cerebellum) of the total thiamine taken up. This is, however, a low-capacity process, because cerebral tissue extracts less than 7% of the plasma thiamine. The other process is nonsaturable, and is most efficient in the cerebral cortex. There is evidence indicating that thiamine can be transported across the blood-brain barrier in the absence of energy-producing metabolism. Changes in dietary thiamine could thus alter the amount of thiamine reaching the brain.

The cerebellum has the highest concentration of thiamine compounds, especially TPP, whereas the sciatic nerve (in periphery) has the lowest. The cerebellum is also highly efficient in performing most of the metabolic steps of thiamine turnover. Cerebral cortex exhibits the least active thiamine metabolism, and brainstem is in an intermediate position. TPP-dependent enzymes are also present in the cerebellum in higher concentrations than in the cerebral cortex and the brainstem.

Several lines of evidence indicate thiamine's importance in neurotransmission, especially in cerebellum. There are three extrinsic afferent indoleamine axonal systems in the cerebellar cortex: (1) parallel fibers to the molecular layer; (2) mossy fibers to the granular layer; and (3) diffusely branching axons to all layers. In thiamine-deficient animals, autoradiograms show a dramatic decline in all indoleamine-labelled structures. Thiamine deficiency also changes the responses of cerebellar cells to iontophoretically applied serotonin. Normally, Purkinje cells respond to serotonin in excitatory, inhibitory, or biphasic ways. In deficient animals, responses are solely inhibitory, and neurons are more sensitive to inhibitory effects of serotonin. It was suggested, on the basis of these results, that thiamine deficiency, by decreasing serotonin innervation in the cerebellum, increases the number of serotonin receptors, thereby providing a different response to any remaining serotonin.

Thiamine deficiency, induced either by diet or by treatment with an antagonist, results in alterations in cholinergic muscarinic binding in several brain regions. Muscarinic binding, primarily in the low-affinity site, increases in corpus callosum, lamina VI of parietal cortex, striatum, ventral thalamus, strata lacunosum moleculare and oriens of the hippocampus, and the dentate gyrus. There is also decreased muscarinic binding in the ventromedial hypothalamus. It is interesting that administration of a thiamine derivative—sulbutiamine—in nondeprived mice increases high–affinity uptake of choline in the hippocampus. These results suggest not only that deficiency impairs cholinergic innervation in several brain sites but also that excess thiamine may actually increase cholinergic proliferation.

Thiamine may also interact with NE systems. Thiamine deficiency results in a significant reduction in NE content in cortex, hippocampus, and olfactory bulb, but not in other regions of the brain. Thiamine, however, does not affect all neurotransmitters; dopamine and serotonin levels remain unaltered in many brain regions. This result is also interesting in contrast to the loss of serotonin innervation of the cerebellum. There appears to be some regional specificity to thiamine's interaction with serotoninergic systems.

*D*iet and Behavior

Ascorbic Acid

It is well known that citrus fruits and vegetables contain relatively high amounts of ascorbic acid. Broccoli contains very high concentrations of the vitamin. (There is, by the way, a fair degree of evidence that microwave cooking, by reducing cooking time and exposure to water, is the best method for preserving the active content of heat-labile and water soluble vitamins.) Table A10, produced by Koplan and others (1986) from the National Health and Nutrition Examination Survey, shows the daily dietary intake of selected nutrients (including ascorbate and thiamine) for persons 18-74 years of age in the United States, from 1976 to 1980.

Cultural and socioeconomic factors play a role in determining ascorbate intake in the United States. In the San Antonio Heart Study, it was shown that Mexican-Americans consume less ascorbate, calcium, and vitamin A than Anglo-Americans. In this same study, it was shown that Anglo-Americans consume less thiamine and riboflavin than Mexican-Americans. If the effects of culture are held constant, the lower the socioeconomic status, the less ascorbate was consumed.

For most animals, ascorbate is not required in the diet per se, as it is synthesized in a biochemical sequence that begins with glucose. In humans and other primates, flying mammals (fruit bats), guinea pigs, and passeriform birds, there is a strict requirement for ascorbate in the diet, since these animals lack one of the enzymes in ascorbate's synthetic sequence: l-gulono-gamma-lactone oxidase.

The actual requirement for ascorbate in a species unable to synthesize it is difficult to determine. This is because the need may change with physiological status, daily variations in activity or diet, stress, and disease. In fact, the margins of safety differ between the United States and Great Britain, leading these two societies to recommend different daily allowances: 30 mg in Great Britian and 60 mg in the United States.

The calculations take into account "buffer" time provided by the body pool to prevent scurvy if the individual were to cease consumption of the vitamin. Clinical scurvy occurs when the body pool of ascorbate is less than 300 mg. Ingestion of as little as 10 mg ascorbate/day can cure or prevent scurvy, but this amount leads to a body pool that is not substantially greater than 300 mg. If the individual were to alter activity levels, or any other factor that increases turnover of ascorbate (including ascorbate intake), ingestion of 10 mg/day may not prevent scurvy. If an individual were to consume 60 mg/day, the body pool would rise to 1500 mg, which is enough to protect against scurvy for at least 30 days if ascorbate ingestion ceases. But, as we previously discussed, there is no clear relationship between the biochemical roles of ascorbate and the deficiency disease. The amount necessary to buffer against the development of scurvy may not be equivalent to the amount that would satisfy diverse enzymatic, antioxidant, and neuromodulator roles for the vitamin.

There is yet another way of viewing the problem. If we correct for body weight, the amount of ingested ascorbate necessary to buffer against scurvy in humans is approximately 0.9 mg/kg/day. Yet the range of ascorbate synthesis in most other mammals is 40-275 mg/kg/day, which is over 40 times the recommended human intake even at the lower value. Even admitting the argument that no simple comparison can be made (though every species measured synthesizes higher amounts), we must take into account that biochemical and organ uses of ascorbate in humans and other animals are indeed comparable. For example, organs with the highest measured ascorbate in both rat (which synthesizes ascorbate) and human are adrenal and pituitary. Organs with a middle range amount in both species include liver, spleen, kidney, and brain. These data suggest roles for ascorbate more far-reaching than the prevention of scurvy.

The data showing a clear role for ascorbate in behavior are still meager, but evidence is growing for ascorbate's involvement in motor activity. For example, voltammetric measurements of ascorbate in the striatum indicate a nocturnal rise in the ascorbate signal, with subsequent peaks that produce a strong correlation with natural motor activity of the animal. These signals were measured in the striatum, as well as in frontal cortex, accumbens, and hippocampus.

In behavioral terms, ascorbate appears to act as a DA antagonist. Administration of ascorbate decreases stereotypy produced by relatively large doses of amphetamine. Ascorbate also appears to enhance catalepsy induced by haloperidol, and will enhance the antiamphetamine effects of the DA antagonist. Similarly to ascorbate, haloperidol increases the firing rate of neostriatal neurons.

In humans, ascorbic acid status has been evaluated in running and sedentary men. In this study (Fishbaine & Butterfield, 1984), there was a positive relationship between activity level (length of daily run) and serum ascorbate levels that was not attributable to differences in intake. Suggestions for the difference included a change in the distribution of vitamin within the tissues leading to its increased metabolic turnover. The authors concluded that exercise may induce a change in the handling of ascorbic acid such that serum levels are maintained high as a consequence of decreased urinary excretion.

A study appointed by the Swedish Sports Federal (Bruce et al., 1985) examined the effects of extra intake of ascorbate on competitive racing over long or short distances. Essentially, there was no effect; however, an increase in the aerobic working capacity was found after a 2 week regimen of 1 g/day ascorbic acid. The problem with this study was that a "training effect" could not be excluded as a factor. The investigators concluded that ascorbate has no beneficial effects in meeting the additional stress imposed by exercise in healthy subjects.

The author is aware of little evidence of nutrient regulation for ascorbate. In an unpublished paper submitted by a student, ratings of taste palatability for a source of ascorbic acid were examined. Both male and female undergraduates participated in this study. Subjects were presented with an array of four food items: a peeled section of a fresh orange, a soda cracker, shelled peanuts, and a slice of cheddar cheese. Subjects were asked to rate the taste palatability of each of these items presented in a random order, and were required to "rinse" and "spit" after each taste. The ratings were presented on a 10-point scale, 5 being "typical," 10 being "much better than usual," and 1 being "worse than usual."

After the ratings were collected, subjects were asked to record everything eaten or drunk, including vitamins, the day prior to the experiment. These listings, taken after the ratings so as not to elicit an expectation, were then examined for sources of vitamin C. Those subjects (n = 10) who had consumed less than 20 mg ascorbate the day before had significantly higher ratings of the orange slice than those subjects (n = 7) who had consumed more than 20 mg ascorbate. Ratings of the other food items were not affected. It was interesting that choices among the high-ascorbate subjects varied extensively, including broccoli, citrus fruits and juices, and vitamins, but still produced relative uniform low ratings. Although this study was not ideal in controlling every factor, it suggests that prior consumption of ascorbate influences an individual's palatability for a subsequent food that contains high amounts of ascorbate.

Thiamine

Although Table A10 gives the thiamine status among a large sample of adults in the United States, it does not provide information on cultural variation, of which there is some. In a study of Jamaican children, thiamine deficiency was found in 7% of the normal children and 36% of malnourished children, which was higher than anticipated values.

Richter's early analysis provided much of the empirical justification for examining intake of thiamine. He and his collaborators (1938) noted that survival of animals depends upon their ability to select from a variety of beneficial, useless, and even harmful substances. When he provided rats with a cafeteria of various nutrient sources, the animals would choose regularly from each source, maintaining health and reproductive abilities at or exceeding levels of animals reared on a "complete" lab chow diet. Yeast as a source of B vitamins (including thiamine) was regularly sampled by the rats. In a separate experiment, Richter (1937) showed that normal as well as deficient rats evidence great interest in dried baker's yeast. Moreover, there is an "overwhelming appetite" for thiamine in a pure crystalline form. The odor of the vitamin as well as its taste aroused great interest in the animals. In fact, the investigators noted great difficulty in stopping the animals from ingesting the substance once they had tasted it. The conclusion was that there existed a powerful craving for the essential nutrient.

Recent genetic studies hint at different needs for thiamine, though there is room for other interpretations. McFarland (1985), examining different mouse phenotypes, showed that a reduction in spontaneous motor activity induced by thiamine deficiency was greater in C57 than in Balb and Nylar mice, though there were no differences in spontaneous alternation or spatial discrimination learning.

Subsequent examinations of behavioral mechanisms that "explain" the nutrient hunger for thiamine were conducted principally by Paul Rozin and his collaborators. In one of the earlier studies (1969), thiamine-deficient rats showed a marked preference for diets containing any of three concentrations of thiamine over diets that lacked thiamine. The preferences appeared whether arbitrary cues were paired with the thiamine or not. Moreover, fewer than half of the animals showed an immediate preference for the thiamine diet. Preferences for the vitamine-rich diet became *greater* as the concentration of the vitamin *increased*, which argued against a notion of "drive reduction" and hinted at the idea that the preference may not be innate as Richter's work had suggested. Furthermore, parallel studies with thiamine in water, in contrast to Richter's findings, showed no such preferences in deficient animals, suggesting that mode of intake (i.e., food when hungry, and water when thirsty) is important in specific hunger for a vitamin.

Need for thiamine apparently plays a minimal role in the development of a thiamine hunger. Deficient animals choose a diet loaded with thiamine over a deficient diet. If these animals are given an injection of thiamine so that they recover from the deficiency, they still choose a diet enriched with thiamine. Recovery from deficiency by ingestion of thiamine also has no significant effect in eliminating preference. The only time animals show no such preference is when they are "naive;" that is, they have never experienced a thiamine deficiency. Thus, something other than a "postingestional effect" is probably involved in the development of a thiamine hunger.

To test whether this "something" was related to "novelty" in food choice, Rodgers and Rozin (1966) offered thiamine-deficient animals a choice between a novel diet and a familiar diet. The deficient animals showed a marked preference for the novel diet. If the novel diet contained thiamine, the preference was maintained over a 10-day period. If the novel diet was deficient in thiamine, and thiamine was added to the familiar diet, animals switched after 3-4 days from an initial preference for the novel diet to one for the familiar diet. Naive controls showed no such preferences. The investigators, arguing from these and previous data, suggested that one difficulty with "innate recognition" as an explanation for deficient animals' preference for thiamine is the failure of a reliable immediate response to the vitamin. The exclusive initial ingestion of a novel diet, they suggested, could facilitate the development of a sustained learned preference: ingestion of thiamine-rich foods makes a deficient rat "feel" better, thus reinforcing the animal's choice.

There were difficulties with this interpretation. One was that there is no such preference for thiamine in water, though it produces the same effect. Another is that rats injected with thiamine still showed preferences despite the loss of stimulus consequences of the food; that is, it no longer is directly linked to the association. Still another difficulty was the long delay in conditioning; most kinds of conditioning were based on shorter time intervals.

Garcia and colleagues (1967) were able to provide insight into the problem with delays in conditioning. They made rats deficient in thiamine and gave them a nonnutritive saccharin solution to drink. If animals were given an injection of thiamine to provide the physiological basis for conditioning, they increased their intake of the saccharin solution, which response had now been conditioned. Delay of the injection up to 30 minutes had no effect on the acquisition of this conditioning. Garcia argued that because the ultimate effects of food are delayed, there is a need for gustatory/visceral associations to span longer times than telereceptor/cutaneous associations. As he illustrated, no one would expect conditioning in rats to the onset of a light, if 30 minutes later an electric shock was delivered to the feet.

Rozin (1968) later argued that long-delay conditioned aversions were not mediated by an aftertaste, which would have made them merely special cases of a classically conditioned response. He was able to show that rats can learn to avoid one of two concentrations of the *same substance* when ingestion of one is followed after 30 minutes by an injection of apomorphine, which produces nausea. Thus, he argued, conditioned aversions are a new form of conditioning in which memory of the relevant taste is stored centrally over a period of at least half an hour.

Rozin also argued that the "neophilia"—choice of novelty—of vitamin-deficient rats may really be explained as a "paleophobia"—an aversion to the old familiar diet. The behavior of deficient rats toward a familiar deficient diet is similar to the behavior of normal rats toward highly unpalatable food. There is a generalized avoidance of the food and frequent spilling. If rats are made deficient on a given diet, and then recover on a new diet, they will avoid the familiar diet even when it is presented alone. This avoidance will occur even if they are food-deprived (hungry) and perfectly healthy. Paleophobia, produced by a conditioned aversion, could explain why animals continue to eat a thiamine-enriched food even after the deficiency is ameliorated. They are still avoiding the food that made them deficient. Deficient animals therefore engage in adaptive feeding behavior.

The question remained, however, whether the choice of a novel diet would be specific for the vitamin. Rodgers showed that it was not. Thiamine-deficient and recovered animals did not prefer a diet supplement in thiamine when given the choice of two forms of the same novel diet mixture or two distinct novel diet mixtures. Furthermore, in tests with thiamine-deficient and pyridoxine-deficient animals, thiamine-deficient animals preferred a diet supplemented with thiamine over a doubly deficient diet. But pyridoxine-deficient animals also showed a preference for the diet supplemented with thiamine. Conversely, pyridoxine-deficient animals prefer a diet supplemented with pyridoxine over a doubly deficient diet, but so do thiamine-deficient animals. Thus, unlike sodium hungers, vitamin-specific hungers are not initially based on a specific taste of the needed vitamins, but on the novelty of their taste or smell. Choice of novelty, conditioned preferences, and conditioned aversions all combine to produce an adaptive response for deficient animals.

Rozin (1969) further explored the food-sampling patterns of vitamin-deficient rats. He showed that thiamine-deficient rats, faced with a choice of four diets, only one of which contains thiamine, often develop strong preferences for the enriched choice. To do so, the deficient rats sample foods systematically, and tend to eat only one type of food in any single meal. This behavior pattern would facilitate the development of a conditioned preference for the "correct" food. Rozin suggested that this would be quite adaptive for an omnivore, who could not be expected to be faced with a simple choice between a familiar deficient food and a novel enriched food.

*B*ehavioral Pathology

A number of conditions caused by vitamin deficiency exist, but in keeping with the scope of this work, any pathologic condition induced by vitamin deficiency will be discussed within the realm of its impact on brain and behavior.

The Wernicke-Korsakoff syndrome is a mental disorder characterized by anterograde amnesia, and a period of retrograde amnesia. It is thought to result from thiamine deficiency secondary to chronic alcoholism. This occurs not only because an alcoholic's diet is typically deficient in thiamine but also because ethanol has been shown to interfere with absorption and utilization of thiamine in experimental animals.

It is particularly important that some of the memory deficits and acute confusional states that result from alcoholism can often be reversed by administration of thiamine. As we previously discussed, deficiencies of thiamine result in alterations in cholinergic muscarinic binding in several regions of the brain when acetylcholine is thought to participate in processes of memory (see Chapter 5). Although it is still conjecture at this time, muscarinic binding may be altered as a result of decreased synthesis of acetylcholine from reduced conversion of pyruvate to acetyl-CoA. Administration of thiamine or its derivatives may thus potentially alleviate deficits by restoring acetylcholine synthesis. There is also evidence that memory deficits could result from the dramatically reduced levels of ACTH, which has been shown to play a role in learning and memory formation.

Alcoholics also have reduced levels of ascorbic acid, and several lines of evidence indicate that ascorbate protects rats from the toxic effects of alcohol. Ethanol preference, however, is not altered by acute dietary deficiency of this vitamin.

Thiamine deficiencies also lead to the appearance of neurologic signs, probably attributable to neurochemical changes in pons, midbrain, and cerebellum. Some of these include loss of righting reflex, convulsions, ataxia, piloerection, and paresis, and are ameliorated by restoration of thiamine, which presumably restores a relatively normal balance of neurochemistry. Memory impairments, however, seem to be a long-term feature of thiamine deficiency in animal models, often remaining long after vitamin administration has normalized the neurologic signs.

One other major feature of thiamine deficiency is a profound anorexia. Speculation as to its cause has focused on neurochemical changes in the hypothalamus: there is reduced NE activity and altered muscarinic binding in ventromedial regions. Other ideas revolve around data showing reduced cerebral glucose utilization, perhaps giving the CNS an inappropriate satiety signal, leading to reduced food intake. It is appropriate, however, that any nutrient deficiency anorexias be considered not only in the light of conditioned aversions but also for how they might model the underlying neurochemical status of anorexia nervosa (see Chapter 9 and previous discussion in this chapter on conditioned aversions).

Summary

Vitamins are usually part of the structures of coenzymes. Dietary intake of many vitamins is necessary to prevent deficiency diseases. Considerable evidence indicates that vitamins interact with CNS transmitters and play an important role in behavioral control, although it is not clear whether specific CNS mechanisms to regulate vitamin intake exist.

Ascorbic acid (vitamin C) plays an important role in mono-oxygenase (hydroxylase) reactions. One of these reactions involves the conversion of dopamine to norepinephrine, which links ascorbate to CNS and sympathetic nervous system function. Ascorbate is also active in the posttranslational modification of peptides. Its influence thus extends to peptides that are important for nervous function. Some of these include calcitonin, corticotropin-releasing factor, substance P, and vasopressin. Ascorbate is also involved in adrenal steroid physiology, and it has an uneven distribution in the brain. Evidence is accruing for ascorbate's interaction with dopamine and glutamate systems and for ascorbate's involvement in behavior.

Thiamine (vitamin B₁) participates in several important biochemical reactions, which include those involved in the metabolism of carbohydrates and the formation of acetylcholine. The brain has relatively high concentrations of thiamine in an uneven distribution. The cerebellum has particularly high concentrations of the vitamin. Dietary variation in thiamine affects the brain's content of thiamine in these specific areas. Thiamine interacts with serotonin, acetylcholine, and norepinephrine systems.

The behavioral regulation of thiamine intake has been intensively studied. The earliest studies indicated that animals have a specific, innate regulatory system for the vitamin, but later studies showed that mechanisms of conditioning were important. Need for thiamine plays a minimal role in the development of a thiamine hunger.

Behavioral pathologic conditions that result from vitamin deficiencies include amnesia and confusional states, neurologic signs, and anorexia. Many of these conditions are ameliorated by treatment with the missing vitamin. Anorectic states can be probed by an analysis of the neurochemical changes that occur during vitamin deficiency.

References

Bruce, A., Ekblom, B., & Nilsson, I. The effect of vitamin and mineral supplements and health foods on physical endurance and performance. *Proceedings of the Nutrition Society, 44*, 1985, 283–295.

Englard, S. & Seifter, S. The biochemical functions of ascorbic acid. *Annual Review of Nutrition, 6*, 1986, 365–406.

Fishbaine, B. & Butterfield, G. Ascorbic acid status of running and sedentary men. *International Journal for Vitamin and Nutrition Research, 54*, 1984, 273.

Garcia, J., Ervin, F.R., Yorke, C.H., & Koelling, R.A. Conditioning with delayed vitamin injections. *Science, 155*, 1967, 716–718.

Koplan, J.P., Annest, J.L., Layde, P.M., & Rubin, G.L. Nutrient intake and supplementation in the United States (NHANES II). *American Journal of Public Health, 76*, 1986, 287–289.

Kratzing, C.C., Kelly, J.D., & Kratzing, J.E. Ascorbic acid in fetal rat brain. *Journal of Neurochemistry, 44*, 1985, 1623–24.

Kratzing, C.C., Kelly, J.D., & Oelrichs, B.A. Ascorbic Acid changes in brain. *International Journal of Vitamin & Nutrition Research, 54*, 1984, 349–353.

Lehninger, A.L. *Biochemistry*, New York: Worth Publishers, 1975.

McFarland, D.J. Mouse phenotype modulates the behavioral effects of acute thiamine deficiency. *Physiology & Behavior, 35*, 1985, 597–601.

Richter, C.P., Holt, L.E., & Barelare, B. Nutritional requirements for normal growth and reproduction in rats studied by self-selection method. *American Journal of Physiology, 122*, 1938, 734–744.

Richter, C.P., Holt, L.E., & Barelare, B. Vitamin B1 craving in rats. *Science, 86*, 1937, 354–355.

Rodgers, W. & Rozin, P. Novel food preferences in thiamine-deficient rats. *Journal of Comparative and Physiological Psychology, 61*, 1966, 1–4.

Rozin, P. Adaptive food sampling patterns in vitamin deficient rats. *Journal of Comparative and Physiological Psychology, 69*, 1969, 126–132.

Rozin, P. Specific aversion and neophobia resulting from vitamin deficiency or poisoning in half-wild and domestic rats. *Journal of Comparative and Physiological Psychology, 66*, 1968, 82–88.

*S*uggested Readings

Butterworth, R.F., Giguere, J-F., & Besnard, A.M. Activities of thiamine-dependent enzymes in two experimental models of thiamine-deficiency encephalopathy: 1. The pyruvate dehydrogenase complex. *Neurochemical research, 10*, 1985, 1417–1428.

Chan-Palay, V., Plaitakis, A., Nicklas, W., & Berl, S. Autoradiographic demonstration of loss of labeled indoleamine axons of the cerebellum in chronic diet-induced thiamine deficiency. *Brain Research, 138*, 1977, 380–384.

Dolinsky, Z.S. & Shaskan, E.G. Dietary ascorbic acid deficiency in guinea pigs: No effect on ethanol preference, spiroperidol binding, or monoamine oxidase activity. *Life Sciences, 34*, 1984, 2159–2164.

Dreyfus, P.M. The quantitative histochemical distribution of thiamine in deficient rat brain. *Journal of Neurochemistry, 8*, 1961, 139–145.

Gardiner, T.W., Armstrong-James, M., Caan, A.W., Wightman, R.M., & Rebec, G.V. Modulation of neostriatal activity by iontophoresis of ascorbic acid. *Brain Research, 344*, 1985, 181–185.

Gehlert, D.R., Morey, W.A., & Wamsley, J.K. Alterations in muscarinic cholinergic receptor densities induced by thiamine deficiency: Autoradiographic detection of changes in high- and low-affinity agonist binding. *Journal of Neuroscience Research, 13*, 1985, 443–452.

Gibson, G.E., Ksiezak-Reding, H., Sheu, K-F.R., Mykytyn, V., & Blass, J.P. Correlation of enzymatic, metabolic, and behavioral deficits in thiamin deficiency and its reversal. *Neurochemical Research, 9*, 1984, 803–814.

Glembotski, C.C., Manaker, S., Winokur, A., & Gibson, T.R. Ascorbic-acid increases the thyrotropin-releasing hormone content of hypothalamic cell cultures. *The Journal of Neuroscience, 6*, 1986, 1796–1802.

Greenwood, J., Luthert, P.J., Pratt, O.E., & Lantos, P.L. Transport of thiamin across the blood-brain barrier of the rat in the absence of aerobic metabolism. *Brain Research, 399*, 1986, 148–151.

Hadjiconstantinou, M. & Neff, N.H. Ascorbic acid could be hazardous to your experiments: A commentary on dopamine receptor binding studies with speculation on a role for ascorbic acid in neuronal function. *Neuropharmacology, 22*, 1983, 939–943.

Hailemariam, B., Landman, J.P., & Jackson, A.A. Thiamin status in normal and malnourished children in Jamaica. *British Journal of Nutrition, 53*, 1985, 477–483.

Hakim, A.M. & Pappius, H.M. The effect of thiamine deficiency of local cerebral glucose utilization. *Annals of Neurology, 9*, 1981, 334–339.

Hoffman, C.J. & Zabik, M.E. Effects of microwave cooking/reheating on nutrients and food systems: A review of recent studies. *Journal of the American Dietetic Association, 85*, 1985, 922–926.

Hornsby, P.J., Harris, S.E., & Aldern, K.A. The role of ascorbic acid in the function of the adrenal cortex: Studies in adrenocortical cells in culture. *Endocrinology, 117*, 1985, 1264–1271.

Knapp, J.A., Haffner, S.M., Young, E.A., Hazuda, H.P., Gardner, L. & Stern, M.P. Dietary intakes of essential nutrients among Mexican-Americans and Anglo-Americans: The San Antonio Heart Study. *American Journal of Clinical Nutrition, 42*, 1985, 307–316.

Lawrence, A.W. Taste palatability of a vitamin C source for low- and high-intake subjects. Research project submitted in partial fulfillment for Motivation Class, Spring, 1985, Tulane University.

Lee, R-S., Strahlendorf, H.K. & Strahlendorf, J.C. Enhanced sensitivity of cerebellar Purkinje cells to iontophoretically-applied serotonin in thiamine deficiency. *Brain Research, 327*, 1985, 249–258.

Levine, M. New concepts in the biology and biochemistry of ascorbic acid. *The New England Journal of Medicine, 314*, 1986, 892–902.

Levine, M. & Morita, K. Ascorbic acid in endocrine systems. *Vitamins & Hormones, 42*, 1985, 1–64.

Mair, R.G., Anderson, C.D., Langlais, P.J., & McEntee, W.J. Thiamine deficiency depletes cortical norepinephrine and impairs learning processes in the rat. *Brain Research, 360*, 1985, 273–284.

Micheau, J., Durkin, T.P., Destrade, C., Rolland, Y., & Jaffard, R. Chronic administration of sulbutiamine improves long term memory formation in mice: Possible cholinergic mediation. *Pharmacology, Biochemistry, & Behavior, 23*, 1985, 195–198.

O'Neill, R.D. & Fillenz, M. Circadian changes in extracellular ascorbate in rat cortex, accumbens, striatum and hippocampus: Correlations with motor activity. *Neuroscience Letters, 60*, 1985, 331–336.

Overbeek, G.A. Hormonal regulation of ascorbic acid in the adrenal of the rat. *Acta Endocrinologica, 109*, 1985, 393–402.

Rebec, G.V., Centore, J.M, White, L.K., & Alloway, K.D. Ascorbic acid and the behavioral response to haloperidol: Implications for the action of antipsychotic drugs. *Science, 227*, 1985, 438–440.

Reggiani, C., Patrini, C., & Rindi, G. Nervous tissue thiamine metabolism in vivo.

I. Transport of thiamine and thiamine monophosphate from plasma to different brain regions of the rat. *Brain Research, 293*, 1984, 319–327.

Rindi, G., Comincioli, V., Reggiani, C., & Patrini, C. Nervous tissue thiamine metabolism in vivo. II. Thiamine and its phosphoesters dynamics in different brain regions and sciatic nerve of the rat. *Brain Research, 293*, 1984, 329–342.

Rodgers, W.R. Specificity of specific hungers. *Journal of Comparative and Physiological Psychology, 64*, 1967, 49–58.

Rozin, P. Central or peripheral mediation of learning with long CS-US intervals in the feeding system. *Journal of Comparative and Physiological Psychology, 67*, 1969, 421–429.

Rozin, P. Specific hunger for thiamine: Recovery from deficiency and thiamine preference. *Journal of Comparative and Physiological Psychology, 59*, 1965, 98–101.

Rozin, P., Wells, C., & Mayer, J. Specific hunger for thiamine: Vitamin in water versus vitamin in food. *Journal of Comparative and Physiological Psychology, 57*, 1964, 78–84.

Schenk, J.O., Miller, E., Gaddis, R., & Adams, R.N. Homeostatic control of ascorbate concentration in CNS extracellular fluid. *Brain Research, 253*, 192, 353–356.

Stamford, J.A., Kruk, Z.L. & Millar, J. Ascorbic acid does not modulate stimulated dopamine release: In vivo voltammetric data in the rat. *Neuroscience Letters, 60*, 1985, 357–362.

Subramanian, N. On the brain ascorbic acid and its importance in metabolism of biogenic amines. *Life Sciences, 20*, 1977, 1479–1484.

Summers, J.A., Pullan, R.T., & Kurnow, D.W. Effect of thiamine deficiency on adrenocorticotrophin and vasopressin in the rat hypothalamus. *Hormone and Metabolic Research, 18*, 1986, 280.

Thorn, N.A., Christensen, B.L., Jeppesen, C., & Nielsen, F.S. Ascorbic acid uptake to isolated nerve terminals and secretory granules from ox neurohypophysis. *Acta Physiologica Scandinavia, 124*, 1985, 87–92.

Waddington, J.L. & Crow, T.J. Drug-induced rotational behaviour following unilateral intracerebral injection of saline-ascorbate solution: Neurotoxicity of ascorbic acid and monoamine-independent circling. *Brain Research, 161*, 1979, 371–376.

Wagner, G.C., Carelli, R.M., & Jarvis, M.F. Ascorbic acid reduces the dopamine depletion induced by methamphetamine and the 1-methyl-4-phenyl pyridinium ion. *Neuropharmacology, 25*, 1986, 559–561.

Wilson, R.L., Kamata, K., Bigelow, J.C., Rebec, G.V., & Wightman, R.M. Crus cerebri lesions abolish amphetamine-induced ascorbate release in rat neostriatum. *Brain Research, 370*, 1986, 393–396.

Appendix

Nutrient Intake in the United States

Dietary data were acquired from about 12,000 American respondents in the second National Health and Nutrition Examination Survey (NHANES II). These data were used to provide quantitative information about the contribution of specific foods to the intake of several essential nutrients. In Chapter 10 on vitamins, the total intake of vitamins and minerals is reported. In this appendix, a compilation by researchers at the National Cancer Institute shows the intake of essential nutrients from the foods most frequently eaten by respondents (Tables A1-A14). The sample of respondents was obtained using a highly stratified multistage probability design to make it representative of a noninstitutionalized U.S. population. The percent contribution of a nutrient provided by a particular food is given as:

$$\frac{\text{Total nutrient from particular food}}{\text{Total nutrient from all foods}} \times 100$$

Since the wheat kernel is a major contributor to several sources of the U.S. diet, a breakdown of the nutrients from wheat is provided.

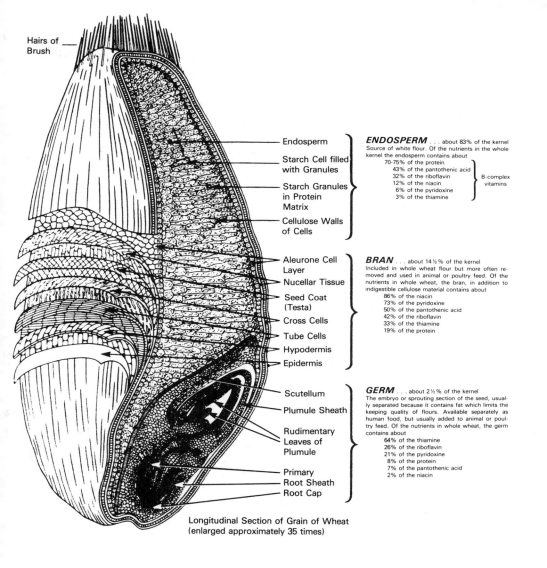

Hairs of Brush	

Endosperm	**ENDOSPERM** . . . about 83% of the kernel
	Source of white flour. Of the nutrients in the whole
	kernel the endosperm contains about
	  70-75% of the protein
	     43% of the pantothenic acid
	     32% of the riboflavin } B-complex
	     12% of the niacin } vitamins
	      6% of the pyridoxine
	      3% of the thiamine

Starch Cell filled with Granules	
Starch Granules in Protein Matrix	
Cellulose Walls of Cells	

Aleurone Cell Layer	**BRAN** . . . about 14½% of the kernel
	Included in whole wheat flour but more often re-
	moved and used in animal or poultry feed. Of the
	nutrients in whole wheat, the bran, in addition to
	indigestible cellulose material contains about
	  86% of the niacin
	  73% of the pyridoxine
	  50% of the pantothenic acid
	  42% of the riboflavin
	  33% of the thiamine
	  19% of the protein

Nucellar Tissue	
Seed Coat (Testa)	
Cross Cells	
Tube Cells	
Hypodermis	
Epidermis	

Scutellum	**GERM** . . . about 2½% of the kernel
	The embryo or sprouting section of the seed, usual-
	ly separated because it contains fat which limits the
	keeping quality of flours. Available separately as
	human food, but usually added to animal or poul-
	try feed. Of the nutrients in whole wheat, the germ
	contains about
	  64% of the thiamine
	  26% of the riboflavin
	  21% of the pyridoxine
	    8% of the protein
	    7% of the pantothenic acid
	    2% of the niacin

Plumule Sheath	
Rudimentary Leaves of Plumule	
Primary Root Sheath	
Root Cap	

Longitudinal Section of Grain of Wheat
(enlarged approximately 35 times)

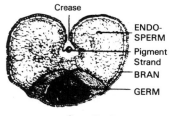

Crease

ENDO-SPERM

Pigment Strand

BRAN

GERM

Cross Sectional View

Figure A.1 Breakdown of the nutrient contribution from a kernel of wheat. (From Nelson, 1985.)

TABLE A1   Major contributors of calories in the US diet: data from the NHANES II survey, 1976-1980

Rank	Description	% of total calories	Cumulative % of calories	Persons per 10,000 population
1	White bread, rolls, crackers	9.59	9.59	7,666
2	Doughnuts, cookies, cake	5.70	15.28	4,085
3	Alcoholic beverages	5.60	20.88	2,663
4	Whole milk, whole milk beverages	4.72	25.60	4,139
5	Hamburgers, cheeseburgers, meat loaf	4.39	29.99	2,618
6	Beef steaks, roasts	4.14	34.13	2,276
7	Regular soft drinks	3.63	37.75	3,908
8	Hot dogs, ham, lunch meats	3.19	40.95	2,959
9	Eggs	2.53	43.48	3,137
10	French fries, fried potatoes	2.53	46.01	1,730
11	Cheeses, excluding cottage cheese	2.45	48.46	3,287
12	Pork, including chops, roast	2.28	50.74	1,443
13	Ice cream, frozen desserts	1.71	52.45	1,429
14	Whole wheat, rye, other dark breads	1.70	54.15	2,326
15	Mayonnaise, salad dressings	1.67	55.82	3,124
16	2% milk	1.67	57.49	1,402
17	Margarine	1.64	59.13	4,196
18	Spaghetti with tomato sauce	1.64	60.77	959
19	Sugar	1.48	62.25	4,067
20	Potatoes, excluding fried	1.47	63.72	2,583
21	Salty snacks	1.41	65.13	1,580
22	Orange juice	1.38	66.51	2,263
23	Coffee, tea	1.35	67.86	7,994
24	Pies, excluding pumpkin	1.31	69.16	747
25	Pinto, navy, other dried beans	1.17	70.34	1,070
26	Chicken or turkey, excluding fried	1.12	71.46	1,151
27	Cornbread, grits, tortillas	0.99	72.44	991
28	Salad and cooking oils	0.94	73.38	1,610
29	Fried fish	0.91	74.29	585
30	Peanuts, peanut butter	0.89	75.19	994
31	Butter	0.87	76.06	1,875
32	Pizza	0.87	76.93	360
33	Cold cereals excluding bran or superfortified types	0.86	77.79	1,177
34	Candy (chocolate)	0.85	78.64	868
35	Fried chicken	0.84	79.47	701
36	Skim milk, buttermilk	0.78	80.25	1,211
37	Chili	0.77	81.02	339

continued

TABLE A1 (Continued)

Rank	Description	% of total calories	Cumulative % of calories	Persons per 10,000 population
38	Other fruit juices not listed here	0.73	81.75	841
39	Bacon	0.64	82.40	1,141
40	Rice	0.64	83.04	915
41	Soups other than vegetable, tomato	0.60	83.64	936
42	Bran and granola cereals	0.59	84.23	661
43	Sausage	0.57	84.80	589
44	Apples, applesauce	0.57	85.37	1,164
45	Mixed dishes with cheese	0.54	85.91	364
46	Beef stew, pot pie	0.53	86.44	278
47	Gravy, other meat sauces	0.53	86.97	938
48	Fortified fruit drinks	0.52	87.49	614
49	Tuna, tuna salad, tuna casserole	0.51	88.00	611
50	Jellies, jams, honey	0.48	88.48	1,722

From Block et al. 1985b.

TABLE A2 Major contributors of protein in the US diet: data from the NHANES II survey, 1976-1980

Rank	Description	% of total protein	Cumulative % of protein	Persons per 10,000 population
1	Beef steaks, roasts	12.59	12.59	2,276
2	Hamburgers, cheeseburgers, meat loaf	8.90	21.49	2,618
3	White bread, rolls, crackers	6.88	28.38	7,666
4	Whole milk, whole milk beverages	6.34	34.71	4,139
5	Pork, including chops, roast	4.79	39.50	1,443
6	Hot dogs, ham, lunch meats	4.57	44.07	2,959
7	Eggs	4.30	48.37	3,137
8	Chicken or turkey, excluding fried	3.96	52.32	1,151
9	Cheeses, excluding cottage cheese	3.81	56.13	3,287
10	2% milk	3.01	59.14	1,402
11	Fried chicken	2.91	62.05	701
12	Spaghetti with tomato sauce	2.08	64.14	959
13	Doughnuts, cookies, cake	1.93	66.06	4,085
14	Skim milk, buttermilk	1.83	67.90	1,211
15	Fried fish	1.71	69.61	585
16	Whole wheat, rye, other dark breads	1.61	71.22	2,326
17	Pinto, navy, other dried beans Fish, broiled, baked, canned	1.52	72.74	1,070
18	Tuna, tuna salad, tuna casserole Chili	1.24	73.98	378
19	Pizza Peanuts, peanut butter	1.24	75.21	611
20	French fries, fried potatoes	1.05	76.27	339
21	Potatoes, excluding fried	1.02	77.29	360
22	Beef stew, pot pie	1.01	78.30	994
23	Ice cream, frozen desserts	1.00	79.30	1,730
24	Cottage cheese	0.95	80.24	2,583
25	Soups other than vegetable,	0.95	81.19	278
26	tomato	0.86	82.05	1,429
27	Bacon	0.81	82.86	508
28	Shellfish Veal, lamb	0.77	83.63	936
29	Cornbread, grits, tortillas	0.74	84.38	1,141
30	Alcoholic beverages	0.73	85.11	310
31	Liver	0.68	85.79	171
32	Sausage	0.68	86.47	991
33	Mixed dishes with cheese	0.67	87.14	2,663
34	Mixed dishes with chicken	0.63	87.77	173
35	Orange juice	0.59	88.36	589

continued

TABLE A2   (Continued)

Rank	Description	% of total protein	Cumulative % of protein	Persons per 10,000 population
36	Cold cereals excluding bran or	0.56	88.92	364
37	superfortified types	0.54	89.46	282
38	Salty snacks	0.51	89.97	2,263
39	Bran and granola cereals			
	Vegetable, tomato, minestrone	0.51	90.48	1,177
40	soups	0.51	90.98	1,580
41	Mixed dishes with beef	0.44	91.42	661
42	Venison, gizzard, other unusual			
	meats	0.44	91.86	483
43	Pies, excluding pumpkin	0.43	92.29	161
44	Tomatoes, tomato juice			
	Green salad	0.41	92.69	99
45	Corn	0.40	93.09	747
46	Candy (chocolate)	0.40	93.49	2,552
47	Rice	0.39	93.86	4,030
48		0.39	94.27	852
49		0.33	94.60	868
50		0.32	94.92	915

From Block et al., 1985b.

TABLE A3   Major contributors of carbohydrate in the US diet: data from the
NHANES II survey, 1976-1980

Rank	Description	% of total carbohydrate	Cumulative % of carbohydrate	Persons per 10,000 population
1	White bread, rolls, crackers	15.03	15.03	7,666
2	Regular soft drinks	8.55	23.58	3,908
3	Doughnuts, cookies, cake	7.52	31.10	4,085
4	Sugar	3.54	34.63	4,067
5	Whole milk, whole milk beverages	3.53	38.17	4,139
6	French fries, fried potatoes	3.28	41.45	1,730
7	Alcoholic beverages	3.28	44.73	2,663
8	Whole wheat, rye, other dark breads	3.08	47.81	2,326
9	Orange juice	3.01	50.82	2,263
10	Potatoes, excluding fried	2.35	53.17	2,583
11	Coffee, tea	2.30	55.47	7,994
12	Spaghetti with tomato sauce	1.90	57.37	959
13	Ice cream, frozen desserts	1.85	59.22	1,429
14	Other fruit juices not listed here	1.76	60.98	841
15	Cold cereals excluding bran or superfortified types	1.70	62.68	1,177
16	Pies, excluding pumpkin	1.60	64.28	747
17	Pinto, navy, other dried beans	1.58	65.87	1,070
18	2% milk	1.58	67.45	1,402
19	Cornbread, grits, tortillas	1.47	68.92	991
20	Salty snacks	1.36	70.28	1,580
21	Apples, applesauce	1.32	71.60	1,164
22	Rice	1.29	72.89	915
23	Fortified fruit drinks	1.18	74.08	614
24	Jellies, jams, honey	1.16	75.24	1,722
25	Candy (chocolate)	1.04	76.28	868
26	Corn	1.01	77.29	852
27	Skim milk, buttermilk	1.00	78.29	1,211
28	Bran and granola cereals	0.98	79.27	661
29	Pizza	0.98	80.25	360
30	Grapefruit, grapefruit juice	0.94	81.19	671
31	Bananas	0.89	82.08	860
32	Syrup, molasses	0.88	82.97	599
33	Hamburgers, cheeseburgers, meat loaf	0.73	83.70	2,618

continued

TABLE A3   (Continued)

Rank	Description	% of total carbohydrate	Cumulative % of carbohydrate	Persons per 10,000 population
34	Candy (nonchocolate)	0.63	84.33	592
35	Tomatoes, tomato juice	0.61	84.94	2,552
36	Soups other than vegetable, tomato	0.61	85.54	936
37	Cooked cereals	0.58	86.12	436
38	Chili	0.57	86.69	339
39	Oranges, tangerines	0.56	87.25	670
40	Green salad	0.50	87.76	4,030
41	Mixed dishes with cheese	0.50	88.26	364
42	Vegetable, tomato, minestrone soups	0.49	88.75	483
43	Peaches	0.45	89.21	526
44	Noodles, macaroni	0.45	89.66	329
45	Pancakes, waffles, French toast	0.45	90.11	329
46	Fried fish	0.40	90.51	585
47	Puddings	0.39	90.91	268
48	Cheeses, excluding cottage cheese	0.38	91.28	3,287
49	Beef stew, pot pie	0.35	91.64	278
50	Pears	0.31	91.94	263

From Block et al., 1985b.

TABLE A4 Major contributors of total fat in the US diet: data from the
NHANES II survey, 1976-1980

Rank	Description	% of total fat	Cumulative % of fat	Persons per 10,000 population
1	Hamburgers, cheeseburgers, meat loaf	7.02	7.02	2,618
2	Hot dogs, ham, lunch meats	6.39	13.41	2,959
3	Whole milk, whole milk beverages	5.98	19.38	4,139
4	Doughnuts, cookies, cake	5.98	25.36	4,085
5	Beef steaks, roasts	5.45	30.82	2,276
6	White bread, rolls, crackers	4.88	35.69	7,666
7	Eggs	4.63	40.33	3,137
8	Cheeses, excluding cottage cheese	4.54	44.86	3,287
9	Margarine	4.50	49.36	4,196
10	Mayonnaise, salad dressings	4.30	53.66	3,124
11	Pork, including chops, roast	3.97	57.64	1,443
12	French fries, fried potatoes	2.70	60.34	1,730
13	Salad and cooking oils	2.59	62.93	1,610
14	Butter	2.39	65.32	1,875
15	Ice cream, frozen desserts	2.05	67.37	1,429
16	Salty snacks	2.02	69.39	1,580
17	Peanuts, peanut butter	1.86	71.26	994
18	Pies, excluding pumpkin	1.53	72.79	747
19	Bacon	1.38	74.16	1,141
20	2% milk	1.37	75.53	1,402
21	Spaghetti with tomato sauce	1.32	76.85	959
22	Sausage	1.26	78.11	589
23	Chicken or turkey, excluding fried	1.23	79.35	1,151
24	Fried fish	1.22	80.57	585
25	Gravy, other meat sauces	1.06	81.63	938
26	Candy (chocolate)	1.04	82.67	868
27	Chili	0.96	83.63	339
28	Potatoes, excluding fried	0.91	84.54	2,583
29	Fried chicken	0.86	85.40	701
30	Pizza	0.77	86.17	360
31	Pinto, navy, other dried beans	0.73	86.89	1,070
32	Tuna, tuna salad, tuna casserole	0.66	87.55	611
33	Cornbread, grits, tortillas	0.64	88.19	991
34	Mixed dishes with cheese	0.64	88.83	364
35	Beef stew, pot pie	0.62	89.46	278
36	Green salad	0.62	90.07	4,030
37	Soups other than vegetable, tomato	0.60	90.68	936

continued

TABLE A4   (Continued)

Rank	Description	% of total fat	Cumulative % of fat	Persons per 10,000 population
38	Cooking fat, lard	0.54	91.22	576
39	Mixed dishes with chicken	0.51	91.73	282
40	Nondairy coffee creamers	0.51	92.24	1,553
41	Whole wheat, rye, other dark breads	0.47	92.71	2,326
42	Cream, half and half	0.44	93.15	729
43	Nuts (excluding peanuts)	0.43	93.59	301
44	Veal, lamb	0.39	93.97	171
45	Coleslaw, cabbage	0.38	94.35	944
46	Fish, broiled, baked, canned	0.35	94.71	378
47	Mixed dishes with beef	0.31	95.02	161
48	Bran and granola cereals	0.30	95.32	661
49	Pancakes, waffles, French toast	0.29	95.61	329
50	Vegetable, tomato, minestrone soups	0.27	95.87	483

From Block et al., 1985b.

TABLE A5   Major contributors of sodium in the US diet: data from the
NHANES II survey, 1976-1980

Rank	Description	% of total sodium	Cumulative % of sodium	Persons per 10,000 population
1	White bread, rolls, crackers	12.09	12.09	7,666
2	Hot dogs, ham, lunch meats	9.76	21.84	2,959
3	Cheeses, excluding cottage cheese	5.37	27.21	3,287
4	Soups other than vegetable, tomato	4.04	31.25	936
5	Spaghetti with tomato sauce	3.61	34.86	959
6	Doughnuts, cookies, cake	3.57	38.42	4,085
7	Potatoes, excluding fried	3.28	41.71	2,583
8	Vegetable, tomato, minestrone soups	2.64	44.35	483
9	Eggs	2.56	46.90	3,137
10	Whole milk, whole milk beverages	2.47	49.38	4,139
11	Whole wheat, rye, other dark breads	2.35	51.73	2,326
12	Chili	1.94	53.67	339
13	Hamburgers, cheeseburgers, meat loaf	1.93	55.60	2,618
14	Mayonnaise, salad dressings	1.85	57.45	3,124
15	French fries, fried potatoes	1.80	59.26	1,730
16	Salty snacks	1.71	60.96	1,580
17	Margarine	1.70	62.66	4,196
18	Cornbread, grits, tortillas	1.66	64.32	991
19	Pizza	1.66	65.97	360
20	Rice	1.49	67.47	915
21	Pork, including chops, roast	1.33	68.80	1,443
22	Pinto, navy, other dried beans	1.30	70.10	1,070
23	Cold cereals, excluding bran or superfortified types	1.28	71.38	1,177
24	2% milk	1.19	72.57	1,402
25	Bacon	1.18	73.75	1,141
26	Beef steaks, roasts	1.14	74.89	2,276
27	Tuna, tuna salad, tuna casserole	1.11	76.01	611
28	Mixed dishes with cheese	1.08	77.09	364
29	Pies, excluding pumpkin	1.02	78.11	747
30	Catsup, other products with tomatoes	0.99	79.10	805
31	Gravy, other meat sauces	0.96	80.06	938
32	Sausage	0.92	80.98	589
33	Corn	0.87	81.85	852
34	Coleslaw, cabbage	0.85	82.70	944

continued

TABLE A5 (Continued)

Rank	Description	% of total sodium	Cumulative % of sodium	Persons per 10,000 population
35	Butter	0.83	83.53	1,875
36	Skim milk, buttermilk	0.81	84.34	1,211
37	Fish, broiled, baked, canned	0.72	85.06	378
38	Mixed dishes with beef	0.69	85.75	161
39	Beef stew, pot pie	0.62	86.37	278
40	Mixed dishes with chicken	0.60	86.97	282
41	Cooked cereals	0.60	87.57	436
42	Cottage cheese	0.57	88.15	508
43	Pancakes, waffles, French toast	0.57	88.71	329
44	Green beans	0.56	89.27	992
45	Chicken or turkey, excluding fried	0.55	89.82	1,151
46	Tomatoes, tomato juice	0.55	90.37	2,552
47	Bran and granola cereals	0.54	90.91	661
48	Ice cream, frozen desserts	0.50	91.41	1,429
49	Fried fish	0.49	91.90	585
50	Peanuts, peanut butter	0.48	92.38	994

From Block et al., 1985a.

TABLE A6   Major contributors of potassium in the US diet: data from the
NHANES II survey, 1976-1980

Rank	Description	% of total potassium	Cumulative % of potassium	Persons per 10,000 population
1	Coffee, tea	8.63	8.63	7,994
2	Whole milk, whole milk beverages	8.18	16.81	4,139
3	French fries, fried potatoes	5.67	22.48	1,730
4	Orange juice	4.53	27.01	2,263
5	Potatoes, excluding fried	4.29	31.30	2,583
6	2% milk	3.92	35.21	1,402
7	Beef steaks, roasts	3.90	39.11	2,276
8	Hamburgers, cheeseburgers, meat loaf	3.17	42.28	2,618
9	Tomatoes, tomato juice	2.72	45.00	2,552
10	White bread, rolls, crackers	2.67	47.67	7,666
11	Skim milk, buttermilk	2.61	50.28	1,211
12	Green salad	2.52	52.80	4,030
13	Spaghetti with tomato sauce	2.42	55.22	959
14	Alcoholic beverages	2.20	57.42	2,663
15	Pinto, navy, other dried beans	2.10	59.51	1,070
16	Hot dogs, ham, lunch meats	2.09	61.60	2,959
17	Pork, including chops, roasts	1.63	63.24	1,443
18	Chicken or turkey, excluding fried	1.53	64.76	1,151
19	Eggs	1.50	66.26	3,137
20	Ice cream, frozen desserts	1.38	67.64	1,429
21	Doughnuts, cookies, cake	1.34	68.98	4,085
22	Salty snacks	1.30	70.28	1,580
23	Bananas	1.28	71.56	860
24	Grapefruit, grapefruit juice	1.16	72.72	671
25	Beef stew, pot pie	1.11	73.83	278
26	Fried chicken	1.10	74.93	701
27	Whole wheat, rye, other dark breads	1.04	75.97	2,326
28	Chili	0.98	76.95	339
29	Fried fish	0.94	77.89	585
30	Cheeses, excluding cottage cheese	0.87	78.76	3,287
31	Peanuts, peanut butter	0.77	79.54	994
32	Oranges, tangerines	0.74	80.28	670
33	Bran and granola cereals	0.74	81.02	661
34	Vegetable, tomato, minestrone soups	0.73	81.75	483
35	Apples, applesauce	0.73	82.48	1,164

continued

TABLE A6   (Continued)

Rank	Description	% of total potassium	Cumulative % of potassium	Persons per 10,000 population
36	Soups other than vegetable, tomato	0.70	83.18	936
37	Fish, broiled, baked, canned	0.68	83.87	378
38	Corn	0.64	84.51	852
39	Coleslaw, cabbage	0.51	85.02	944
40	Cantaloupe	0.51	85.53	181
41	Other fruit juices not listed here	0.49	86.02	841
42	Peaches	0.46	86.48	526
43	Tuna, tuna salad, tuna casserole	0.45	86.93	611
44	Carrots, peas and carrots	0.41	87.34	811
45	Cold cereals, excluding bran or superfortified types	0.40	87.74	1,177
46	Candy (chocolate)	0.40	88.14	868
47	Pizza	0.40	88.53	360
48	Cornbread, grits, tortillas	0.38	88.91	991
49	Pies, excluding pumpkin	0.36	89.27	747
50	Yogurt	0.36	89.63	237

From Block et al., 1985a.

TABLE A7   Major contributors of phosphorus in the US diet: data from the
NHANES II survey, 1976-1980

Rank	Description	% of total phosphorus	Cumulative % of phosphorus	Persons per 10,000 population
1	Whole milk, whole milk beverages	10.46	10.46	4,139
2	Cheeses, excluding cottage cheese	6.04	16.50	3,287
3	White bread, rolls, crackers	5.69	22.19	7,666
4	Beef steaks, roasts	5.58	27.77	2,276
5	2% milk	5.00	32.77	1,402
6	Hamburgers, cheeseburgers, meat loaf	4.68	37.45	2,618
7	Eggs	4.36	41.80	3,137
8	Alcoholic beverages	4.15	45.96	2,663
9	Skim milk, buttermilk	3.38	49.33	1,211
10	Doughnuts, cookies, cake	2.94	52.27	4,085
11	Pork, including chops, roast	2.86	55.13	1,443
12	Hot dogs, ham, lunch meats	2.54	57.67	2,959
13	Whole wheat, rye, other dark breads	2.00	59.67	2,326
14	Chicken or turkey, excluding fried	1.97	61.64	1,151
15	Pinto, navy, other dried beans	1.74	63.38	1,070
16	Coffee, tea	1.73	65.10	7,994
17	Spaghetti with tomato sauce	1.69	66.79	959
18	Ice cream, frozen desserts	1.61	68.40	1,429
19	French fries, fried potatoes	1.52	69.92	1,730
20	Fried chicken	1.47	71.39	701
21	Potatoes, excluding fried	1.38	72.77	2,583
22	Fried fish	1.20	73.97	585
23	Bran, and granola cereals	1.18	75.15	661
24	Chili	1.07	76.22	339
25	Cornbread, grits, tortillas	1.04	77.26	991
26	Peanuts, peanut butter	0.94	78.20	994
27	Fish, broiled, baked, canned	0.92	79.12	378
28	Regular soft drinks	0.79	79.91	3,908
29	Orange juice	0.77	80.67	2,263
30	Cold cereals, excluding bran or superfortified types	0.75	81.43	1,177
31	Pizza	0.75	82.18	360

continued

TABLE A7 (Continued)

Rank	Description	% of total phosphorus	Cumulative % of phosphorus	Persons per 10,000 population
32	Salty snacks	0.75	82.92	1,580
33	Tuna, tuna salad, tuna casserole	0.69	83.61	611
34	Beef stew, pot pie	0.67	84.28	278
35	Soups other than vegetable, tomato	0.66	84.94	936
36	Corn	0.66	85.60	852
37	Mixed dishes with cheese	0.63	86.23	364
38	Green salad	0.61	86.84	4,030
39	Cottage cheese	0.60	87.44	508
40	Tomatoes, tomato juice	0.59	88.02	2,552
41	Liver	0.57	88.60	173
42	Bacon	0.53	89.13	1,141
43	Candy (chocolate)	0.50	89.63	868
44	Shellfish	0.49	90.12	310
45	Cooked cereals	0.48	90.60	436
46	Pancakes, waffles, French toast	0.47	91.07	329
47	Rice	0.45	91.52	915
48	Yogurt	0.43	91.94	237
49	Fortified fruit drinks	0.34	92.29	614
50	Sausage	0.34	92.63	589

From Block et al., 1985a.

TABLE A8   Major contributors of iron in the US diet: data from the NHANES II
survey, 1976-1980

Rank	Description	% of total iron	Cumulative % of iron	Persons per 10,000 population
1	White bread, rolls, crackers	11.43	11.43	7,666
2	Beef steaks, roasts	9.04	20.47	2,276
3	Hamburgers, cheeseburgers, meat loaf	6.90	27.37	2,618
4	Eggs	4.16	31.53	3,137
5	Coffee, tea	4.05	35.58	7,994
6	Pork, including chops, roast	3.59	39.17	1,443
7	Doughnuts, cookies, cake	3.34	42.51	4,085
8	Hot dogs, ham, lunch meats	3.26	45.77	2,959
9	Cold cereals, excluding bran or superfortified types	3.11	48.88	1,177
10	Pinto, navy, other dried beans	2.66	51.54	1,070
11	Spaghetti with tomato sauce	2.52	54.06	959
12	French fries, fried potatoes	2.44	56.50	1,730
13	Whole wheat, rye, other dark breads	2.41	58.91	2,326
14	Superfortified cold cereals	2.13	61.04	210
15	Bran and granola cereals	2.02	63.06	661
16	Green salad	1.80	64.86	4,030
17	Liver	1.34	66.20	173
18	Chili	1.32	67.51	339
19	Potatoes, excluding fried	1.31	68.83	2,583
20	Chicken or turkey, excluding fried	1.23	70.06	1,151
21	Cooked cereals	1.18	71.24	436
22	Tomatoes, tomato juice	1.13	72.37	2,552
23	Fried chicken	1.03	73.40	701
24	Beef stew, pot pie	1.01	74.41	278
25	Cornbread, grits, tortillas	1.00	75.41	991
26	Pizza	0.91	76.32	360
27	Cheeses, excluding cottage cheese	0.81	77.13	3,287
28	Soups other than vegetable tomato	0.79	77.92	936
29	Salty snacks	0.79	78.70	1,580
30	Pies, excluding pumpkin	0.68	79.38	747
31	Rice	0.68	80.06	915
32	Fried fish	0.63	80.69	585
33	Shellfish	0.61	81.31	310
34	Tuna, tuna salad, tuna casserole	0.61	81.92	611
35	Vegetable, tomato, minestrone soups	0.55	82.47	483

continued

TABLE A8   (Continued)

Rank	Description	% of total iron	Cumulative % of iron	Persons per 10,000 population
36	Green beans	0.55	83.01	992
37	Grapefruit, grapefruit juice	0.55	83.56	671
38	Orange juice	0.54	84.09	2,263
39	Peas	0.53	84.62	553
40	Corn	0.47	85.10	852
41	Peanuts, peanut butter	0.46	85.56	994
42	Bananas	0.45	86.01	860
43	2% milk	0.44	86.45	1,402
44	Breakfast bars and drinks	0.44	86.89	192
45	Sausage	0.43	87.33	589
46	Apples, applesauce	0.43	87.76	1,164
47	Mixed dishes with beef	0.42	88.18	161
48	Fish, broiled, baked, canned	0.41	88.59	378
49	Mixed dishes with cheese	0.41	89.00	364
50	Prunes	0.40	89.40	130

From Block et al., 1985a.

TABLE A9   Major contributors of calcium in the US diet: data from the NHANES II survey, 1976-1980

Rank	Description	% of total calcium	Cumulative % of calcium	Persons per 10,000 population
1	Whole milk, whole milk beverages	21.97	21.97	4,139
2	Cheeses, excluding cottage cheese	12.01	33.98	3,287
3	2% milk	10.55	44.53	1,402
4	White bread, rolls, crackers	8.39	52.92	7,666
5	Skim milk, buttermilk	6.88	59.79	1,211
6	Ice cream, frozen desserts	3.34	63.13	1,429
7	Eggs	2.38	65.52	3,137
8	Doughnuts, cookies, cake	1.91	67.42	4,085
9	Whole wheat, rye, other dark breads	1.62	69.04	2,326
10	Spaghetti with tomato sauce	1.47	70.51	959
11	Coffee, tea	1.44	71.95	7,994
12	Alcoholic beverages	1.28	73.23	2,663
13	Cornbread, grits, tortillas	1.19	74.43	991
14	Hamburgers, cheeseburgers, meat loaf	1.18	75.61	2,618
15	Mixed dishes with cheese	1.18	76.79	364
16	Pizza	1.15	77.94	360
17	Pinto, navy, other dried beans	1.00	78.94	1,070
18	Green salad	0.99	79.93	4,030
19	Yogurt	0.90	80.83	237
20	Potatoes, excluding fried	0.83	81.66	2,583
21	Soups other than vegetable, tomato	0.76	82.43	936
22	Orange juice	0.75	83.17	2,263
23	Candy (chocolate)	0.65	83.82	868
24	Pancakes, waffles, French toast	0.65	84.47	329
25	Cream, half and half	0.64	85.11	729
26	Greens (mustard, turnip, collards)	0.58	85.69	244
27	Puddings	0.55	86.24	268
28	Beaf steaks, roasts	0.55	86.78	2,276
29	Oranges, tangerines	0.53	87.32	670
30	Tomatoes, tomato juice	0.50	87.81	2,552
31	Cottage cheese	0.48	88.29	508
32	Chili	0.45	88.75	339
33	Coleslaw, cabbage	0.41	89.15	944
34	Green beans	0.40	89.55	992
35	Fish, broiled, baked, canned	0.39	89.94	378

continued

TABLE A9   (Continued)

Rank	Description	% of total calcium	Cumulative % of calcium	Persons per 10,000 population
36	Breakfast bars and drinks	0.38	90.32	192
37	Shellfish	0.37	90.69	310
38	Grapefruit, grapefruit juice	0.36	91.04	671
39	Pies, excluding pumpkin	0.35	91.39	747
40	Fortified fruit drinks	0.34	91.74	614
41	Salty snacks	0.32	92.06	1,580
42	French fries, fried potatoes	0.32	92.38	1,730
43	Cooked cereals	0.29	92.67	436
44	Hot dogs, ham, lunch meats	0.29	92.96	2,959
45	Vegetable, tomato, minestrone soups	0.29	93.25	483
46	Spinach	0.26	93.51	237
47	Fried fish	0.26	93.77	585
48	Cold cereals, excluding bran or superfortified types	0.26	94.03	1,177
49	Peanuts, peanut butter	0.25	94.28	994
50	Rice	0.24	94.52	915

From Block et al., 1985a.

TABLE A10   Major contributors of thiamine in the US diet: data from the
NHANES II survey, 1976-1980

Rank	Description	% of total thiamine	Cumulative % of thiamine	Persons per 10,000 population
1	White bread, rolls, crackers	17.81	17.81	7,666
2	Pork, including chops, roast	8.78	26.59	1,443
3	Hot dogs, ham, lunch meats	5.37	31.95	2,959
4	Cold cereals, excluding bran or superfortified types	4.48	36.43	1,177
5	Orange juice	3.86	40.29	2,263
6	Doughnuts, cookies, cake	3.45	43.74	4,085
7	Whole milk, whole milk beverages	3.43	47.17	4,139
8	Whole wheat, rye, other dark breads	2.90	50.07	2,326
9	Hamburgers, cheeseburgers, meat loaf	2.71	52.78	2,618
10	Breakfast bars and drinks	2.26	55.04	192
11	French fries, fried potatoes	2.12	57.16	1,730
12	Pinto, navy, other dried beans	2.09	59.25	1,070
13	Potatoes, excluding fried	2.01	61.25	2,583
14	Eggs	1.91	63.16	3,137
15	Spaghetti with tomato sauce	1.88	65.04	959
16	Bran and granola cereals	1.87	66.91	661
17	Superfortified cold cereals	1.84	68.75	210
18	Beef steaks, roasts	1.78	70.52	2,276
19	2% milk	1.74	72.27	1,402
20	Tomatoes, tomato juice	1.31	73.58	2,552
21	Skim milk, buttermilk	1.30	74.88	1,211
22	Sausage	1.29	76.17	589
23	Green salad	1.27	77.43	4,030
24	Pizza	1.05	78.49	360
25	Cornbread, grits, tortillas	1.04	79.53	991
26	Bacon	1.01	80.53	1,141
27	Salty snacks	1.00	81.53	1,580
28	Rice	0.93	82.46	915
29	Pies, excluding pumpkin	0.82	83.28	747
30	Cooked cereals	0.77	84.05	436
31	Oranges, tangerines	0.73	84.79	670
32	Peanuts, peanut butter	0.73	85.52	994
33	Corn	0.63	86.15	852
34	Ice cream, frozen desserts	0.56	86.71	1,429
35	Grapefruit, grapefruit juice	0.56	87.27	671
36	Chicken or turkey, excluding fried	0.53	87.80	1,151
37	Beef stew, pot pie	0.52	88.32	278

continued

TABLE A10 (Continued)

Rank	Description	% of total thiamine	Cumulative % of thiamine	Persons per 10,000 population
38	Soups, excluding vegetable, tomato	0.51	88.83	936
39	Peas	0.50	89.33	553
40	Fried fish	0.48	89.81	585
41	Cheeses, excluding cottage cheese	0.46	90.27	3,287
42	Mixed dishes with cheese	0.45	90.72	364
43	Noodles, macaroni	0.45	91.17	329
44	Pancakes, waffles, French toast	0.39	91.56	329
45	Fried chicken	0.37	91.93	701
46	Apples, applesauce	0.37	92.30	1,164
47	Bananas	0.34	92.64	860
48	Candy (chocolate)	0.33	92.96	868
49	Liver	0.33	93.29	173
50	Vegetable, tomato, minestrone soups	0.31	93.60	483

From Block et al., 1985a.

TABLE A11   Major contributors of vitamin C in the US diet: data from the
NHANES II survey, 1976-1980

Rank	Description	% of total vitamin C	Cumulative % of vitamin C	Persons per 10,000 population
1	Orange juice	26.54	26.54	2,263
2	Grapefruit, grapefruit juice	7.20	33.74	671
3	Tomatoes, tomato juice	6.12	39.86	2,552
4	Fortified fruit drinks	5.84	45.70	614
5	Oranges, tangerines	4.90	50.60	670
6	Potatoes, excluding fried	4.20	54.80	2,583
7	French fries, fried potatoes	4.08	58.88	1,730
8	Green salad	3.49	62.37	4,030
9	Other fruit juices not listed here	2.81	65.17	841
10	Broccoli	1.98	67.15	249
11	Coleslaw, cabbage	1.96	69.11	944
12	Spaghetti with tomato sauce	1.88	70.99	959
13	Fortified orange juice substitutes	1.84	72.83	112
14	Cold cereals, excluding bran or superfortified types	1.77	74.60	1,177
15	Hot dogs, ham, lunch meats	1.68	76.28	2,959
16	Cantaloupe	1.66	77.94	181
17	Whole milk, whole milk beverages	1.47	79.41	4,139
18	Greens (mustard, turnip, collards)	1.38	80.78	244
19	Strawberries	1.30	82.08	291
20	Superfortified cold cereals	0.91	82.99	210
21	Bananas	0.86	83.85	860
22	Beef stew, pot pie	0.73	84.59	278
23	Corn	0.70	85.29	852
24	2% milk	0.55	85.84	1,402
25	Lemons, lemon juice	0.53	86.37	335
26	Spinach	0.49	86.85	237
27	Apples, applesauce	0.46	87.32	1,164
28	Liver	0.46	87.77	173
29	Green beans	0.44	88.21	992
30	Bacon	0.42	88.63	1,141
31	Peas	0.42	89.06	553
32	Green peppers	0.41	89.47	129
33	Pinto, navy, other dried beans	0.40	89.87	1,070
34	Pizza	0.39	90.26	360
35	Vegetable, tomato, minestrone soups	0.39	90.65	483
36	Salty snacks	0.39	91.04	1,580
37	Peaches	0.38	91.42	526

continued

TABLE A11   (Continued)

Rank	Description	% of total vitamin C	Cumulative % of vitamin C	Persons per 10,000 population
38	Cauliflower	0.36	91.78	125
39	Watermelon	0.36	92.14	106
40	Bran, and granola cereals	0.34	92.48	661
41	Carrots, peas and carrots	0.30	92.78	811
42	Catsup, other products with tomatoes	0.30	93.08	805
43	Mixed vegetables	0.29	93.37	183
44	Chili peppers, hot chili sauce	0.28	93.64	84
45	Brussels sprouts	0.26	93.90	38
46	Sweet potatoes	0.26	94.16	158
47	Skim milk, buttermilk	0.25	94.40	1,211
48	Jellies, jams, honey	0.25	94.65	1,722
49	Gelatin dessert	0.24	94.90	333
50	Fruit cocktail, fruit salad	0.24	95.13	176

From Block et al., 1985a.

TABLE A12   Major contributors of preformed niacin in the US diet: data from
the NHANES II survey, 1976-1980

Rank	Description	% of total niacin	Cumulative % of niacin	Persons per 10,000 population
1	White bread, rolls, crackers	9.51	9.51	7,666
2	Beef steaks, roasts	8.49	18.00	2,276
3	Coffee, tea	7.93	25.93	7,994
4	Hamburgers, cheeseburgers, meat loaf	7.58	33.50	2,618
5	Alcoholic beverages	5.00	38.51	2,663
6	Chicken or turkey, excluding fried	4.56	43.07	1,151
7	Cold cereals, excluding bran or superfortified types	3.82	46.89	1,177
8	Pork, including chops, roast	3.73	50.62	1,443
9	Fried chicken	3.66	54.28	701
10	Hot dogs, ham, lunch meats	3.33	57.62	2,959
11	French fries, fried potatoes	2.67	60.29	1,730
12	Peanuts, peanut butter	2.10	62.39	994
13	Doughnuts, cookies, cake	1.93	64.32	4,085
14	Potatoes, excluding fried	1.86	66.18	2,583
15	Tuna, tuna salad, tuna casserole	1.86	68.04	611
16	Spaghetti with tomato sauce	1.79	69.83	959
17	Whole wheat, rye, other dark breads	1.75	71.57	2,326
18	Bran and granola cereals	1.55	73.12	661
19	Superfortified cold cereals	1.51	74.63	210
20	Liver	1.32	75.95	173
21	Cheeses, excluding cottage cheese	1.21	77.17	3,287
22	Beef stew, pot pie	1.01	78.18	278
23	Orange juice	1.00	79.17	2,263
24	Tomatoes, tomato juice	0.99	80.17	2,552
25	Breakfast bars and drinks	0.91	81.08	192
26	Fried fish	0.90	81.98	585
27	Fish, broiled, baked, canned	0.84	82.82	378
28	Whole milk, whole milk beverages	0.82	83.63	4,139
29	Pizza	0.78	84.41	360
30	Salty snacks	0.76	85.16	1,580
31	Chili	0.72	85.88	339
32	Skim milk, buttermilk	0.66	86.54	1,211
33	Corn	0.65	87.19	852
34	Rice	0.62	87.81	915
35	Bacon	0.61	88.42	1,141
36	Pinto, navy, other dried beans	0.57	88.99	1,070

continued

TABLE A12   (Continued)

Rank	Description	% of total niacin	Cumulative % of niacin	Persons per 10,000 population
37	Veal, lamb	0.56	89.55	171
38	Soups other than vegetable, tomato	0.53	90.08	936
39	Cornbread, grits, tortillas	0.48	90.56	991
40	Green salad	0.47	91.02	4,030
41	Sausage	0.46	91.48	589
42	Vegetable, tomato, minestrone soups	0.46	91.94	483
43	Pies, excluding pumpkin	0.45	92.39	747
44	Mixed dishes with chicken	0.44	92.83	282
45	Shellfish	0.44	93.27	310
46	Mixed dishes with beef	0.38	93.65	161
47	Candy (chocolate)	0.31	93.96	868
48	Bananas	0.29	94.26	860
49	2% milk	0.27	94.53	1,402
50	Peaches	0.27	94.80	526

From Block et al., 1985a.

TABLE A13 A. Percentage of daily nutrient intake contributed by wheat foods for men and women 19-64 years old

Nutrient	Breads	Breakfast cereals	Crackers	Pasta	Sweet goods	Tot.
Protein	6.6	0.6	0.4	1.2	1.6	10.4
Fat	3.1	0.1	0.6	0.3	4.8	8.9
Carbohydrate	15.8	2.5	1.1	2.8	7.2	29.4
Calcium	10.8	0.4	0.3	0.3	2.2	14.0
Iron	13.0	3.9	0.7	2.5	3.2	23.3
Magnesium	7.3	1.8	0.4	1.6	2.1	13.2
Phosphorus	7.5	1.2	0.4	1.1	2.6	12.8
Vitamin A	0.2	4.0	—	—	0.6	4.8
Thiamin	21.6	4.7	1.0	6.2	3.7	37.2
Riboflavin	10.7	3.8	0.8	2.3	2.9	20.5
Niacin	11.1	4.0	0.9	3.0	1.9	20.9
Vitamin B-6	2.7	4.6	0.1	0.4	0.8	8.6
Vitamin B-12	0.2	5.0	—	—	0.7	5.9
Vitamin C	—	2.8	—	—	0.1	2.9

From Nelson, 1985.

B. % Nutrient distribution in the wheat kernel*

	Endosperm	Aleurone layer	Scutellum	Embryo	Pericarp & testa
Protein	72	15	4.5	3.5	4
Minerals	20	61	8	4	7
Thiamin	3	32	62	2	1
Riboflavin	32	37	14	12	5
Niacin	12	82	1	1	4
Vitamin B-6	6	61	12	9	12
Pantothenic Acid	43	41	4	3	9

*Pomeranz, Y., Ed. Wheat: Chemistry and Technology. AACC: St. Paul, 1978.
From Nelson, 1985.

C. Mineral content of wheat and milled fractions*

	Zn ppm	Fe ppm	Mn ppm	Cu ppm	Se ppm
Wheat	21-63	18-31	24-37	1.8-6.2	0.04
Bran	56-141	74-103	72-144	8.4-16.2	0.10
Germ	100-144	41-58	101-129	7.2-11.8	0.01
Flour	3.4-10.5	3.5-9.1	2.1-3.5	0.62-0.63	0.01

*As adopted from MNF by Turnland. SR Cereal Foods World 27:153, 1982.
From Nelson, 1985.

TABLE A14   Dietary intake recommendations for daily intakes of the micronutrients by the food and nutrition board (national research council)

	Adult men	Adult women	1-year-old infant
Recommended Dietary Allowances, 9th Edition, 1980			
Vitamin A (RE)	1000	800	400
Vitamin D (μg)	5	5	10
Vitamin E (mg)	10	8	4
Thiamin (mg)	1.4	1.0	0.5
Riboflavin (mg)	1.6	1.2	0.6
Niacin (mg)	18	13	8
Vitamin B_6 (mg)	2.2	2.0	0.6
Folic acid (μg)	400	400	45
Vitamin B_{12} (μg)	3.0	3.0	1.5
Vitamin C (mg)	60	60	35
Iron (mg)	10	18	15
Zinc (mg)	15	15	5
Safe and Adequate Dietary Intakes			
Vitamin K (μg)	70-140	70-140	10-20
Biotin (μg)	100-200	100-200	35
Pantothenic acid (mg)	4-7	4-7	2
Copper (mg)	2-3	2-3	0.7-1.0
Manganese (mg)	2.5-5.0	2.5-5.0	0.7-1.0
Fluoride (mg)	1.5-4.0	1.5-4.0	0.2-1.0
Chromium (μg)	50-200	50-200	20-40
Selenium (μg)	50-200	50-200	10-40
Molybdenum (μg)	150-500	150-500	30-60

From Burk & Solomons, 1985.

References

Block, G., Dresser, C.M., Hartman, A.M., & Carroll, M.D. Nutrient sources in the American diet: Quantitative data from the NHANES II survey. I. Vitamins and minerals. *American Journal of Epidemiology, 122*, 1985a, 13–26.

Block, G., Dresser, C.M., Hartman, A.M., & Carroll, M.D. Nutrient sources in the American diet: Quantitative data from the NHANES II survey. II. Macronutrients and fats. *American Journal of Epidemiology, 122*, 1985b, 27–40.

Burk, R.F. & Solomons, N.W. Trace elements and vitamins and bioavailability as related to wheat and wheat foods. *The American Journal of Clinical Nutrition, 41*, 1985, 1091–1102.

Nelson, J.H. Wheat: Its processing and utilization. *The American Journal of Clinical Nutrition, 41*, 1985, 1070–1076.

Glossary

acetylcholine   Neurotransmitter important in memory and motor processes; formed from acetylCoA and choline.

acetylcholinesterase   Enzyme that breaks the ester bond of acetylcholine and degrades it into acetic acid and choline.

adenosine triphosphate (ATP)   Molecular linking agent in the flow of chemical energy. Required in oxidation of fuels (e.g., glycolysis). Used in phosphorylation.

adipose tissue   Fatty tissue. Fat cells are adipocytes.

adrenal gland   Glands located just above kidneys. Cortex secretes glucocorticoids and mineralocorticoids. Medulla secretes epinephrine.

adrenalin   See epinephrine.

afferent   Target direction in which nerve fibers are received. Conducting toward a site of reference.

albumin   A simple, water soluble protein found in egg white, blood serum, milk, and various animal tissues.

aldehyde   Class of organic compounds containing a carbonyl group (carbon double bonded to oxygen), with the carbon attached to one hydrogen.

aldosterone   Steroid secreted by the adrenal cortex important in salt regulation. Mineralocorticoid.

amino acid   Member of a chemical group (mostly) having a free carboxyl group and a free unsubstituted amino group on the alpha carbon atom. Amino acids are the substituents of proteins.

amphetamine   (d,1-phenylisopropylamine) Drug that stimulates catecholamine activity—inhibits MAO, blocks uptake, and stimulates release of catecholamines.

amygdala   Nuclei in lateral subcortical regions of brain. Reciprocally connected to hypothalamus, hippocampus, and thalamus. Important functions in emotions, olfaction, and feeding.

angiotensin   Octapeptide (angiotensin II) that regulates circulatory volume and pressure. In brain, elicits thirst and drinking behavior.

angiotensinogen   Plasma protein degraded by renin to produce angiotensin I, which is further degraded into angiotensin II.

anomer   Same chemical composition, but the bond location of a specific grouping is different and thereby produces a different optical rotation.

anorexigenic   Producing or causing anorexia.

anterior   Directional term—opposite posterior. Toward the front.

antidiuretic hormone (ADH)   See vasopressin.

anxiolysis   Reduction or elimination of anxiety.

apomorphine   Drug that stimulates dopamine receptors.

ascorbic acid   Vitamin C. An antioxidant. Prolonged lack results in scurvy. Less severe deficiency produces alterations in connective tissue and may cause decreased resistance to some infections.

aspartame   The ingredient of NutraSweet. Dipeptide sweetener. 1-methyl-N-L-alpha aspartyl-L-phenylalanine.

aspartate   (Aspartic acid) Acidic amino acid. Acts as excitatory neurotransmitter. Substituent of aspartame.

atrial natriuretic factor   Peptide produced in myocytes of mammalian atria and also found in brain. Has potent natriuretic and diuretic actions. Opposes actions of angiotensin and inhibits saline intake.

atropine   Prototypical anticholinergic drug that blocks muscarinic receptors. Produces increase in sympathetic tone and can produce confusion, amnesia, and hallucinations.

autonomic nervous system   Part of the peripheral nervous system involved in homeostasis. Composed of sympathetic and parasympathetic nervous systems.

basal ganglia   Comprised of three large subcortical masses: caudate nucleus, putamen, and pallidum. Important in the initiation of movement and usually involved in motor dysfunction.

blood-brain-barrier   Filtering system of the central nervous system. Comprised of glial membranes juxtaposed against capillary pores. Molecules must be small enough to fit through capillary pores and lipid (fat) soluble to pass through this system into brain. Weaker in tissue surrounding ventricles.

bulbospinal   Refers to projection of nerve fibers from brain stem into spinal cord.

calcium   Nutrient metal required for bone, muscle, and nerve functions. Involved in neurotransmitter release. Evidence exists for its behavioral regulation.

carbachol   Drug that mimics the action of acetylcholine and is resistant to breakdown by cholinesterases.

carbohydrate   General class of macronutrient that includes sugars and starches. Source of energy upon metabolism. Composed of carbon, hydrogen, and oxygen as $(CH_2O)_n$.

carboxypeptidase   Enzyme that catalyzes the cleavage of amino acids from the C terminal of peptides.

casein   Major nutrient protein of milk. Often used as a dietary protein for experimental animals.

catecholamine   Class of hormones and neurotransmitters derived from tyrosine and having a catechol nucleus with an amine group attached to it on a side chain. Includes dopamine, norepinephrine, and epinephrine.

caudal   Directional term—opposite rostral. Toward the tail.

chelate   The molecular process of holding a metal ion in bond coordination with a molecule. A chelator refers to a drug or agent that attaches to metal ions, usually in an attempt to increase their excretion.

cerebellum   Convoluted bilaterally symmetrical structure located in posterior portion of cranium. Controls timing and pattern of muscles activated during movement. Involved in postural control. Recent evidence for memory involvement.

cholecystokinin (CCK)   Peptide found in brain and gut. A potent satiety agent.

choline   Water soluble dietary substance that is a precursor for the synthesis of acetylcholine.

chorda tympani   Nerve that supplies taste information from anterior two-thirds of the tongue.

choroid plexus   Tissue found in cerebral ventricles. Capillary networks surrounded by cuboidal or columnar epithelium. Functions in secreting cerebrospinal fluid.

circadian   Daily rhythm. A period of about 24 hours.

circumventricular   Refers to brain areas immediately surrounding cerebral ventricles.

citric acid cycle See tricarboxylic acid cycle.

cortex Outer layer of brain tissue. Thought to have developed latest in evolution. Controls higher level perceptions and motor actions.

corticosterone Steroid glucocorticoid secreted by the adrenal cortex important in gluconeogenesis.

corticotropin Pituitary hormone that activates release of adrenal cortical steroids. (e.g., Adrenocorticotropic hormone—ACTH)

cortisol Steroid glucocorticoid secreted by the adrenal cortex important in glucose release from the liver and increased glycogen deposition.

deafferentation Removal of nerve supply to a tissue or brain area—usually by cutting of nerve fibers.

depolarize In this context refers to reducing ionic charge difference across the nerve membrane. Stimulates nerve.

dextrose Another name for one molecular configuration of glucose. The nutrient form of glucose.

diencephalon Comprised of thalamus, hypothalamus, subthalamus, and epithalamus. Key relay to transmit information about sensation and movement, and contains control for important autonomic (homeostatic) functions.

dipeptide Peptide composed of two amino acids.

diuretic Any substance that stimulates the flow of urine.

dopamine Catecholamine neurotransmitter important in motor control, feeding, and sexual behavior. Principal transmitter of the nigrostriatal pathway.

dorsal Directional term—opposite ventral. Toward the back or top.

duodenum First portion of small intestine.

efferent Target direction from which nerve fibers extend. Conduction away from a site of reference.

electrolyte A compound which, when dissolved in water, separates into ions (e.g. salt). Sometimes refers to ionic balance of blood.

epinephrine Catecholamine neurotransmitter important in basic processes of arousal and the liberation of fuels by glycogenolysis. Secreted by adrenal gland and nerves.

extrapyramidal Motor system of brain not directly related to projections of neurons from motor cortex. Includes basal ganglia and connections.

feedback The signal in a control system providing information about the system's output.

fluorophore Fluorescent molecule. Target molecule made by reacting transmitter with fluorescent compound.

gamma amino butyric acid (GABA) Nonprotein amino acid that acts as an inhibitory neurotransmitter.

gastric Pertaining to the stomach.

gavage Feeding by a tube passed into the stomach.

glia Non-neural cells in the nervous system. Have several interactive functions with neurons.

glucagon Peptide hormone secreted by alpha cells in pancreatic islets. Causes liver to break down glycogen to restore blood glucose. Counterbalances insulin.

glucocorticoid Steroids from adrenal cortex participating in gluconeogenesis and important for growth and development.

glucokinase Enzyme in the first stage of glycolysis that catalyzes the phosphorylation of glucose by ATP.

gluconeogenesis The biosynthesis of a "new" sugar from smaller precursor molecules.

glucopenia Scarcity of glucose. Neuroglucopenia is a scarcity of glucose in nerves.

glucoprivation Deprivation of glucose. Usually refers to condition occurring in cells or tissues.

glucose Simple sugar with six carbons (hexose). Major source of energy. May be feedback signal for food intake.

glutamate (Glutamic acid) Acidic amino acid that acts as an excitatory neurotransmitter and is the principal substituent of monosodium glutamate (MSG).

gluten Mixture of plant proteins occurring in cereal grains—mainly corn and wheat. Used as adhesive and as flour substitute.

glycogen A storage form of glucose containing several glucose residues.

glycolysis Refers to the biochemical breakdown of glucose—a major chemical pathway for the release of energy.

glycosuria Abnormally high sugar content in the urine.

gonadotropin Class of pituitary hormones that have stimulatory effects on the gonads.

hexokinase Enzyme that catalyzes the phosphorylation of hexoses (e.g., glucose) by ATP. Differs from glucokinase in specificity.

hippocampus Curved, layered cortical structure. Part of limbic system. Involved in working memory and other limbic functions. Target for several transmitter systems sensitive to dietary precursors. Contains much zinc.

hormone Chemical secreted by a gland into the bloodstream where it has functional effects on any organ or tissue with receptors for it.

hydrolysis Decomposition of a chemical compound by reaction with water.

hyperglycemia Condition of excess glucose in the blood.

hyperinsulinemia Condition of excess insulin in the blood.

hyperphagia Overeating.

hyperpolarize In this context refers to increasing ionic charge difference across nerve membrane. Inhibits nerve.

hyperreactivity Extreme reactions to stimuli.

hypertension A state of abnormally increased blood pressure. High blood pressure.

hypoglycemia   Condition when blood has abnormally low levels of glucose.

hypothalamus   Portion of brain tissue at ventral base of the brain important for homeostatic regulation and motivational processes. Secretes peptides and other molecules that regulate pituitary function. Shown to be important in the control of nutrient intake.

iatrogenic   Resulting from an attitude or action of a physician.

insulin   Peptide hormone secreted by the beta cells in the pancreatic islets. Released after meal in response to blood glucose rise. Regulates blood glucose levels. Facilitates transport of glucose into tissues.

interneuron   Nerve cell in central nervous system that extends its axon only a short distance to connect within its brain region. Often utilizes GABA as neurotransmitter.

intraventricular   Injection into the cerebral ventricles.

iontophoresis   Introductions of ions into the body for therapeutic purposes. In an experimental context, refers to electrical ejection of a charged (ionic) substance.

ketoacidosis   Elevation of ketone bodies with a decrease in blood pH (toward acidity).

lateral   Directional term—opposite medial. Toward the side.

lecithin   Refers to phosphatidylcholine. Often used as a food emulsifier, though commercially it is composed of other phosphoglycerides. A source of choline for the synthesis of acetylcholine in the brain.

limbic system   Brain circuitry elaborated first by Paul Broca and later by James Papez. Limbic structures include hippocampus, amygdala, septum, olfactory tubercle, mammillary bodies, anterior thalamic nuclei, and cingulate gyrus.

locus ceruleus   Brain stem nucleus containing largest aggregate of norepinephrine neurons. Principal source of norepinephrine projections through nervous system.

macronutrient   Nutrient required in large proportion for growth, development, and maintenance.

medial   Directional term—opposite lateral. Toward the middle.

medulla   Most caudal portion brain stem between pons and spinal cord. Contains cell bodies of cranial nerves controlling sensation and movement in head and neck and visceral functions.

metalloenzyme   Enzyme that requires metal ion(s) as cofactor.

mineralocorticoid   Adrenocortical steroid important in regulation of salt (e.g., aldosterone).

monoamine   Usually refers to any transmitter with single amino group (e.g., dopamine, norepinephrine, serotonin).

monoamine oxidase   (MAO) enzyme that catalyzes the oxidation of monoamines. Once the principal treatment for depression. Involved in dietary hypertensive crisis if patients consume some fermented foods during treatment.

muscarinic Pertaining to a type of acetylcholine receptor activated selectively by muscarine.

muscimol Drug that acts as GABA receptor agonist.

myelin The insulating sheath around the axon of some nerve cells. Formed from a glial cell. Facilitates neural conduction.

naloxone Drug that antagonizes the action of opiates.

natriuresis The excretion of sodium in the urine.

neophilia Enjoyment or love of something new. In this context, refers to a preference for new food.

neostriatum See striatum.

neuroglucopenia See glucopenia.

neuroleptic Refers to class of antipsychotic drugs. Chlorpromazine is prototype. Causes motor disturbances in patients.

neuropil A feltwork in nerve tissue formed by interlacing branches of nerve fibers and dendrites.

neurotransmitter A biochemical (or perhaps trace metal) released by a nerve ending that initiates a cellular response in the receiver cell.

norepinephrine Catecholamine neurotransmitter important in arousal, feeding, and memory formation. Norepinephrine fibers penetrate the entire central neuraxis and are the principals in the sympathetic nervous system.

omnivore An animal who will include almost anything edible in its diet.

ouabain Drug that inhibits the sodium pump in nerves. Under its influence, nerves cannot recover by pumping out sodium.

oxytocin Peptide hormone produced in the hypothalamus and released from the posterior pituitary. Has stimulant effects on smooth muscle of uterus. Has role in milk ejection.

parasympathetic nervous system Division of autonomic nervous system important in behavioral quieting and inhibition of arousal.

parathyroid hormone Parathormone. Secreted from parathyroid gland. Regulates blood concentration of calcium and phosphorus. Elevates blood calcium—opposite calcitonin.

pepsin Enzyme useful for hydrolysis of peptide chain. Secreted by chief cells of stomach. Digests proteins.

peptide Relatively short chain of amino acids. Can be hormone or neurotransmitter.

perikarya Pl. A perikaryon is the cell body of a neuron containing the nucleus.

peritoneum In this context refers to the cavity containing the abdominal viscera.

phenylalanine Amino acid with nonpolar phenyl group on the R chain. It acts as precursor to tyrosine and is a substitutent of aspartame.

phosphatidylcholine   Lecithin. Formed from dietary choline or may be ingested as source of choline.

phosphorylation   Process of adding a phosphate group. Often used to give molecule favorable energy configuration.

phytate (phytic acid)   Contains stereoisomer of the plant sugar alcohol inositol. Increases excretion of zinc.

pica   A perversion of appetite in which normally inedible substances are eaten.

pineal gland   Part of epithalamus. Contains highest concentration of serotonin and its metabolites (e.g. melatonin) in the brain. Important in seasonal rhythms of reproduction. Presumably responsive to dietary changes in tryptophan.

pinealocytes   Cells in the pineal gland.

polydipsia   Excessive thirst.

polyphagia   Excessive ingestion of food.

polyuria   Excessive secretion of urine.

pons   Region of brain stem between medulla and midbrain. Contains abundant interconnections with cerebellum and has cell bodies of several cranial nerves.

posterior   Directional term—opposite anterior. Toward the back or rear.

potassium   Nutrient metal important in nerve conduction. Evidence exists for its behavioral regulation.

prolactin   Pituitary hormone. Controls activity of mammary gland during lactation. Involved in sexual and parenting behavior.

protein   General class of macronutrient built as a chain of amino acids.

proteolysis   Digestion of proteins.

Purkinje cells   Golgi type I cells in the cerebellum that contain several dendritic branches.

pyridoxine   Crystalline substance that has vitamin B_6 activity. Coenzyme form is used in transamination.

raphe nuclei   In this context refers to nuclei in brainstem (dorsal and median) that are major sources of serotonin projections throughout brain.

receptor   Usually a membrane protein that interacts with a communicating biochemical—e.g., hormone, neurotransmitter—to initiate or communicate a cellular change.

renin   Enzyme secreted by kidneys and found in brain that degrades angiotensinogen into angiotensin I. Secreted when blood pressure drops.

rostral   Directional term—opposite caudal. Toward the head.

septum   Refers to medial nuclei in rostral area of brain. Part of limbic system. Has importance in emotional behavior.

serotonin   Neurotransmitter derived from tryptophan important in overall organismic sedation.

sodium   Nutrient metal important in nerve conduction and several bodily processes. Considerable evidence exists for its physiological and behavioral regulation. Table salt is composed of sodium chloride.

steroid   One of a class of biochemicals derived from squalene. Steroids usually travel through the bloodstream and have a distinctive function after binding to receptors.

striatum   Collective term usually referring to caudate nucleus and putamen (neostriatum) and globus pallidus (paleostriatum).

sucrose   A sugar composed of glucose and fructose. Table sugar.

sympathetic nervous system   Division of autonomic nervous system important in arousal.

telencephalon   General term referring to cerebral hemispheres. All rostral brain matter developed beyond diencephalon.

thalamus   Part of diencephalon. Nuclei located in center of brain. Functions as key relay for sensory and motor information.

thiamine (also thiamin)   Refers to vitamin B_1. Important in several biochemical reactions. Deficiency causes beriberi.

trace metal   Includes metals like zinc and selenium necessary for growth and health. Often used by enzymes for catabolic function.

transamination   Transfer of alpha amino group in catabolism of at least 12 amino acids.

tricarboxylic acid cycle   Almost universal cyclic sequence of biochemical reactions. Main biochemical pathway for oxidation of carbohydrate in muscle. Biochemical pathway of respiration—releases carbon dioxide.

trigeminal nerve   Supplies primary parasympathetic innervation of viscera. Important in the control of feeding.

tryptophan   Amino acid precursor for the synthesis of serotonin.

tuberoinfundibular   Passing from tuberal region of hypothalamus into pituitary stalk (infundibulum).

tyrosine   Amino acid precursor for the synthesis of catecholamines.

vagus nerve   Complex mixed nerve containing general somatic afferent and visceral afferent and efferent fibers. Receives fibers conveying taste from chorda tympani. Receives information about viscera, interacts with nutrients such as glucose and transmits to solitary nucleus.

vasoconstriction   Decrease in the caliber of blood vessels.

vasopressin   Anti-diuretic hormone (ADH). Peptide hormone produced in hypothalamus and released in posterior pituitary under conditions of water deprivation or depletion of extracellular volume.

ventral   Directional term—opposite dorsal. Toward the bottom or front.

vitamin   Trace substance vital for many important biochemical reactions. Vitamins are water-soluble or fat-soluble.

zinc   Trace metal important for growth and several biological processes. High levels found in hippocampus and other brain areas. Evidence exists for its behavioral regulation.

Index